HYPERTENSION

A Symposium EDITED BY *E. T. Bell,* M.D.

HYPERTENSION

· · · · · · · · · · · · · · · · · · · *A Symposium*

HELD AT THE UNIVERSITY OF MINNESOTA ON

SEPTEMBER 18, 19, AND 20, 1950, IN HONOR OF

Elexious T. Bell, M.D., Benjamin J. Clawson, M.D.,

and George E. Fahr, M.D.

University of Minnesota Press, Minneapolis

LONDON · GEOFFREY CUMBERLEGE · OXFORD UNIVERSITY PRESS

Dr. Elexious T. Bell

ELEXIOUS T. BELL *was born in Ralls County, Missouri, in 1880. He attended the University of Missouri as a premedical student and received his Bachelor of Science degree in 1901 and his Doctor of Medicine degree in 1903. He taught in the Department of Anatomy at the University of Missouri until 1905, when he went to Europe for a year of study at the University of Bonn under Dr. M. Nussbaum. After returning from Europe, he resumed his work at the University of Missouri, where he remained until 1910. At that time he joined the Department of Anatomy at the University of Minnesota. In 1911 he became a member of the staff of the Department of Pathology and in 1921 was named Director of the Department. He became Professor Emeritus in 1949. Although his scientific interests are broad, he has long concerned himself especially with kidney diseases and hypertension. His numerous scientific publications include two books,* Textbook of Pathology *and* Renal Diseases.

Dr. Benjamin J. Clawson

BENJAMIN J. CLAWSON *was born in Dixonville, Pennsylvania, in 1881. He received his Bachelor of Science degree and his Master of Arts degree from the University of Kansas in 1909 and 1911, respectively, having majored in bacteriology. He taught bacteriology at the Oklahoma Agricultural and Mechanical College from 1911 to 1912 and at the University of Kansas from 1912 to 1917. He studied medicine during summer sessions and during a leave of absence from the University of Kansas and received his Doctor of Medicine degree from Rush Medical College in 1917. He was a member of the faculty of the University of Chicago until 1919, when he received his Doctor of Philosophy degree in bacteriology. As professor of pathology and bacteriology, he served the University of North Dakota from 1919 to 1921, when he*

*came to the University of Minnesota Department of Pathology. He
was named full Professor in 1927 and Professor Emeritus in 1949. He
is the author of numerous scientific papers, most of them concerned
with cardiovascular diseases.*

Dr. George E. Fahr

GEORGE E. FAHR *was born in Meadville, Pennsylvania, in 1882. He
received his Bachelor of Science degree from the University of Chicago
in 1904. Except for one year spent at Johns Hopkins University Medical School, his undergraduate medical school years were spent in
Germany, and he received his Doctor of Medicine degree from the
University of Würzburg in 1909. He was a member of the Department
of Physiology in the University of Würzburg from 1907 to 1910 and
at the University of Leyden from 1911 to 1913. Thereafter he studied
in Bad Nauheim, Bern, and Basle. He returned to the United States
in 1916 as resident physician at Montefiore Hospital, New York City.
Service in the University of Michigan Medical School, United States
Army Medical Corps, and the University of Wisconsin Medical School
followed, and in 1921 he came to the University of Minnesota. In 1926
he was named Chief of the Medical Service at Minneapolis General
Hospital, and in 1927 was made full Professor. Professor Emeritus
since June 1950, he is still adding to his many contributions in the
field of cardiovascular disease.*

Table of Contents

· · · · · · · · · · MORNING SESSION · SEPTEMBER 18

PRESIDING, *Maurice B. Visscher*

Greetings and a Word of Explanation

DR. MAURICE B. VISSCHER: It is always a privilege for a student to have an opportunity to pay tribute to his teachers. In the aggregate the three of our beloved colleagues whom we are honoring for their services to the University of Minnesota and to science, particularly in the field of cardiovascular diseases, have spent a total of 95 years in this institution. I am especially happy to be able to open this first meeting of the symposium on the problems of hypertension, because I feel it is a real privilege to be able to say "Thank you" to three of my most stimulating teachers. Twenty-eight years ago I began learning not only about hypertension but about pathological physiology in general under Dr. Bell and Dr. Clawson. Twenty-seven years ago I began learning about the law of the heart and related phenomena from Dr. Fahr. You can well imagine, then, the pleasure it is for me to take part in honoring these three Minnesota scholars.

Dean Harold S. Diehl will speak on behalf of the faculty of the Medical School and for the University Administration.

DR. HAROLD S. DIEHL: Before extending the greetings of the medical faculty, there are one or two brief explanations about this conference that I should like to make. In the first place, I must admit that although I am first on the program, the idea for this symposium did not originate with me. I wish it had, for it is an excellent one. It originated with Dr. Cecil J. Watson. My part in it, after it had been suggested, was to appoint a committee of Dr. George Aagaard and Dr. Watson, who with the advice of Dr. Bell, Dr. Clawson, Dr. Fahr, and Dr. Visscher made the arrangements for the program.

The only other part that I as dean had in this symposium was to find the financial support needed for it—a usual function of deans. And that proved to be a simple task. Not only did President Morrill say that the University of Minnesota would be glad to support a symposium of this sort. The officials of the Mayo Foundation for

3

Medical Education and Research said they too should welcome the opportunity, as did also the officers of the Variety Club of the North-west—the organization that has provided funds for the Special Heart Hospital, which I hope you will see. On behalf of the University, I wish to express our gratitude to these organizations for their generous aid.

I should like to add a word to what Dr. Visscher has said about the function of this symposium in honoring the three distinguished members of our medical faculty who have changed to emeritus status during the past year. They have all been leading and key figures in the development of our medical school for more than a quarter of a century. Individually as well as collectively, they have been distinguished scholars and scientists in their own right. They have been stimulating teachers to both graduates and undergraduates. They have showed a rare capacity to stimulate young men to do original scientific work. Interestingly enough, the major field of all three has been cardiovascular disease. Dr. Bell's research has been directed primarily toward hypertension and kidney disease; Dr. Clawson's toward rheumatic fever and endocarditis of various types; and Dr. Fahr's toward the normal and pathological physiology of the heart and circulation. A symposium on the problems of hypertension seems, therefore, a most appropriate way of paying tribute to them and their work.

Speaking for the medical faculty, I want to say that we are very much pleased by the attendance at this symposium. We are honored to have in the audience so many distinguished guests who themselves have done outstanding work in the field of hypertension. We are glad that so many alert and interested practitioners of medicine are here, for these are the men who must take to the patient and to the bedside the advances made in the laboratory and clinic. We hope you will find these three days both interesting and pleasant.

DR. VISSCHER: By way of introduction, I should like to make a few additional remarks about the method we want to use in carrying out this symposium. Our specially invited guests will present their papers from the platform. We hope, however, that after the papers have been given there will be discussion from the floor. After each presentation, or sometimes after two presentations, where it seems appropriate to consider two together, we shall open up a period for questions and comments. We feel that this symposium is not simply an opportunity to summarize existing knowledge with regard to hypertension and its problems. It is also an opportunity to point the way toward future research—research that may solve many of the problems that will still be unsolved at the end of our three days' discussion.

. . . . *by* HARRY GOLDBLATT

Anatomical Considerations of Hypertension

IT IS a great honor and privilege to be the first speaker on this symposium arranged in honor of three great men of medicine for whom I have the highest regard.

Many years before the existence of a hypertensive state in the vascular system of man was first recognized, the anatomical changes in the blood vessels frequently found associated with this condition had already been the subject of exhaustive study. It seems definitely in order, therefore, that a consideration of these anatomical changes should be the introductory contribution to this symposium. It is certainly fitting, also, that a pathologist should be the one to present this topic, because it was pathologists who first studied the anatomical alterations accompanying this condition. My own reason for choosing this topic was that the basis of our work on the experimental production of hypertension in animals was, in part at least, anatomical. Had I known that Dr. Bell, one of the three men being honored on this occasion, would participate in this program and choose this topic also as the subject of his talk, I certainly should have picked some other subject, but I did not know this until I received a printed copy of the program. In the circumstances, I can only hope that, because our views about the pathogenesis of hypertension are different and because I shall stress the experimental point of view, there will not be too much overlapping and repetition in our separate presentations.

Historical

Before the existence of any form of hypertension had become known and, indeed, even before the blood pressure of man had ever been measured, the large, heavy heart of the hypertensive person had already been observed and described. In 1836 Richard Bright (1), a clinician but also a careful observer at the autopsy table, published his view that some of the large, heavy hearts of his patients with renal

5

disease were not the result of intrinsic heart disease. Without knowing anything about the blood pressure of man, he concluded that there was a direct relationship between renal disease and large, heavy hearts, and he came close to the recognition of the ultimate cause of the hypertrophy of these hearts. By recognizing the probable existence of increased resistance to the flow of blood through the peripheral blood vessels, he came about as close as we are today to the recognition of the primary cause of the elevated blood pressure which we now consider the cause of the cardiac hypertrophy. He even concluded that the renal disease was responsible for the presence of some chemical in the blood which was responsible for the cardiac hypertrophy, but he thought that it had a direct effect on the cardiac muscle.

Bright knew little or nothing about arteriosclerosis, nor did Johnson (2), who in 1868 recognized the existence of thick-walled arteries, both large and small, but who did not recognize the arteriosclerotic nature of the thickening and thought that it was due entirely to hypertrophy of the muscular coats. This condition he considered secondary to the Bright's disease and believed that, when diffuse, such a thickening (hypertrophy of the media) of the blood vessels could constitute a basis for increased peripheral vascular resistance. Widespread organic disease of the arterioles was actually described in 1872 by Gull and Sutton (3), who called it "arterio-capillary fibrosis" and concluded that it was a primary, organic, pathologic basis for increased peripheral vascular resistance. They regarded this vascular disease as independent of renal disease and thought that the pathologic changes in the kidneys of Bright's disease, especially the contracted kidneys, were "but a part of a general morbid condition." The clinical observations of Mahomed, in that same period, led him to the view that high blood pressure precedes the development of any clinical signs of Bright's disease.

Evans (4) in 1921 combined the observations of Johnson and of Gull and Sutton and described diffuse hyperplastic sclerosis, which he found most commonly in the kidney. He regarded the lesion as a manifestation of active inflammation and on the basis of physiological response differentiated it from senile arteriosclerosis. He failed to observe any changes in the muscles. Kernohan, Anderson, and Keith (5), however, in 1929 did describe stenosis of the arterioles due to hypertrophy of the media and thickening of the intima in the muscles of hypertensive persons. Degenerative arteriolar lesions were also found in the muscles of a high percentage of hypertensive persons by Scott, Seecof, and Hill (6) in 1933, and by Andrus (7) in 1936, who described fibrosis in the media without stenosis of the lumen or thickening of the wall.

The Relationship of Hypertension to Vascular Disease and Renal Vascular Disease

As soon as the hypertensive state was fully recognized, those who had begun to theorize about the origin of the elevated blood pressure and of the vascular disease were divided in their opinions about which comes first. Is the involvement of the kidneys part of the generalized vascular disease, and what part, if any, does the disease of the kidneys play in the origin of the hypertension? We still seem to be in the same state of uncertainty.

From the time when Jores (8) first clearly differentiated inflammatory from vascular disease of the kidneys, there has never been much doubt about the renal origin of the hypertension which accompanies the development of inflammation of the kidneys. The same may be said now of a number of other known primary abnormalities of the kidneys that are associated with hypertension. Also, a non-renal origin of the hypertension accompanying diseases of the endocrine organs, such as pheochromocytoma of the adrenal and basophilic adenoma or basophilism of the pituitary, is now generally accepted. But the bone of contention still is the nature of the relationship of vascular disease and especially of arterial and arteriolar sclerosis of the kidneys, or true nephrosclerosis, to the hypertension so frequently found associated with it.

Although it is generally recognized that vascular disease of the kidneys leads to nephrosclerosis, that is, to the scarred kidney so commonly found in cases of benign essential hypertension, yet despite all the work that has been done on the subject, it is still not firmly established whether the hypertension or the renal vascular disease comes first. The main reason for this difficulty is that in benign essential hypertension, by definition, the hypertension is frequently unassociated with any impairment of the renal excretory function detectable by clinical laboratory methods. This is interpreted by some to mean that the hypertension may precede by some time the development of the organic vascular disease in the kidney.

This it is difficult to disprove. Although I, for one, have always been on the side of those who believe that the renal vascular disease precedes the establishment of the fixed hypertension associated with it, yet I have never denied the possible existence of other types of hypertension, such as the purely endocrinogenic, the psycho-neurogenic, and other forms. I have even accepted the existence of a labile or intermittent type of hypertension, on the basis of simple vasomotor instability, which could be called a prehypertensive state, without necessarily implying that this pre-existent elevation of the blood pressure plays any part in the development of generalized vascular disease or nephrosclerosis. There is no reason why some persons with this type of disturbance of the blood pressure should not also develop renal vascular disease and consequent persistent hypertension, while others continue to have only the vasomotor instability. It seems, however, that many develop hypertension without ever going through this preliminary phase.

The views of others. Although Volhard (9) always contended that the malignant type of hypertension, characterized by impaired renal excretion and elevated blood pressure, is of renal origin, yet he, too, refused to accept the benign phase of essential hypertension as being of renal origin and considered that nephrosclerosis is merely part of a primary diffuse vascular disease which causes hypertension. It is true that studies by Fishberg (10), by Bell and Clawson (11), and by Moritz and Oldt (12), indicate the almost invariable presence, at autopsy, of pronounced vascular disease of the kidneys in cases of human essential hypertension, but the criticism usually made of these studies is that the investigators were dealing with the end stage of the condition, when the presence of vascular disease in the kidney did not necessarily mean that it preceded the development of hypertension. As a matter of fact, Bell and Clawson, although they admit that some forms of hypertension are of renal origin, still interpret their own findings as indicating that the hypertension associated with vascular disease is primary—not of renal origin—and actually the cause of the arteriolar sclerosis in the kidneys as well as in the rest of the body. On the other hand, Moritz and Oldt, who found that the incidence of vascular disease in the kidney is much greater than in any other organ, inferred that either the kidney must be more vulnerable than all other organs to the effect of hypertension (and they found no evidence to support this) or the hypertension does not occur unless and until the kidneys are affected by the vascular disease. They came to the latter conclusion, which coincides with my own view.

The author's experiments and views. Before our attempt to produce hypertension in animals was made, I was hopeful enough to believe that the experimental production of hypertension, without an accompanying disturbance of the renal excretory function, by a method which produces interference with the hemodynamics of the kidney in a way simulating the presumed circulatory disturbance in the nephrosclerotic kidney, would go a long way toward proving that obliterative arterial and arteriolar sclerosis of the kidneys does precede, and actually determines, the development of the hypertension. It seemed to me also that if the production of persistent experimental renal hypertension was not followed by the development of generalized arterial and arteriolar sclerosis, then it would be fair to conclude that the vascular disease, whatever may be its cause, comes first, and that the hypertension develops only when the kidneys are also involved.

Well, as you all know, experimental hypertension without accompanying renal excretory functional disturbance was produced by constriction of the main renal arteries (13), and generalized arterial and arteriolar sclerosis did not develop in the animals, even after seven years of persistent hypertension (14); but despite these findings, it has not been generally accepted that the vascular disease comes first. Why? (1) Because in some human beings and in some animals with hypertension, impaired renal blood flow has not been demonstrated. (2) Because perfusion of some of the kidneys of hypertensives, at autopsy, has failed to show a reduction in the flow through those kidneys. (3) Because some observers have failed to find significant vascular disease in small biopsy specimens of the cortex of the kidneys of some human hypertensives.

I question the significance of the failure to find (by indirect methods) a statistically decreased blood flow through the kidney in an occasional hypertensive person or animal, because in man, at least, the prehypertensive renal blood flow of such individuals is not known. I also question the value of most of the perfusion experiments performed on the kidney after death, because I doubt that they really reflect what happens in life, and most of the perfusion fluids have been entirely different from blood, both chemically and physically. Finally, it seems fair to challenge the value of the assessment of the hemodynamic state of a kidney on the basis of the histological examination of a small fragment from the periphery of the cortex. One should keep in mind that obliterative sclerosis of one large intrarenal artery (never seen in such biopsy specimens) can easily account for considerable hemodynamic disturbance in a part of the kidney supplied by a large number of arterioles. Similar obliterative sclerosis of only a few large intrarenal branches of the renal artery could account for great disturbance in the entire renal circulation, although the preglomerular arterioles might not show much obliterative sclerosis.

Such kidneys are not rare. We now know that a reduction in the size of the orifice of one renal artery, due to sclerosis in the wall of the aorta at the site of origin of the renal artery, or in the main renal artery itself; or a congenitally small orifice of only one main renal artery with a correspondingly small main renal artery and a hypoplastic kidney; or obliterative sclerosis or arteritis of any portion of a main renal artery or of the large intrarenal branches; or aneurysm (true or dissecting); or kinking, embolism, or thrombosis of a main renal artery; and even compression and constriction of the main renal artery by neoplasm may all produce the intrarenal hemodynamic effects of intrarenal vascular disease and account for hemodynamic disturbance in the kidney sufficient to induce the development of elevated blood pressure. Certainly none of these conditions can ever be detected by the examination of a small fragment from the periphery of the cortex of a kidney, but the return of the blood pressure to normal after the excision of such a kidney (provided the other kidney is normal) indicates that the unilateral renal disease was the cause of the hypertension.

Vascular Disease: The Lesions of the Benign and Malignant Phases of Essential Hypertension

Many investigators have confused the hyalinizing process of the arterioles, seen in the benign phase, with the necrosis and necrotizing arteriolitis that characterize the malignant phase. There should be no such confusion. Arteriolar necrosis, especially when observed in experimental hypertension, has often been referred to erroneously as arteriolosclerosis. There is no good reason for accepting the view that arteriolar necrosis is merely an exaggeration of arteriolar sclerosis. Anyone who has observed the development of the most pronounced necrosis of the arterioles and of necrotizing arteriolitis in 48 hours, or even less, after constriction of the main renal arteries in a previously normal animal with presumably normal arterioles will be convinced that necrosis and sclerosis of the arterioles are two different processes.

The nearest thing to benign, hyalinizing arteriolar sclerosis that has been produced experimentally is the vascular disease that was observed by Hartroft and Best (15) in rats that had been subjected in early life to a brief period (not more than a week) of choline deficiency and then returned to a normal diet. Those animals that survived and grew well after they were returned to the normal diet gradually developed hypertension and, at autopsy, had the hyalinizing lesion of the arterioles. Hartroft and Best also observed fibrinoid necrosis of the arterioles, like that of the malignant phase, but only in a few rats that had pronounced renal excretory insufficiency as well as hypertension. Sobin and Landis (16) failed to produce either arteriolosclerosis, arteriolar necrosis, or hypertension in animals subjected to prolonged choline deficiency. This was because they did not hit upon the method of a brief period of choline deficiency followed by a long period on the normal diet.

The contribution of Hartroft and Best is an important clue, to be followed up assiduously, because it may possibly lead to the discovery of the cause of hyalinizing arteriolosclerosis in human beings. It has always seemed probable to me that a dietary abnormality, either a deficiency or an excess of one or more constituents, might be found responsible for the development of arterial and of arteriolar sclerosis. The fact that the animals with renal arteriolosclerosis also developed hypertension is of the greatest interest, because it points directly to the renal origin of the hypertension that occurs after the development of vascular disease. It is of great interest also that the only animals that developed fibrinoid necrosis of the arterioles were those with pronounced renal excretory insufficiency accompanying the hypertension. This is certainly in keeping with our own findings in dogs with experimental hypertension due to constriction of the main renal arteries. All of the experimental evidence points directly to the probability that the arterial and arteriolar sclerosis of the benign phase of essential hypertension is primary, and precedes the development of the elevated blood pressure, and that the arteriolar necrosis of the malignant phase is secondary, and frequently a terminal manifestation.

The nature and origin of arteriolosclerosis. Much of the difficulty involved in the whole problem of the pathogenesis of essential hypertension is the lack of knowledge of the nature and origin of obliterative arterial and arteriolar sclerosis. Although hyalinizing arteriolosclerosis bears no close morphologic resemblance to simple intimal arteriosclerosis of the larger arteries, yet it has been pretty generally accepted that it is, nevertheless, the counterpart of obliterative endarterial proliferation and atheromatosis of the larger arteries. This is based in great part on the fact that some lipoidal deposits can be demonstrated in some of the hyalinized arterioles and that proliferation of the arteriolar intima does occur. This may all be correct, but it has not been established beyond question that the two are pathogenetically identical. It may be that the work of Hartroft and Best has opened the way to the elucidation of this perplexing problem, and the more recent contribution of Gofman and collaborators (17) may hasten its solution.

Periarteritis nodosa. A matter that requires clarification is the question of the identity of panvasculitis (periarteritis nodosa) and the necrotizing lesion of the arterioles seen in the malignant phase of essential hypertension. The occurrence of periarteritis in the contralateral kidney and especially in other sites in rats with hypertension as a result of constriction of only one main renal artery, as well as in rats, especially unilaterally nephrectomized ones, treated with desoxycorticosterone acetate and a high salt diet (Selye and collaborators, 18), has brought this question to the fore. The work of Loomis (19), in Dr. Oliver's laboratory, has focused attention on the possible significance of the absorption of breakdown products of infarcted, necrotic renal substance in the pathogenesis of this type of vascular lesion. The studies of Holman (20) with uranyl nitrate and mercuric chloride, because of the known necrobiotic effects of these chemicals on renal parenchyma, tend in the same direction. As a matter of fact, many years earlier Dominguez (21) also studied the effect of uranyl nitrate on the vascular system of rabbits. It is interesting that in dogs Holman observed necrotizing arteritis only in the heart and lung, whereas in rabbits Dominguez observed degeneration, including calcification but not periarteritis nodosa, even in the smaller arteries and arterioles of many organs, especially the kidney, with atrophy of the kidney and with hypertension in at least one of his animals. He attributed all these lesions to the direct effects of the poison. Yet Cromartie (22), who induced the development of hypertension in rats by the perinephritis method, reported the development of periarteritis nodosa in many organs, presumably as a direct result of hypertension. There was no necrosis in the kidneys.

Dr. Talia Bali and I (23) have been working on this subject for more than a year, during which time we have studied more than 500 rats. We can certainly confirm the development of periarteritis nodosa in many rats with hypertension from unilateral renal ischemia, but we can also assert, without equivocation, that massive necrosis from infarction of the renal tissue is not a necessary condition for the development of these lesions. The work of Selye (18) with his so-called endocrine kidney is in complete accord with our view. This does not exclude parenchymatous degeneration of the kidney from playing a part in this phenomenon.

We have been greatly interested in the healing process of periarteritis nodosa. Although the acute and subacute stages are easily and definitely distinguishable from simple intimal arteriosclerosis, yet we have become convinced that there is at least a superficial resemblance between the end stage of the healing process of periarteritis nodosa and obliterative arteriosclerosis, especially of the type without atheromatous intimal deposits and calcification. One cannot help wondering whether, in some cases at least, the two have not been confused. Much work still remains to be done on this subject for the purpose of elucidating the possible relationship between these two conditions.

The probability that they are closely related is not great, for a number of reasons: In the first place, the occurrence of definitely recognizable acute or subacute periarteritis nodosa in individuals with hypertension is infrequent. It can be said with certainty, therefore, that in man, at least, hypertension per se is not a sufficient condition for the production of periarteritis nodosa. The same applies to the dog. In about 1300 dogs, we have seen this condition in only 2, and in these, only in the large branches of the coronary arteries. In the second place, the healing stage of periarteritis nodosa does show definite morphologic differences from simple intimal arteriosclerosis, the most striking ones being the scarring of the media, which is not a common accompaniment of simple intimal arteriosclerosis. There is also much less elastosis in periarteritis nodosa than there is in arteriosclerosis. As a matter of fact, even Dorothy Loomis spoke mostly of the destruction of the elastica in periarteritis nodosa, but because she observed a few larger vessels with elastosis, she attributed this to the healing of the inflammatory process of periarteritis nodosa instead of concluding that these vessels were also the seat of simple intimal arteriosclerosis. Still another difference between simple intimal arteriosclerosis and healed periarteritis nodosa is that although lipid material is found at times in vessels that are the seat of periarteritis nodosa, yet it is situated mainly at the site of the degenerating internal elastic lamina, where it is deposited diffusely between the fibers, and lipid is also present in the inflammatory nodules in the adventitia, but mostly within large mononuclear foam cells. This distribution is entirely different from the lipid deposits found in simple intimal arteriosclerosis.

The unusual susceptibility of the rat and rabbit to periarteritis nodosa may yet prove to have been merely a source of confusion, especially in relation to the vascular changes of the malignant phase. The latter involves a decision whether the necrotizing lesion of the smallest arterioles is identical with periarteritis nodosa. A typical arteriolar lesion of the malignant phase is characterized either by necrosis of the arteriole—just a naked, necrotic vessel—or by necrosis with slight perivascular infiltration of some lymphocytes and a few polymorphonuclear leucocytes, but not with proliferation of the ad-

ventitia or diffuse lymphocytic infiltration of the wall. The distinguishing conditions are as follows: Periarteritis nodosa occurs naturally in
old, presumably otherwise normal, rats, while the malignant arteriolar
lesions do not occur naturally in young or old rats. As a matter of fact,
although the old rats are referred to as normal, yet the incidence of
hydronephrosis, focal interstitial nephritis, and arteriosclerosis in such
rats is great, so that the connection with renal disease is still there.
Periarteritis nodosa occurs with no greater frequency in young animals
with elevated blood pressure, without impairment of renal excretion,
than in old rats with normal blood pressure. Table 1, however, shows
that the occurrence of periarteritis nodosa is much greater in young
and old rats with elevated blood pressure and renal excretory insufficiency, as indicated by elevated blood creatinine, than in those with
normal blood pressure and normal renal function. The definitely
greater incidence of malignant vascular lesions than of periarteritic
lesions in such animals is at least an indication that although they
may occur together, yet the two may not be identical and perhaps not
even caused by the same condition. It is my earnest hope that the
discussion will help to clear up some of these problems.

   The effect of hypertension alone in the pathogenesis of vascular

TABLE 1. The Occurrence of Periarteritis Nodosa and of Arteriolar Necrosis in Rats
with Experimental Renal Hypertension, with or without Uremia *

	Periarteritis Nodosa	Arteriolar Necrosis	Periarteritis Nodosa and Arteriolar Necrosis
Normal blood pressure, normal creatinine, left kidney ischemic (37 rats)..10.8% (= 4 rats)		0	0
Elevated blood pressure, normal creatinine, left kidney ischemic (92 rats)..10.8% (= 10 rats)		0	0
Elevated blood pressure, elevated creatinine, left kidney ischemic, right kidney hydronephrotic (31 rats) ....41.9% (= 13 rats)		64.5% (= 20 rats)	25.8% (= 8 rats)

*In the three groups, the aorta was contricted between the origins of both main
renal arteries. Periarteritis occurred with the same frequency in the two groups that
showed no impairment of renal excretory function, with or without hypertension. The
incidence of periarteritis nodosa is much greater in the group with hypertension and
renal functional impairment. In this group the incidence of arteriolar necrosis was
greater than the incidence of periarteritis nodosa.

lesions. There are those who hold the view that in man hypertension per se is a sufficient condition for the production of arterial and arteriolar sclerosis (24). The best example of arteriosclerosis presumably caused by hypertension alone is the unusual amount of sclerosis seen in the pulmonic artery in association with chronic mitral stenosis. It is supposed that the stretching of the thin-walled blood vessel, by reason of the hypertension in the lesser circulation, is the direct cause of the pathologic change; but this can hardly be regarded as proved, and other conditions, even the chemical state of the blood in this vessel, must be taken into consideration. Phlebosclerosis is usually mentioned as another example of the effect of hypertension alone on a blood vessel, but again, other conditions, such as stasis and the consequent chemical state of the blood, cannot be ignored. On the contrary, I have failed to find convincing reports of simple intimal arteriosclerosis in the vascular tree proximal to aortic coarctation in young persons in whom such a degree of arteriosclerosis could not be expected under ordinary conditions. The vessels are large and thick, to be sure, by reason of hypertrophy of the media, but they are not sclerotic. Similarly, I have failed to find a convincing report of simple intimal arteriosclerosis in a young person with pheochromocytoma of the adrenal; yet such persons frequently have the highest blood pressures ever recorded, and it may even be of the persistent type. Thus at least two pathologic conditions which in man are usually associated with hypertension, without renal disease, fail to afford any evidence that elevated blood pressure alone may cause arteriosclerosis.

The Significance of Hypertension Alone in the Development of Vascular Lesions in Experimental Hypertension

Experimental renal hypertension. Many investigators of experimental hypertension have held the view that elevated blood pressure alone is a sufficient condition for the determination of experimental sclerosis and arteriolar necrosis, and experimental evidence has been adduced for this view. How well this evidence will stand the test of time remains to be seen. Wilson and Pickering (25), for example, although they did not study renal excretory function in most of their animals, still determined that in rabbits either with one kidney removed and the main renal artery constricted or with both renal arteries constricted, acute arterial lesions developed structurally identical with those of the malignant phase in man, and they concluded that the effect was the result of the raised intra-arterial pressure alone. In a later study. Wilson and Byrom (26) came to a similar conclusion based upon a study carried out on rats. In these animals, the only tests of renal excretory function were determinations of blood urea in some of the animals. It is interesting to note that many rats with the highest blood pressures they recorded, but without renal excretory insufficiency, had no vascular lesions. Despite this, however, the investigators concluded that elevated blood pressure alone is a sufficient condition for the determination of these vascular lesions. The reasoning is not clear.

Finally, Byrom and Dodson (27) recently reported the production of typical, necrotic arterioles and necrotizing arteriolitis in the kidneys of normal rats subjected simply to the forcible injection of Ringer's solution under pressure through one carotid artery (about 15 times in quick succession) into the systemic circulation. When the animals were killed several days later, some showed vascular lesions. From this they concluded that increased intravascular tension alone is directly concerned in causing arteriolar necrosis in a hypertensive animal and, by inference, in human hypertensives. They found that neither uremia nor toxic absorption from injured renal tissues was a constant or necessary factor in the process, but suggested that either one may possibly facilitate the production of these lesions. They even went so far as to reason, teleologically, "that the lesions probably represent a vigorous attempt to repair a threatened breach due to local death and lysis of over-stretched medial muscle fibres in the terminal arteries and arterioles." Their idea is that brief, artificial distention of the arterial tree in normal rats causes the typical focal arteriolar necrosis, the smaller arteries of the kidney being selectively vulnerable, and that the same procedure causes more widespread but transient focal spasms of the small renal arteries. No one, so far, has published a refutation or confirmation of this work, and it should be kept in mind that it deals with the pathogenesis of arteriolar necrosis and not arteriolar sclerosis.

Neurogenic hypertension. I have had the opportunity of studying the tissues from our own and other dogs with neurogenic hypertension on the basis of excision of the carotid sinuses and a section of the aortic depressor nerves, but in none did I observe arterial or arteriolar sclerosis or necrosis, although some of the dogs had had this type of hypertension for more than two years. I have never learned whether the rats in which Visscher and his collaborators (28) produced hypertension by exogenous neurogenic stimuli developed vascular lesions or, if they did, what the nature of these lesions was. The end result of this experiment would be of great interest.

Bilateral nephrectomy in vascular disease. Finally, there is the work of Winternitz (29), of Holman (30), and of Grollman and collaborators (31) on the vascular changes in animals with bilateral nephrectomy. Grollman and his collaborators demonstrated that in nephrectomized dogs treated with either cross transfusion, peritoneal lavage, or the artificial kidney, an elevation in blood pressure may develop. The animals also had profound azotemia. At autopsy, the investigators found pathologic changes which they interpreted as characteristic of malignant hypertension in such animals. I have seen some of these sections, and although in most of them the pathologic changes in the blood vessels were not typical of the malignant lesion usually seen in dogs with both renal arteries constricted to excess, yet in some there were undoubtedly lesions of the arterioles characterized by necrosis of the wall and extravasation of blood into the wall, typical of the malignant phase of experimental renal hypertension. It must be remembered, however, that these animals were not just bilaterally nephrectomized animals. They were *treated* bilaterally nephrectomized animals, and they were both hypertensive and azotemic. The exact cause of the elevated blood pressure is not known, but there is at least a reasonable possibility that it was plethoric in origin. No determinations of the blood volume or of the amount of tissue fluid were given in the publication. What the significance of all this work will prove to be remains to be seen.

Pathologic Changes in Special Organs

The heart. Little new has been learned in recent years about cardiac hypertrophy, one of the classical anatomical manifestations of the hypertensive state. This condition also develops in animals with experimental renal hypertension, especially in the rat and rabbit, in which it occurs rapidly and in which it has been used as a measure of hypertension.

There is certainly no evidence on the basis of the work on experimental renal hypertension for accepting the general view that coronary arteriosclerosis is a consequence of hypertension, although it must be admitted that it occurs with greater frequency and severity in hypertensive than in normotensive human beings. Certainly, no one can assert that hypertension is a necessary condition for the development of coronary arteriosclerosis, for severe coronary arteriosclerosis occurs in persons with normal blood pressure and nothing resembling true intimal arteriosclerosis has been observed in dogs with persistent experimental renal hypertension of the benign type, even after 7 years of hypertension. Periarteritis nodosa has been found in the coronary arteries as well as in the arteries of other organs in human beings and in dogs with normal or elevated blood pressure.

The adrenals. Simple or nodular hyperplasia and even true adenoma of the adrenal cortex have been reported in association with human essential hypertension (32). These findings have not been widely confirmed (33). In our own experience, at the Institute of Pathology, Western Reserve University, these changes were by no means a constant finding at autopsy in cases of essential hypertension. It remains to be seen what significance is to be attached to these alterations. Further studies of cortical hormones may help to clear up this matter. It is now generally accepted that pheochromocytoma of the medulla causes paroxysmal hypertension, but the significance of hyperplasia of the medulla and muscular hypertrophy of the adrenal veins, described by Goldzieher in hypertensive individuals, is now discredited.

Selye, on the basis of his work with desoxycorticosterone acetate, has reported that hyperplasia of the adrenal cortex with depletion of the lipid material in the cortex occurs in rats with experimental hypertension on the basis of administration of this material or as a result of renal ischemia. According to Selye, overdosage with desoxycorticosterone acetate induces the development of nephrosclerosis and hypertension in rats receiving sodium chloride, especially if they are unilaterally nephrectomized. He has reported the development of hyaline necrosis in the arterioles of the kidneys of such animals. The main vascular lesion found, however, was periarteritis nodosa. The fact that the ablation of the adrenals interferes with experimental renal hypertension is another indication that these glands probably play an important part in the pathogenesis of hypertension.

The hypophysis. An increase in the number of basophilic cells in the anterior lobe of the hypophysis and basophilic invasion of the posterior lobe have been reported in a high percentage of all cases of essential hypertension, but especially in patients in the malignant phase. This change, however, has also been found in chronic glomerulonephritis in some forms of obesity, and in other conditions. It is practically always associated with hyperplasia or adenoma, or both, of the adrenal glands. There is a tendency now to regard these alterations of the pituitary body as merely secondary. The fact that there is no basophilism whatsoever in many cases of essential hypertension minimizes the possible significance of this manifestation in the pathogenesis of essential hypertension. The recent studies of experimental hypertension have not helped to unravel the part played by the pituitary in the pathogenesis of the elevated blood pressure.

The brain. Hypertensive encephalopathy is recognized as a manifestation of the benign and malignant phases of essential hypertension and, according to Scheinker (34–36), is the result of changes brought about by cerebral vascular disease. He has described alterations of cerebral capillaries, veins, and arterioles in this condition which seem previously to have escaped observation. Changes of a similar nature have not been described in the experimental animal. He draws attention to an acute form of hypertensive brain disease characterized in the gross and histologically by findings characteristic of cerebral swelling. According to him, this is caused by acute vasomotor disturbances, followed by vasoparalytic distention of the veins and capillaries and associated with increased permeability of the vessel walls for serous fluid. This alteration is considered reversible, in the early stage.

Scheinker has also directed attention to the early stage of cerebral vascular change in cases of human arterial hypertension in which vascular alterations are characterized by a combination of proliferative and degenerative changes confined to the capillaries. He found no direct parallelism between the cerebral vascular changes and those of the kidneys. The pathologic changes consisted of hyaline degeneration and fibrotic thickening of the walls, associated with a narrowing or obliteration of the lumen. He considered these a special form of arteriolopathy typical of hypertension and different from those found in the usual cases of arteriosclerosis. He believes that these characteristic arteriolar changes may be due to functional vascular disturbance of prolonged duration or of repeated occurrence. The changes in the remainder of the brain consist of diffusely scattered, circumscribed, small foci of old and recent softening, perivascular hemorrhage, small or massive hemorrhage, and diffuse or localized edema of the brain. He believes that the alteration of the brain is secondary to the arteriolar lesions.

He also studied the venous alteration associated with hypertensive disease of the brain in 65 cases. The lesions were of two types: (1) reversible changes, manifested by venous stasis, resulting in tremendous distention; and (2) structural alterations of the vessel walls characterized by an extreme degree of atrophy and advanced signs of degeneration and necrosis. He draws attention to the predominantly venous origin of cerebral hemorrhage, which he considers the terminal phase in a sequence of events which have their beginning in reversible vascular disturbance. In a later stage structural alteration of the cerebral veins occurs and, terminally, degeneration and necrosis of the vessel wall are present. He believes that in the presence of far advanced venular atrophy, an elevation of the venous pressure would appear to be an essential precursor of the massive escape of blood.

More studies of this kind are still necessary before the significance of the cerebral manifestations described by Scheinker can be properly evaluated.

The conjunctival capillaries. The most recent contribution to our knowledge of the anatomical changes associated with the hypertensive state in man is a study of the conjunctival vessels by the method of biomicroscopy, utilizing magnifications up to 200 times, which has been carried out by Dr. Lack and his collaborators (37). They have observed a hypertensive pattern of abnormality in the capillaries of the conjunctiva. This pattern is characterized by pronounced narrowing, elongation, and looping of the capillaries, which in addition show fixed angularities or tortuosities, tubular thickening of the walls, and loss of normal distensibility.

They found that 98 per cent of all hypertensive patients showed significant capillary changes of this type. There was a direct correlation between the severity of this abnormal capillary pattern and the rise in diastolic pressure. A correlation between capillary vascular damage and sex or age was not established. In 80 per cent of the series of hypertensives they also found pathologic changes in the arterioles. No capillary involvement was found in 72 per cent of non-hypertensive hospital patients who composed a control series. Some changes, usually slight and of bizarre type, were present in 28 per cent, but none showed the hypertensive pattern of capillary abnormality. In 96 per cent of the hypertensive series, they found intravascular clumping of the red cells. This was also found in 67 per cent of the control series.

Their conclusion was that the results of their study indicate it may be worth while clinically to evaluate by this method the role of the capillary in hypertension and to direct efforts toward systemic evaluation of the pathologic changes in the capillary bed as it relates to the process of hypertension. Inasmuch as from the studies on man it is impossible to arrive at any conclusion about the causative relationship between the changes in the capillaries and hypertension, Dr. Lack, Dr. Schwartz, and I have undertaken a similar study in dogs before and after the development of experimental renal hypertension. This may afford the answer to this important problem.

Thus, although the anatomical changes associated with the hypertensive state have been the subject of study for more than a century, I hope it has become abundantly clear from this brief survey that the causative relationship between vascular disease and hypertension still remains to be established.

· · · · · · · · · · · · · · · *by* ARTHUR GROLLMAN

Experimental Studies on Hypertension

THE present paper summarizes some of the experimental studies which have been carried out by the author and his associates during the last decade on the general subject of hypertension. These studies have touched upon various aspects of the problem of experimental hypertension as it is induced in the laboratory animal and as it occurs clinically in the human patient; they will be discussed with reference to the generally accepted notions as well as the work of others in the same field. It may be stated at the outset that despite the often repeated statement that experimental and clinical hypertension may have little in common, this view is not supported by the available data. In fact, the resemblances between the condition as induced experimentally and as occurring spontaneously in man are so close as to justify the working hypothesis that the two are fundamentally related and that a study of the experimentally induced disease will help to elucidate the disorder as observed in human beings.

The Induction of Hypertension in the Experimental Animal

Attempts to induce hypertension in the experimental animal by manipulations of the kidney date from the last century. Much of the earlier work, however, was based on observations of the immediate effect on the blood pressure of various manipulations of the kidney and hence either demonstrated an acute rise in pressure which has no relationship to hypertension as a disease or else failed to note the subsequent development of hypertension after the lapse of some time following the procedure. The first demonstration that hypertension could be induced by interference with the blood flow through the kidney was that of Dr. E. T. Bell (1), in whose honor this symposium is being held. In association with A. H. Pedersen (2), Dr. Bell in 1930 demonstrated the development of hypertension in a rabbit by occlusion of the renal vein and the application of a membrane around the kidney to prevent the development of a collateral circulation. This was the first clear-cut demonstration that interference with the blood supply to the kidney might result in hypertension and that a similar condition was perhaps responsible for the disorder as it occurs in man. Chanutin and Ferris (3) in 1932 induced cardiac hypertrophy which reflected the rise in blood pressure occurring in rats subjected to subtotal nephrectomy, a procedure used subsequently by others to induce hypertension.

Goldblatt and his collaborators (4) in 1934 introduced the procedure of partially clamping the renal artery by means of a specially devised clamp. This method was an advance over those previously used in that it did not involve drastic measures with the kidney and led to much more uniform responses than had been previously obtained. Subsequently, others utilized the application of collodion, cellophane, silk, cotton (5), and more recently, a plastic, to attain the same result. It was discovered later, however, that mere constriction of the renal parenchyma by application of a figure-of-eight ligature (6) offered a simple means of inducing hypertension that was more certain than any of the above described measures. The method has been adapted to the rat, rabbit, and dog and used throughout our subsequent work. It avoids the too drastic constriction of the artery that is possible with the method of Goldblatt *et al.* and the infection apt to occur when enveloping the kidney, and it is technically simpler than these measures.

It must be emphasized here that hypertension occurs in only a small proportion of animals when one kidney is interfered with by the above described procedures. In most cases, it requires the removal of the opposite kidney before hypertension is induced. The significance of this will be referred to again later.

In addition to the operative procedures outlined, hypertension can be induced in animals in a variety of ways, including bilateral nephrectomy (to be referred to in detail later), the use of various toxic agents —for example, lead and other metallic poisons, and dietary insufficiency. All of these have in common the fact that they either remove kidney tissue, induce obvious damage to the renal parenchyma, or interfere with the blood flow through the organ. In the last-named procedure there is no obvious morphologic change in the kidney as determined by the usual methods of histologic examinations. In the disorder of the human being, we also encounter the disease without obvious morphologic damage (the so-called benign hypertension), as well as with renal damage, as in the hypertension secondary to infections (nephritides), to vascular disturbances (nephrosclerosis), etc. Assuming that hypertension is of renal origin, one may conclude, therefore, that either functional (i.e., without demonstrable anatomic change) or organic damage to the kidney may, if it involves the proper segment of the nephron, result in the disorder designated as hypertensive cardiovascular disease. This is characterized by an elevation in the diastolic blood pressure, an increased peripheral resistance, and other changes in the heart, eyes, brain, blood vessels, etc.

The Determination of the Blood Pressure in the Experimental Animal

The level of the blood pressure in different laboratory animals in which hypertension is induced is essentially the same as it is in human beings with the disease. The particular animal species to be used in a given study will be determined by the nature of the experiment at hand. For most purposes the rat offers many advantages, and for this reason we have used this species in many of our experimental studies. It was necessary, however, to find a procedure for determining the blood pressure in the rat, and a plethysmographic method (7), which has been widely used, was devised. There have been several modifications of this procedure, but in our hands, at least, none of these has offered any advantages and in general suffers from certain disadvantages. When proper precautions are taken, reproducible and accurate values may be readily obtained. The preliminary heating necessary in this procedure, if properly done, does not lead to error in the determination. Heating, however, may be limited to the rat's tail, but this renders the method unnecessarily tedious. Others have devised various electrical procedures for replacing the plethysmograph (8), but in our hands these methods lack the ease and accuracy of our original procedure, being dependent upon acoustic changes that are harder to detect than are the visual changes used in the plethysmographic method.

In the dog direct puncture of the femoral artery is easy and leads to unequivocal values for the mean blood pressure (9). We have therefore used this method exclusively in our studies. In the rabbit the method of McGregor (10), devised in Dr. E. T. Bell's laboratory, has proved satisfactory. This consists of the application of a small armcuff around the abdominal aorta and the detection of the auscultatory Korotkow sounds, as in determinations made on the human being.

Is a Pressor Agent Responsible for the Elevation in the Blood Pressure in Hypertension?

It is generally accepted that the elevation in the blood pressure observed in experimental hypertension is humoral in origin, but the nature of this humoral agent has been the subject of dispute. Earlier workers accepted renin, a pressor agent first observed in renal extracts by Tigerstedt and von Bergmann (11) in 1895, as responsible for the observed rise in blood pressure following manipulation or disease of the kidney. Subsequently angiotonin or hypertensin, produced by activation of renin, was accepted as the pressor responsible for the elevation in blood pressure. As work has progressed, however, this view has become increasingly untenable, so that most workers in the field have gradually wavered in their acceptance of this relatively simple and obvious explanation of the role of the kidney in the pathogenesis of hypertension. Others have sought in blood and kidney tissue for other pressor agents.

In earlier publications we have pointed out the invalidity of the pressor hypothesis (12, 13, 14). It must be remembered that kidney tissue or blood subjected to any chemical procedure may readily result in the development of either pressor or depressor substances and that it is unjustifiable to conclude from the presence of such agents that they actually play a physiological role in the organism. This objection can be raised to the more recently described claims that pressor agents have been isolated from the blood or from kidney tissue in hypertension. However, the most convincing argument against the existence of a pressor agent derived from the kidney is afforded by experiments on the effect of nephrectomy on the blood pressure, and these will, therefore, be discussed in greater detail later. The induction of hypertension by bilateral nephrectomy could be explained as due to a circulating pressor agent only by assuming that such a pressor agent is of extrarenal origin and that it is inactivated or excreted normally by the kidney.

The Effects of Unilateral Injury or Unilateral Nephrectomy on Hypertension

As already indicated, hypertension results when at least one kidney is injured and the contralateral one removed. Occasionally, however, the manipulation of a single kidney will result in hypertension. Apparently the same is true in the human being, where it has long been known that unilateral nephrectomy does not usually result in the development of hypertension. But sometimes, for reasons to be discussed later, such an operation may result in a rapidly progressive malignant hypertension if the patient already manifests some degree of hypertension before the removal of the kidney. In the dog (9) only rarely does the application of a Goldblatt clamp to one renal artery result in hypertension unless the contralateral kidney is removed. In our experience, it has occurred in less than 2 per cent of our animals. In the rabbit (15) the application of a figure-of-eight ligature unilaterally results in the development of hypertension in approximately 5 to 10 per cent of animals, whereas in the rat the effect of a unilateral operation is more variable. In well-nourished animals, raised on an ample and adequate diet and maintained in good condition, the incidence of hypertension following unilateral operation is much lower than in animals less well maintained. In some groups of animals, as high as 20 per cent may develop hypertension after the application of a figure-of-eight to one kidney without removal of the contralateral one.

As demonstrated by Halpern and the author (16), the incidence of hypertension following either the application of a unilateral figure-of-eight or unilateral nephrectomy is dependent on the status of the opposite kidney at the time of the removal of or operation on the other. If lesions are present, hypertension develops; if absent or minimal, the animal remains normotensive. Apparently the same thing is true of other animals, including man. If injury has already occurred in both kidneys, although this may be minimal and result in no great elevation in the blood pressure, the removal of one kidney may then result in a rapid elevation in the blood pressure to hypertensive levels. It is apparently a matter of the degree of renal disturbance or the percentage of the total available functional kidney tissue that determines whether or not hypertension develops. In the perfectly normal animal unilateral nephrectomy will result in little change in the blood pressure since the contralateral kidney can maintain the animal in normal condition. However, if the contralateral kidney already manifests some imperfection in function, although this may not be manifested by an elevation in the blood pressure, removal of or interference with the opposite kidney suffices to induce hypertension.

In the small percentage of animals in which hypertension is induced by operative manipulation of one kidney, the other one remaining intact, the removal of the first kidney after the induction of hypertension fails to cure the hypertension (9, 15). This result is opposed to the exceptional one observed in human beings, where removal of a hydronephrotic kidney or non-functional atrophic kidney has apparently brought about a decline in blood pressure (1). Why this should at times occur has not been adequately explained. Does the presence of the defective kidney prevent compensatory hypertrophy with increased function of the contralateral one? Unfortunately the occurrence of this condition is relatively rare, and no comparative study has as yet been made between the small group of patients responding to unilateral nephrectomy and the much larger group that fail to do so.

The Effects of Bilateral Nephrectomy on the Blood Pressure

One of the difficulties involved in determining experimentally the exact role which the kidney plays in the pathogenesis of hypertension has been the impossibility of ablating this organ without introducing the fatal effects of interference with its excretory functions. It has been impossible to apply the simple experimental procedure of extirpation, which has proved so important in elucidating the function of other organs. The earliest attempts at determining the effect of bilateral nephrectomy on the blood pressure led to the conclusion that this operation resulted in no change or a decline in the blood pressure. However, these experiments were invalidated by the fact that the animals survived for so short a period following the operation. In the hypertensive animal it has been demonstrated that the removal of the kidneys does not result in an immediate decline in the blood pressure (9, 15) but that this remains elevated until the animal becomes moribund. It has also been demonstrated in parabiotic rats in which the kidneys are removed from one of the pair that hypertension develops in the parabiont deprived of its kidneys, whereas the twin remains normotensive (17).

We have recently devised procedures which enable one to maintain nephrectomized dogs alive for extended periods in a relatively normal state of health. Originally an artificial kidney (18) was utilized, but this procedure has been superseded by intermittent peritoneal lavage, which has proved much more effective and convenient not only with experimental animals but with human patients as well (19). The details of this method are described elsewhere, but suffice it to say here that nephrectomized dogs have been maintained in good condition for from 30 to 70 days (Fig. 1). This enables one to study the effect of the absence of renal tissue in the body on the level of the blood pressure. The results of this study have shown that when the kidneys are removed from dogs, hypertension ensues and blood pressure levels comparable to those seen in hypertension develop (18). Contrariwise,

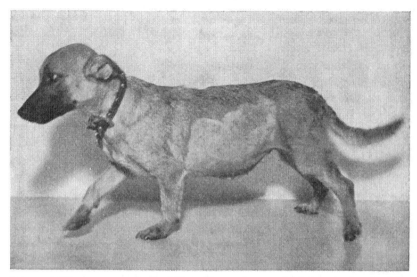

FIGURE 1. The appearance of a bilaterally nephrectomized dog (maintained by peritoneal lavage twice daily) 6 weeks following nephrectomy. Note the normal appearance of this animal, which was sacrificed 1 month after the above photograph was taken.

when the renal excretory function is excluded by ligature of the ureters or implantation of the ureters into the gut or vena cava (the kidneys being allowed to remain in the body), no elevation in the blood pressure results except in a few animals in which the destruction of the renal parenchyma by an infected hydronephrosis occurs (18, 19). Apparently, then, the presence of renal tissue in the body is necessary for the maintenance of a normal blood pressure; its absence results in the development of hypertension. Animals which have been nephrectomized and in which the blood pressure gradually rises to hypertensive levels reveal, at autopsy, pathological changes (to be referred to later) which we believe are the result of the development of malignant hypertension.

The induction of hypertension by bilateral nephrectomy is of fundamental importance in arriving at a general concept regarding the pathogenesis of this disorder. If hypertension is induced by the removal of the kidneys, obviously theories based upon the assumption that the kidney produces some pressor agent are entirely untenable. One might assume, of course, that peritoneal lavage or other artificial measures used to remove excretory products from the body fail to remove some agent normally excreted by the kidney, but such an assumption is rendered invalid by the observation that bilateral ureteral ligation or implantation of the ureter into the gut or vena cava, with excretory products being removed by the same artificial measures, results in no hypertension.

Several objections might be raised against the validity of the observations in the bilaterally nephrectomized animal, but these have been refuted by our more recent experiments (19). It might be objected, for example, that the moderate degree of uremia occurring in nephrectomized animals subjected to artificial measures for the removal of waste products suffices to cause an elevation in the blood pressure and the pathological lesions observed. However, a similar degree of uremia in animals with ureters ligated or implanted into the gut or vena cava fails to do so. The level of the blood pressure attained in the nephrectomized animal is also independent of the urea level of the blood. It might also be objected that the removal of the kidney results in an increased cardiac output or that the methods used result in an increased blood volume, which in turn increases the cardiac output and thus results in an elevation in the blood pressure. However, the invalidity of these objections has also been demonstrated (19). We have shown, for example, that the cardiac output is not materially affected but is actually decreased in the nephrectomized animal at a time when its blood pressure is markedly elevated. The blood volume and venous pressure are also not appreciably affected by this procedure. The level of urea and non-protein nitrogenous constituents of the blood does not apparently affect the level of the blood pressure, since this may be normal in animals with a high urea and non-protein nitrogen content—for example, in animals with a ureter implanted into the vena cava or duodenum. On the other hand, by subjecting animals to intermittent peritoneal lavage at 2-hour intervals, the blood urea content will remain below 100 mg. per cent. Despite this, one observes the usual elevation in the blood pressure (19).

Pathological Findings in Experimental Renal Hypertension

The pathological findings observed in animals suffering from experimental renal hypertension have been the subject of much study, with results that have been variously interpreted. There has been much conjecture regarding the relationship of the observed lesions to those seen in human hypertension. In 1938 Child (21) noted the presence of "innumerable petechial hemorrhages, diffuse in distribution, though predominating in the cardiac musculature and in the gastrointestinal tract." The source of these hemorrhages was the capillary bed, but there were no variations from normal in the arterioles and the walls of the larger arteries. Child noted the appearance of acute arteritis with thromboses and myocardial infarcts, hyaline degeneration of the media, edema, and fragmentation of the intima with diminution of the lumen and periarterial fibrosis. The arterioles in the liver of one dog showed marked intimal thickening with all but complete obliteration of the lumen. Goldblatt (22) in the same year demonstrated the appearance of diffuse arteriolar hyalinization and necrosis in dogs with experimental hypertension in which the malignant phase with renal insufficiency had been induced. Grossly these also showed petechiae, some of which were confluent with the extravasation of blood. Microscopically there was a degenerative disease of varying severity with hyalinization and necrosis of the arterioles and fresh extravasations of blood into the tissues.

According to Goldblatt, the degenerative and necrotizing arteriolar lesions which he observed were not distinguishable from those found in most cases of malignant hypertension in man as described by Moritz and Oldt (23) except that they were more severe and more widespread. The hyalinization and necrosis of the arterioles were also more severe and more widespread in animals which had suffered from a period of benign hypertension before the onset of renal insufficiency. In one animal which had previously suffered from a long period of benign hypertension, there was thickening of the arterioles with or without hyalinization of the intima.

We have demonstrated the occurrence of necrosis of the arteries, arterioles, and myocardium, similar to that observed by previous authors, in animals subjected to bilateral nephrectomy (20). In an attempt to elucidate the pathogenesis of these lesions, a variety of manipulations on the kidney were performed, including (1) removal of both kidneys, life being prolonged by dietary restriction in which diffusible salts were excluded from the diet, by use of the artificial kidney, by exchange transfusion, or by peritoneal irrigation; (2) ligation of the ureters; (3) implantation of one ureter into the small intestine, with contralateral nephrectomy; (4) implantation of one ureter into the vena cava, with or without contralateral nephrectomy; (5) section of the ureters, with drainage of the urine into the intraperitoneal; and (6) the injection intraperitoneally of concentrated dialyzed urine. The results of these experiments demonstrated that arterial, arteriolar, and myocardial necroses are dependent neither on an elevation of the blood pressure nor on an accumulation of the usual catabolites, but may occur even when the blood pressure is not elevated or in the absence of a severe degree of uremia.

The vascular lesions seen in dogs differ considerably from those seen in patients dying from hypertension as ordinarily observed. However, they do resemble those seen in patients with acute renal insufficiency in which hypertension has developed over a relatively short period, for example, as a result of blockage of the renal artery by a growing tumor or in the acute anuria of the so-called lower nephron nephrosis (24). The vasculitis occasionally seen in patients dying from malignant hypertension is usually associated with more cellular response than that observed in experimental animals. The changes observed in the myocardium resemble those seen as a result of potassium deficiency,* a resemblance that raises the question whether the latter changes are not induced by the kidney damage known to result from acute potassium deficiency. The observed changes in the myocardium of the hypertensive have an important bearing on the occurrence of myocardial damage in people suffering from hypertension.

It is not unexpected that lesions induced in the dog in the course of a week should differ from those encountered in man, in whom hypertension in a benign form may exist for many years before death. That the duration of the disease and the extent of the renal damage may determine the morphological appearance of the arterial and arteriolar lesions is well illustrated in a patient reported by Muirhead and the author (24) in whom a rapidly developing hypertension secondary to widespread tubular damage was followed by death within 10 days. The lesions in the blood vessels in this patient were identical with those observed in dogs following bilateral nephrectomy. As pointed out by Goldblatt (22), only in a dog which he had maintained with an elevated blood pressure for several years were the arteriolar lesions comparable to those observed in man. Goldblatt concluded that the "combination of increased vascular tension and the effect of a chemical substance of renal origin, the result of interferences with the circulation of the kidney, are necessary conditions for the production of arteriolar necrosis and the associated hemorrhages." However, the lesions are producible with or without an elevation in the blood pressure and with or without "uremia." The combination of the two is nevertheless most effective in their production.

* I am indebted to Dr. Benjamin Castleman of the Massachusetts General Hospital for his comments and suggestions regarding these observations.

Water and Electrolyte Disturbances in Hypertension

Water and electrolyte disturbances in hypertension are of considerable interest not only from an experimental standpoint but also from a practical clinical one, in view of the demonstrated effect of drastic sodium restriction in the treatment of hypertension (25). It is now generally conceded that drastic sodium deprivation results in a lowering of the blood pressure and an amelioration of symptoms in many patients manifesting hypertensive cardiovascular disease. This procedure has been widely applied clinically (26), either by means of diets in which the sodium content is reduced to from 200 to 500 mg. per day or more drastically in the so-called rice diet, the efficacy of which depends, we believe, upon its low salt content (27), although the low protein content may also play a part in bringing about the observed hypotensive effects.

The mechanism whereby the restriction of salt induces its hypotensive action is still the subject of study. However, that some disturbance in the salt and water metabolism occurs in chronic hypertension is clear not only from the effect of drastic salt restriction on the level of the blood pressure but also from the different reactions of normal and hypertensive persons to salt restriction (28), the increased antidiuretic content of the urine in hypertension (29), and, as demonstrated by Eichelberger (30) and by Laramore and the author (31), the change in the water and salt content of the tissues in hypertension. The latter authors have demonstrated that in the late stages of the disease in rats the water content is greatly increased, as is also the sodium content, while the potassium content of the tissues is decreased. The chloride content of the muscular tissues (the heart, gut, striated muscle, and spleen) is also increased, while that of other tissues (the blood, brain, liver, and skin) is decreased. These findings offer histochemical evidence of the systemic effects of hypertensive disease, effects demonstrated also by the widespread pathological lesions observed in this disorder.

Despite the apparent abnormality of the salt and water metabolism in hypertension, it is unjustifiable to conclude that this is the basic dysfunction responsible for the manifestations of this disorder. It is equally unjustifiable to conclude that the adrenal cortex, despite its well-known action in the regulation of the salt and water metabolism, plays an important role in the pathogenesis of the disorder. Cortisone and ACTH, incidentally, even in the unphysiological doses in which these drugs are administered, exert relatively minor effects on the blood pressure of the normal or hypertensive rat or dog (32).

The Alleviation of Hypertension in the Experimental Animal

In order to apply the same procedures to human beings, many attempts have been made to lower the elevated blood pressure in animals rendered hypertensive. The experimental animal offers a great advantage in the study of this problem because of the marked variability shown by the human hypertensive. As has been often demonstrated, the course, particularly the blood pressure, of the human hypertensive, is subject to marked fluctuations, which it is difficult to obviate unless the patient is hospitalized and repeated measurements are made over periods of many months. Unfortunately this is not always practicable, and many of the data cited in the literature are inconclusive because sufficiently long control studies were not made before the patient was subjected to a given procedure. In the experimental animal, on the other hand, one can rigidly maintain a base line of control pressures and evaluate the effect of a given procedure in the course of several weeks. Moreover, by using the rat as the experimental animal, one can deal with a sufficient number of individuals to overcome the inevitable effects of biological variation and can utilize amounts of materials sufficiently small to permit their experimental study and chemical fractionation.

Applying the above methods, we have studied the various drugs used in the treatment of human hypertension or advocated in the past, as well as other procedures. However, it must be emphasized that noxious material will lower the blood pressure in experimental hypertension just as infections, myocardial infarction, and other debilitating effects tend to lower it in the human. This has not always been taken into account by investigators, and one finds in the literature references to procedures such as the implantation of dead kidney tissue or the injection of turpentine or of crude renal extracts exerting a pyrogenic effect, as procedures that lower the blood pressure. Such noxious influences in lowering the blood pressure obviously have no therapeutic application and are misleading. Before attributing any significance to a lowering of the blood pressure in the experimental animal or man, it is necessary to demonstrate that the material is not exerting a purely noxious influence, that the duration of life is extended, and that the general well-being of the animal is ameliorated by the therapeutic measure.

Applying the above procedures to the rat with experimental hypertension, one finds that many of the drugs advocated from time to time for the treatment of hypertension exert little or no effect on the blood pressure except when used in excessively large doses and that when so used the effects are deleterious, resulting usually in a short-ened period of survival for the animal. This is true, for example, of the nitrites, thiocyanate, the veratrum alkaloids, histamine, and other vasodepressor agents which have been advocated for use in human hypertension (33).

In experimental hypertension the only consistently effective agents for lowering the blood pressure that we have encountered and that have not induced evidence of deleterious action but on the contrary have prolonged the survival of the hypertensive animals in better con-dition than the untreated controls are (1) drastic sodium restric-tion (27), (2) certain renal extracts (34), and (3) certain oxidation products obtained from marine oils (35). The effect of drastic salt restriction has already been discussed in the preceding section. The effectiveness of renal extracts administered orally was first reported over a decade ago, and consistently, in our hands, the method has proved effective in lowering the blood pressure in the experimental animals and in the few patients on whom it has been tried. It must be emphasized that these extracts differ from those described by others who have utilized dialyzed extracts (dialysis results in discarding the principle we consider to be effective), crude extracts rich in pressor agents, or crude kidney tissue, all of which, we believe, lower the blood pressure through their pyrogenic and other noxious influences. Renal extracts prepared by alcohol extraction of fresh kidneys may be sub-jected to further purification to give a water-clear solution contain-ing a minimum of solid material, and when administered orally they result in an appreciable lowering of the blood pressure, although this does not reach the normal level in animals with long-standing chronic hypertension.

Results comparable to those obtained with renal extracts have also been obtained through the oral administration of certain oxidized marine oils. A striking clinical response on a single patient has been reported where such an extract was used (35). This patient was hos-pitalized for a period of 16 months and alternately treated twice with renal extract and a comparable oil which was inactive. In each ob-servation period extending over several months, the administration of the active oil resulted in a marked lowering of the blood pressure, which later returned to its initial level while the patient was receiving the placebo.

That the administration of renal extracts or marine oils induces no noxious effect has been demonstrated by the long survival of animals so treated compared to untreated controls whose blood pressure was allowed to remain at a high level (36). We feel, therefore, that the lowering of the blood pressure by this means unlike that obtained by other procedures cannot be considered a deleterious effect. The possibility of lowering the blood pressure by such means is of greatest practical and theoretical importance.

The effective principles present in renal and oxidized marine-oil extracts have not been isolated or identified. However, that they are identical has been demonstrated to be highly probable by absorption studies of highly purified preparations.

Neurogenic Hypertension

It is possible to induce a type of hypertension, which has been designated as "neurogenic hypertension," by removing the pressor mechanisms in the neck through the cutting of the vagus and the removal of the carotid sinus on the opposite side, thereby eliminating the accelerator fibers (37). This often results in an elevation of the blood pressure, which, however, differs entirely from that observed following interference with the kidney. For example, the hypertension induced by the above operative procedure is often temporary; there is a return to normal after a lapse of days or weeks, as is not true in renal hypertension, which is permanent and increases progressively. The existence of permanent neurogenic hypertension does not appear to shorten the life of the animal, which remains in good condition. One of the dogs of our series, for example, survived for a period of over 5 years. A striking characteristic of this type of neurogenic hypertension, too, is the fact that exercise often brings about a reduction to normal levels, something not true of renal hypertension.

It is a widely current notion that hypertension in man is the result of nervous influences induced by the stress and strain of daily life; although the elevation is at first only paroxysmal in nature, eventually a permanently elevated blood pressure ensues. Despite the general acceptance of this view and its superficial reasonableness, there are, in fact, no convincing data to support it. In favor of this hypothesis, however, are the experimental studies of Farris, Yeakel, and their collaborators (38), who, by air-blasting, claim to have induced hypertension in rats. But some of their control animals also developed hypertension, although in a smaller percentage of the total than in the experimental group. We have repeated these experiments, with negative results (19). Of the usual laboratory rats only a few will react by convulsive seizures to the air-blast for extended periods, but even in these few hyperreactors no sustained elevation in the blood pressure has resulted. On the other hand, the viciousness of the wild grey rat (*Mus norvegicus*), with which Yeakel *et al.* obtained their most impressive results, necessitates such violent handling that any results obtained are inconclusive since they may be attributed to extraneous causes rather than directly to psychic stimulation.

The effectiveness of total sympathectomy in man in reducing the blood pressure, like the effectiveness of drastic sodium restriction, does not necessarily imply that nervous influences were the initial cause of the hypertension. Against the view that they are responsible are the recent studies of Wheeler *et al.* (40), who showed that the incidence of hypertension in a group of subjects diagnosed as suffering from neurocirculatory asthenia was no greater than in control subjects. Of great significance also are the independent observations of Dubois (41) and of Hartnett and Ratcliffe (42). The former found the incidence of hypertension in the natives of the Congo living in their primitive environment to be 35 per cent. The latter noted an incidence of 16 per cent in the southern Negro of the U.S.A., which is essentially that found by others in the Negro living under the more stressful environment of the North. Apparently, then, such diversities in environment as are encountered among native Africans, their North American descendants in Chicago, or those in Mississippi are of no importance in determining the incidence of hypertension. Must we conclude, therefore, that some intrinsic and hereditary defect rather than external environmental influences are responsible for the occurrence of hypertension in man? Such a view would be logical on the basis of our known facts, both experimental and clinical. The hereditary nature of "essential" hypertension is generally accepted, and it is only necessary to assume that in man, as in the experimental animal, a deficiency of function may occur in the kidney without morphologic damage manifestable by the routine procedures of pathology.

Conclusion

The preceding summary may appear to the reader to deal with unrelated and disjointed aspects of the problem of hypertension. However, they may be correlated and synthesized into a single concept which is in accord with the available experimental and clinical data. Although the statement is often made that experimental and clinical hypertension do not represent the same disorder, the resemblance between the two is most striking in many respects and is much greater than for other disorders reproducible in the laboratory animal. As a working hypothesis, we are certainly justified in assuming that the two conditions represent the same fundamental disorder.

The renal origin of hypertension in the experimental animal is established beyond question, as is also the fact that this hypertension may be present with or without morphologically evident disturbances. Likewise in man hypertension may occur either secondary to obvious renal disease or, as in essential hypertension, as a result of a congenital hereditary functional disturbance involving a non-excretory activity of the kidney. The nature of the mechanism is not established, but the effectiveness of renal extracts would suggest that it may be incretory.

Although much still remains to be learned about experimental as well as clinical hypertension, the available data point the way to the possibility of ultimately controlling this widespread and devastating disease without resort to such unsatisfactory procedures as the rice diet, drastic salt restriction, sympathectomy, the use of depressant drugs, or psychiatric procedures.

Questions and Discussion

DR. MAURICE B. VISSCHER: We have had two sides of the problem of hypertension presented to us this morning. The problem has more than two phases, as I am sure you will all agree after we have heard the papers on the remainder of our three-day program. At this point, however, we have a few minutes in which to begin our discussion. Does anyone among our guests wish either to ask a question of our first two speakers or comment on their material or the points of view they have expressed?

DR. EPHRAIM SHORR: I should like to ask Dr. Grollman a question about the interesting data he has presented on the electrolytic pattern in the tissues of the hypertensive animal. Were the animals on which the experiments were conducted made hypertensive by nephrectomy, perinephritis, or clamping? It would seem of the highest importance to his thesis to ascertain whether the electrolytic pattern in the animals made hypertensive by procedures such as perinephritis or constriction of the renal artery is identical with, or differs from, that in the animal which develops hypertension following nephrectomy.

DR. VISSCHER: Before calling on Dr. Grollman to answer this question, I should like to put another question of the same general sort to him. I wonder, Dr. Grollman, whether you have blood volume studies on your animals after sympathectomy, and whether the blood pressure changes are related to those in the blood volume, quantitatively.

Are there other questions before I call on Dr. Grollman?

DR. L. L. WATERS (YALE UNIVERSITY): I should like to comment on Dr. Goldblatt's statement that necrosis of the arterioles in malignant hypertension and arteriolosclerotic lesions are very different. The anatomical differences are obvious. What we want to know is whether or not these result from the same etiological and pathogenetic factor. That is important.

In commenting on Dr. Grollman's paper, I should like to say that

38

necrotizing arteriolar lesions follow in normal dogs the injection of pressor (renin) extracts of kidney protein, without any evidence of renal excretory failure.

DR. ELEXIOUS T. BELL: I am glad that issue was raised. I am glad it has been raised early in the symposium. That is, which comes first, the hypertension or the renal vascular disease? This is the most fundamental problem before the symposium. Is the hypertension initiated by organic vascular changes in the kidneys? Or is it a spastic change in these vessels which brings about the hypertension?

Now let us separate sharply, secondary from primary hypertension. Primary hypertension is the thing we are talking about here. Secondary hypertension, as we all know, is associated with diseases of the kidneys such as glomerulonephritis, polycystic renal disease, and the occasional instances of occlusion of the renal arteries or veins which Dr. Goldblatt referred to. There is no doubt that there is an occasional human case which resembles the Goldblatt kidney in its etiology, e.g., thrombosis of the main renal artery or vein.

I have the highest regard for my distinguished colleague, Dr. Goldblatt, and I think that his brilliant researches have shown beyond any doubt that kidneys may initiate hypertension. But I must disagree with him on his implication that what he has produced is comparable to human essential hypertension. I think he has reproduced the things which we call secondary hypertension of renal origin in man. I hope to present a little evidence that I have supporting the idea that primary hypertension is spastic in origin and not primarily due to organic changes in the renal blood vessels.

DR. GROLLMAN: I regret that the 25 minutes that was assigned for my presentation did not permit me to give more detailed data in support of my conclusions. The points raised in the questions which have been asked are very pertinent and have been taken into consideration.

In answer to Dr. Shorr, the analyses which were presented of the water and electrolyte content of tissues were made on rats rendered hypertensive by the application of a figure-of-eight ligature to one kidney and the removal of the contralateral kidney. These animals were subjected to no form of treatment, and hence any alteration in the composition of their tissues was taken to represent the effects of the induced chronic hypertension, which in every case had been present for at least several months. As controls, unoperated normotensive animals of approximately equal size and age were used. Eichelberger has also reported changes in the composition of the skeletal muscle of hypertensive dogs comparable to those which we have observed in a variety of tissues in the rat.

In answer to Dr. Visscher's question, blood volume determinations were made on the dogs prior to nephrectomy and subsequently, when an elevation in the blood pressure had occurred. The results of these studies indicated that the observed rise in the blood pressure could not be attributed to any increased blood volume, to peripheral circulatory failure (as evidenced by changes in the venous pressure), or to an increased cardiac output. In short, the hemodynamic factors in the nephrectomized dog are comparable to those observed in the animal with hypertension induced by manipulation of the kidneys. It is quite easy, of course, to induce edema, an increased blood volume, and other abnormalities in the nephrectomized dog by the injudicious application of such measures as the artificial kidney and peritoneal lavage, but under such conditions any elevation in the blood pressure is only transient and the animal soon succumbs to the abnormal circulatory condition induced. It is only in the animal in which a relatively normal state of the circulatory hemodynamics is maintained that an elevation in the blood pressure is observed and survival for such prolonged periods as I have reported is made possible.

Finally, concerning Dr. Waters' comment, we made only a semiquantitative estimate of the distribution of the lesions observed in the nephrectomized dogs at autopsy. However, I wish to correct any unintentional implication as to the significance of the acute necrotizing lesions which we have observed, for one may question justifiably their relation to the state of malignant hypertension. We have noted, for example, that comparable lesions may be obtained in the absence of any elevation in the blood pressure (for example, after cutting the ureters and allowing the urine to drain into the peritoneal cavity) or in the absence of azotemia. To be sure, a combination of azotemia and hypertension may, as claimed by Goldblatt, contribute to their appearance, but neither factor is essential to their presence. Incidentally, microscopic study of the dogs which have survived for longer periods (from 1 to 2 months) after nephrectomy reveals the proliferative changes of the media characteristic of the hypertensive state.

DR. GOLDBLATT: I am usually misquoted on my ideas about the causative relationship between hypertension, azotemia, and vascular lesions of the malignant phase, and Dr. Grollman has been similarly guilty. I did not state that all animals that develop vascular lesions have to have azotemia, but I did mention that some animals have azotemia, without implying that azotemia was a necessary condition. What I did say was that hypertension and impairment of renal function are necessary. Some form of renal injury is involved. That is quite different from the statement that "azotemia is a necessary condition."

Another matter that I should like to refer to is the question of hypertension per se causing arteriosclerosis. I had the opportunity of examining the tissues of a goodly number of dogs that had hypertension from ablation of the carotid sinuses and denervation of the aorta. These animals had the intermittent type of hypertension that occurs in this condition. I examined the tissues of these animals with great care and found no signs whatsoever of arteriosclerosis or arteriolosclerosis in those that had had this type of hypertension for 2 or more years. I should be greatly interested to learn what vascular changes Dr. Visscher and his group found in the blood vessels of animals with hypertension produced by exogenous neurogenic stimuli. If those animals, with hypertension obviously not directly of renal origin and without azotemia, showed changes resembling arteriolosclerosis, it would be of great interest. I doubt that they found any significant alterations in the blood vessels.

· · · · · · · · · · · · · · · ·*by* GEORGE W. PICKERING

Experimental Hypertension in the Rabbit

TEN years ago it looked as though hypertension produced by constriction of the renal artery was due to the release of renin from the kidney into the renal vein. In the dog it had been shown that hypertension could be produced in the sympathectomized animal, by constricting the artery to a kidney grafted in the neck or groin (4, 5). The Buenos Aires school had found an excess of a pressor substance in the blood (6). The only known renal pressor substance was renin, discovered by Tigerstedt and von Bergmann in 1898 (16), subsequently entombed, and disinterred by many workers between 1936 and 1938 (9, 11, 13). Renin would produce the same kind of gross circulatory changes as were found in experimental hypertension (10, 11). It acted by splitting a plasma protein into a smaller molecule, angiotonin, or hypertensin, and this had properties similar to the substance found in the blood by the Buenos Aires group (6, 8). Since then an increasing body of evidence has accumulated to show that the release of renin by the kidney is not the only factor involved. I want to summarize this evidence as presented to us in the rabbit.

In the autumn of 1936 Prinzmetal and I began trying to repeat Tigerstedt and von Bergmann's observations on renin. Having found that renin existed, we set out to try and assay it in the kidneys with a view to finding out if it was increased in experimental hypertension. As a standard we prepared an alcohol-dried powder of rabbits' kidneys and defined one unit as the amount of renin in 100 mg. of standard powder,* assaying unknowns by trying to match their effects on the

---

* This was the first attempt to carry out a biological assay of renin. Since then there have been many others, each employing a different unit. All these different units are most confusing. The method originally proposed was sound in principle in (1) using as a unit a given weight of a given substance which proved stable, at least for some years, and (2) assaying the unknown by trying to find the amount that would produce the same effect as a given amount of standard. One of the most urgent needs is to agree to a unit of renin, which should be defined as a certain weight of a standard stable preparation of renin kept in a central depot.

blood pressure of the unanesthetized rabbit with solutions of the standard. The error of this method is substantial, certainly of the order of 25 per cent. But variations in the renin content of rabbits' kidneys exceed this error. Restricting our enquiry to animals with one kidney, we found that in animals with the renal artery constricted, (1) renin was greatly reduced when the constriction was severe and the kidney infarcted. In these animals hypertension existed for only 2 or 3 days before the blood pressure fell below normal, prior to death. (2) Renin was increased in animals developing hypertension without renal infarction, provided the kidney was obtained in the first week. (3) Renin was normal in animals having hypertension lasting 2 months or more (14) (Fig. 1).

The second observation came my way by chance. In 1939 Miss Hill and I had shown that we could maintain hypertension by renin infusions lasting 4 hours, and I was anxious to obtain figures comparing the rate of the decline of hypertension after stopping an infusion and after removing the sole ischemic kidney. So in a number of animals the kidney was exteriorized when the renal artery was constricted and, at the end of a week, excised. The blood pressure fell to normal in about 4 hours, taking the same time to do so as after the stopping of a renin infusion. Now in 1938 Dr. Kelsall and I had shown that where all visible nerves were removed from the pedicle of the sole ischemic kidney* of the rabbit, hypertension persisted. To make the demonstration even more convincing, we then removed the kidney, expecting the blood pressure to fall. To our surprise it did not. After our assays were complete and I had had time to think about these results, the possible implications of these differences in the effects of nephrectomy became apparent, and I set out to confirm and extend them. I published the results in 1945 (12).

Briefly, in 10 out of 11 rabbits, excising the sole ischemic kidney 1 week after constricting the renal artery reduced the blood pressure to normal in a few hours, the pressure staying down till the animal died of uremia in 3–4 days (Fig. 2). In 8 rabbits, excising the sole ischemic kidney 2 months or more after constricting the renal artery did not abolish the hypertension, the pressure staying essentially un-altered till the animal died (Fig. 3). Extraction of the tissues of these animals showed no source of renin other than the kidney. Injection of renin showed that the response of the chronically hypertensive nephrectomized animal was unusually intense and prolonged, prob-

*To avoid confusion "sole ischemic kidney" throughout signifies that the renal artery has been constricted after removing the opposite kidney.

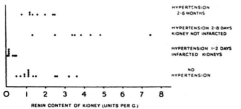

FIGURE 1. The renin content of the kidney, in units per gram, in rabbits from which one kidney had been removed. In those animals with no hypertension the kidney was either intact or had had the renal artery exposed but not clamped. In animals in which the renal artery was clamped, the hypertension lasted up to 2 days and then subsided; the kidney was found infarcted and contained little renin. In animals with maintained hypertension, the kidney showed increased renin from 2 to 8 days after clamping and a normal renin content from 2 to 6 months after clamping. (Pickering, Prinzmetal, and Kelsall: Clin. Sc. 4:401, 1942. This figure and the following three are reproduced by permission of the copyright owner.)

FIGURE 2. Rabbit 185. Right kidney removed (R.N.) 10/17/38. Left renal artery clamped (L.C.) 10/31/38. Left kidney removed 11/8/38. The arterial pressure returned to normal after nephrectomy. (Pickering: Clin. Sc. 5:229, 1945.)

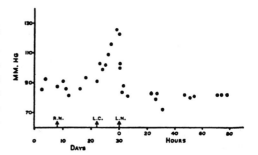

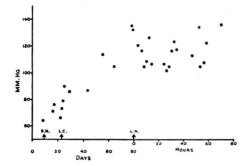

FIGURE 3. Rabbit 513. Right nephrectomy (R.N.) 7/28/43. Left renal artery constricted (L.C.) 8/11/43. Left kidney removed (L.N.) 10/7/43. The arterial pressure did not return to normal after nephrectomy. (Pickering: Clin. Sc. 5:229, 1945.)

44

ably a summation of the effects severally of nephrectomy and chronic hypertension, but the blood pressure returned to the preinjection level in all animals. The persistence of the hypertension in the absence of the source of renin thus suggests unmistakably that the hypertension is due to a cause other than renin.

Organic vascular lesions were not the cause. Moreover, Drs. Blacket and Sellers (3) have recently shown that removing the clamp from the renal artery abolishes the hypertension quickly if of short duration, more slowly if of long duration. The implication of these observations seems perfectly clear. The mechanism of hypertension is essentially different early and late after the constriction of the renal artery. In the early stages, the hypertension must be due to something coming out of the kidney, since removing the kidney abolishes it. It cannot be due to the secretion by the kidney of a depressor substance or to the accumulation of a pressor substance normally excreted or destroyed by the kidney. In the late stages, the hypertension cannot be due to something coming out of the kidney, since removing the kidney does not affect it, unless it is a long-acting pressor substance such as that described by Shipley and others (15). It must be due to an activity of the kidney, since removing the clamp abolishes it. It might obviously be due to the accumulation of a pressor substance probably of extrarenal origin, normally slowly excreted or destroyed by the kidney, or to an accumulated deficit of a depressor substance normally secreted by the kidney. The terms "depressor" and "pressor substances" are used in rather a wide sense, since the activity of the kidney in changing the milieu interne is strikingly slow and cumulative in chronic hypertension. Our conclusions as to the changing mechanism are similar to those reached by Ogden and his colleagues on quite different grounds, though I cannot go all the way with them on the part played by the central nervous system. The conclusions as to chronic hypertension are similar to those reached by Grollman, again on very different evidence.

My conception of the mechanism of hypertension in the rabbit is that the two factors are concerned from the outset, but that at first the secretion of the renal pressor substance, probably renin, is the more important. Later the other factor is the more important. This conception would explain a fact that has troubled me ever since I saw it in Goldblatt's first paper and observed it myself repeatedly in the rabbit. Frequently after the constricting of the renal artery the arterial pressure rises progressively over weeks or months. Now whatever the stimulus within the kidney that evokes the hypertensive response, it is difficult to imagine that it is not maximal soon after constricting the artery, since later the general arterial pressure rises and collateral vessels may grow in from the capsule. This slow rise is compatible with the slow intervention of the new factor that dominates the chronic stages.

In the effort to imagine to what extent the secretion of renin from the ischemic kidney may contribute to experimental hypertension, there has hitherto been one very material barrier, namely, ignorance of the properties of renin hypertension. In 1939 Miss Hill and I succeeded in maintaining hypertension with renin infusions lasting 4 hours, provided the dose was not too large. But it seemed vitally important to maintain infusions for much longer periods. Drs. Blacket and Sellers and I began such observations 3 years ago and eventually succeeded in keeping infusions running into the external jugular vein of the conscious rabbit for periods up to 3 weeks, by attending to such details as the maintenance of absolute asepsis in the infusion apparatus. We and our subsequent colleagues have established the following points:

1. Hypertension is maintained throughout infusions of renin lasting up to 18 days (Fig. 4).

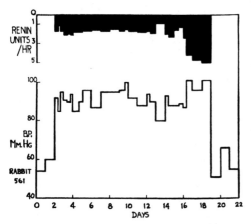

FIGURE 4. The daily average arterial pressure during a continuous intravenous infusion of saline for 2 days, renin for 17 days, and then saline for 3 days. Note that while the dose of renin is left constant, the arterial pressure fluctuates without any tendency to rise or fall. After the infusion was stopped, the arterial pressure fell to normal in 2 hours. (Blacket *et al.*: Clin. Sc. 9: 223, 1950.)

2. Provided the dose remains constant, there is no recognizable tendency for the hypertension to rise or fall over periods up to 10 days.

3. Increasing doses produce progressively smaller increments of arterial pressure, response being approximately linearly related to the logarithm of the dose.

4. The maximum degree of hypertension produced was 40 to 45 mm. Hg. This is the order of the hypertension that can be produced

in the same time by constricting the renal artery. It is less than that often found 2 months or more after constricting the renal artery.

5. The responsiveness to renin does not seem to be altered by removing 1 or 1⅓ kidneys.

6. When the infusion is stopped after periods up to 18 days, the blood pressure returns to normal or below in a few hours in all animals. There is no tendency for hypertension to persist after stopping renin.

7. While we were able with renin to produce maintained hypertension in all animals, we were unable to do so for more than two or three days with noradrenaline or adrenaline or mixtures of the two.

I should feel in a stronger position to comment on the implications of these observations on the problem of experimental hypertension in the rabbit if we had been able to continue infusions up to 2 months. But while the spirit was willing, the flesh, both human and rabbit, was weak, for these did prove most exacting experiments. With this reservation I think we can say that the results are consistent with the idea that the release of renin from the renal vein may be the chief factor in producing hypertension in the early stages after renal artery constriction. They provide no support for the idea that the mechanism that later intervenes is set in motion by the secretion of renin; it must be initiated by the changes in renal function occurring as a result of renal artery constriction. I regard the identification of this mechanism intervening in chronic hypertension as the most important outstanding problem in the field of hypertension.

· · · · · · · · · · · · · · · · · · · *by* IRVINE H. PAGE

The Renin-Angiotonin Pressor System

This symposium marks the formal acknowledgment, though certainly not a final conclusion, of the work of three men, Dr. Bell, Dr.
Fahr, and Dr. Clawson. Their retirement we must regret, though it
is in tune with the orderly course of nature which we all must serve,
and whose workings they have so diligently explored. Their varied
contributions have been wrought with great skill and favored at times
with good fortune. Hence they will endure. No man can wish for more.

It has seemed to me that a symposium such as this serves a highly
important function if it is used to air opinions derived from experience
and compiled with what wisdom we can. As concerns the renin-angiotonin system, I must confess with regret that our original hopes have
not been met and our goals have changed repeatedly. It has not been
shown that angiotonin is the mediator of either renal hypertension
in animals or essential hypertension in man, despite much testimony
in favor of this point of view. Nor has it been shown that it is not.
The final resolution of this problem remains for discovery. In saying
this, I do not in any way wish to minimize the importance of all the
experiments and observations that have been made, but rather to state
the goal clearly in front of us.

It is one of the prerogatives of getting older to have opinions. I
shall utilize this fully in my discussion in the hope that by showing
some to be wrong and some to be right, we shall all emerge from the
somewhat *iffy* position in which we now find ourselves. We have all
been guilty of covering up and, unwittingly, adding to the complexity
of the problem by such devices as giving names to uncertain phenomena, of drawing too sweeping conclusions, and of giving undue
importance to isolated phenomena. But without this immature and
youthful approach, we should not find ourselves with so many vistas
which can now be explored with more thoroughness, equal resolution,
and, I hope, greater equanimity. None of us, I believe, would pretend
now to give final answers on this key problem in hypertension. We

have lived long enough to recognize some of our shortcomings, but not long enough to get the facts on which must be based a satisfying solution of the problem. Perhaps others with even fewer inhibitions than we will find the key while we are still busy raking over debris created by our more youthful efforts. In the words of Bishop Berkeley, "We have first raised a dust and then complain that we cannot see." Let us hope that, at least, we can quit complaining.

Renin

Nature. The story of renin begins in 1898, when Tigerstedt and von Bergmann (1) showed that saline extracts of fresh rabbits' kidneys when injected into anesthetized rabbits produced a rise in the blood pressure. The active material was unstable to heat and non-dialyzable. It was not until 1909 that the work was confirmed by Bingel and Strauss (2), who further showed that much of the pressor activity was precipitable by ammonium sulfate between $\frac{1}{3}$ and $\frac{7}{12}$ saturation. Press juice from most other organs, regardless of the type of animal source, with the possible exception of the spleen, produced a fall in the arterial pressure rather than a rise as observed with kidneys. Then followed a period of years during which these results were in part confirmed but mostly denied. For example, Pearce (3) was unable to obtain pressor extracts from dogs' kidneys, whereas rabbits' kidney extract was active. Press juice gave only depressor effects.

Vincent and Sheen (4) recognized as early as 1903 that the problem was no simple one. They found evidence that kidney tissue contains both pressor and depressor substances. But most other tissues as well contain both, a view that was endorsed many years later by Collip (5). Vincent and Sheen concluded that, in general, pressor substances are extractable by saline solutions at ordinary temperatures, while depressor agents are extractable by boiling saline, which destroys pressor substances.

The next significant, but somewhat faltering, attempt to further the renin problem is described in Batty-Shaw's book, *Hyperpiesia and Hyperpiesis*, published in 1922. He attempted to repeat Tigerstedt and von Bergmann's original results with only moderate success. But the kidney extract from his hypertensive patients, extracted with saline, gave only depressor effects. Using animals freshly killed, however, he was able to find fairly marked pressor effects from kidney extracts, especially when compared with extracts of liver and brain, which were uniformly and strongly depressor.

In 1924 James Cash published his important work showing that hypertension could be produced in dogs by reducing the total kidney substance, but that, in addition, hypertension did not occur unless a portion of the kidney which had been deprived of its circulation had been allowed to remain *in situ*. This observation was confirmed in 1929 by Hartwick and provided the impetus for the work in Volhard's laboratory by Hessel (6) on renin, the first publication of which appeared in 1932.

Fresh pig kidney and spleen press juice was found almost always depressor, an observation which we have been able repeatedly to confirm. The depressor was dialyzable. It was only after autolysis that pressor activity appeared. But Hartwick and Hessel (7) found an ultrafiltrable pressor substance and concluded that both the depressor and pressor substances were of small molecular weight. If these observations were to prove true, prior concepts of the nature of renin would have to be radically revised. Their work has never been repeated by others so far as I am aware. Thauer confirmed the observation that depressor substance could be separated by dialysis, but the pressor substance, as Bingel had shown, he found to be precipitable by ammonium sulfate and its activity to disappear on complete deproteinization.

Hessel's (8) last publication in 1938 summarizes his more recent results and views. Unfortunately, many claims are unsupported by evidence. My personal experience with Dr. Hessel leads me to believe that probably most of the claims have some, although not complete, validity. In short, he found that long autolysis of the kidneys reduced the amount of renin, and the amount was independent of the blood contained in the kidneys. He defined a unit of renin as that amount of renin required to raise the blood pressure 30 mm. Hg in a 10-kilogram dog under pernocton narcosis. His preparations required from 0.1 to 0.2 mg. of dry substance for a unit. He prepared renin from kidneys frozen in liquid air, showing that post-mortem autolysis was not necessary for the formation of renin. On sterile autolysis, he was unable to show an increase in the renin content.

Our own work was begun in 1931, stimulated by Hessel and later by the announcement of the production of reproducible hypertension without a reduction in renal function by Goldblatt in 1934.

Preparation. The usual procedure for the preparation of renin consists of drying kidney cortex with acetone and ether and then extracting the stable dried powder with cold saline, or the ground cortical material is extracted directly with saline. The filtrate is brought to pH 4.5, the precipitate discarded and the filtrate adjusted to pH 6.5. After centrifugation, the supernatant fluid is brought to a concentration of 2 M. potassium phosphate. The precipitate is again brought into solution and reprecipitated. After re-solution, the addition of salt and acetic acid precipitates large amounts of inactive protein and pigment. Dialysis and the adjustment of the pH to 6.5 precipitate further inactive protein.

A wide variety of modifications of this method, and others somewhat different, are currently employed. They are all dependent on treating renin as though it were a labile protein. The method now used in our own laboratory by Dr. Arda Green consists of grinding frozen kidneys into 0.4 M. ammonium sulfate at pH 2.0 as the initial step. By repeated fractionation at different concentrations of ammonium sulfate and at different hydrogen ion concentrations, a highly active renin is obtained.

It would serve no purpose to present in detail any of the methods available for the preparation of renin. The original articles should be consulted (9). There is as yet no way which all investigators are agreed on of comparing quantitatively the different preparations of renin. About the best that can be said is some preparations are far more active in terms of milligrams of protein nitrogen than others when tested on dogs, cats, or rabbits. But no one has so far determined which steps in the preparation of renin are most efficient. Doubtless many of the precautions which are now recommended are needless.

Properties. Until 11 years ago, renin was regarded as a pressor substance, but no one had any idea what sort of substance it was. I think the first clue to its nature came from the observation of Kohlstaedt, Helmer, and Page in 1938 (10) that purification led to a marked increase in pressor activity when tested in the intact animal but that when perfused along with Ringer's solution in a dog's tail, constriction became progressively weaker and finally disappeared. It was only when we added plasma to the perfusing mixture of purified renin and Ringer's solution that full activity was restored. Clearly something in plasma was necessary for the activity of renin, and thinking we were being ultraconservative, we named the substance in plasma "renin activator" to indicate that in its absence renin was inactive. This subsequently proved an unfortunate choice, which a few of our scientific colleagues have been at very considerable pains not to let us forget.

In the late fall of 1938 Helmer and I (11, 12) found that after incubating renin with plasma and then ultrafiltering the mixture, we had a highly active pressor substance in the ultrafiltrate. From this observation our hitherto muddy thinking clarified, and it became obvious that an enzymatic reaction was involved, with the formation of a new substance. Evidently it became equally obvious to Muñoz, Braun-Menendez, Fasciolo, and Leloir (13), for they published simultaneously with ours a preliminary note in *Nature* suggesting that renin is an enzyme.

This justly famous group, under the brilliant direction of Braun-Menendez, has continued ever since to build the foundations of our knowledge of the renin-angiotonin system.

I need not pursue the testimony which makes it altogether probable that renin is a proteolytic enzyme acting on a protein contained in plasma to produce a third substance. Plentl and I (14) have tried to characterize this proteolytic property by comparing it with the similar action of enzymes and substrates of a known constitution. Bergmann and Fruton classified these intracellular enzymes as pepsinases, trypsinases, aminopeptidases, and carboxypeptidases, because of their analogies to the enzyme of the gastrointestinal tract. It might have been expected that renin would be homospecific with pepsin from the important observations of the two Croxattos that pepsin acting on substrate produces a pressor substance. This did not prove true. Renin is heterospecific when compared to pepsin or intracellular pepsinases. Prolonged dialysis of renin resulted in the elimination of the carboxypeptidase component, and other evidence gives but little support to the view that renin activity and trypsinase or aminopeptidase activity are homospecific. Thus renin seems to belong to a separate category of intracellular proteolytic enzymes, cathepsins 1 to 4. This evidence has been recently strengthened by Schales, Holden, and Schales (15).

Renin is also highly specific in that a pressor substance is produced only when the substrate and enzyme are of special sorts. As Fasciolo, Leloir, Muñoz, and Braun-Menendez (16) first showed, human renin yields angiotonin when acting on the plasma of men, pigs, and dogs; but pig renin produces none when incubated with human serum. Others have further amplified our knowledge of renin and substrate (Bean, 44; Helmer and Page, 45).

There are many other specific chemical and physical characteristics of renin which are partially known. But much of the work is clouded by the fact that renin has so far not been got out pure. Until this has been accomplished, we are forced to accept with reserve conclusions drawn from its study.

Now we shall consider even more briefly the problem of the substrate on which renin acts.

Renin-substrate (hypertensinogen). I have already described how we arrived at the conclusion that renin itself is not a pressor substance but requires the presence of another protein contained in plasma for its vasoconstrictor and pressor action. Helmer and I and, independently, Braun-Menendez, Fasciolo, Leloir, and Muñoz found the product of this reaction to be a dialyzable, heat-stable substance of much lower molecular size than either of the other constituents of the reaction.

Fractionation of hog serum with ammonium sulfate by Plentl, Page, and Davis (17) showed that the alpha$_2$ globulin component contained the material that acted as the substrate for the production of angiotonin. Euglobulins were entirely inactive. While renin-substrate moves with the alpha$_2$ globulin fraction in the electrophoresis apparatus, it has not as yet been prepared in an entirely pure form, and much too little of its chemistry is known.

About 10 years ago we (18) investigated the origin of this substance in the body and showed, not wholly conclusively, that the liver was its source. In our experiments hepatectomy was performed, and the progressive loss of response to renin shown. Leloir *et al.* (19), however, pointed out rightly that the kidneys should first have been removed, and then the liver, to prevent the discharge of renin during the operation of hepatectomy. We have adopted Leloir's suggestion and confirmed our previous observations. Unless some other objection arises, it seems safe to assume the liver as the source of renin-substrate.

There have been published a number of papers dealing with the concentration of renin-substrate in the blood. It may well be that the results will ultimately turn out to be correct, at least in a semi-quantitative sense, but I strongly fear that some of this work will require revision when better methods are available.

It is, then, with hesitancy, that I state that the pituitary has no part in its production, that nephrectomy elevates the blood concentration, and that renin injections reduce it, as does also the onset of shock. After adrenalectomy renin-substrate is said to disappear from the blood. Since most of us here have been responsible for some part of these observations, I do not dare point the finger of scorn. It is quite obvious that just as in the measurement of renin, the environment in which the enzyme must work is entirely uncontrolled, and the product of the reaction must be determined by bio-assay. Pure standards are not available. Interfering substances have not been recognized and steady-state reactions have been entirely ignored. Having confessed our sins, I am sure future investigators will do better. The least we can now do is re-examine the current methods to determine whether they are faulty.

Angiotonin (Hypertensin)

With the recognition that renin protein was not itself a pressor substance but required a protein in plasma, the possibility arose that renin was really an enzyme. In 1939 we (11) wrote: "It is suggested that renin is an enzyme—not a pressor substance—which acts on a substrate ('renin-activator') to produce a pressor substance, 'angiotonin'." As I have already pointed out, Helmer and I had found a strong pressor agent in the ultrafiltrate after the reaction of renin with renin-substrate, and simultaneously Braun-Menendez and his group announced that they had found a similar substance. I think from personal communication that both groups were quite well aware that an enzymatic reaction was involved, though somewhat clumsy efforts have been made to stress the differences rather than the uniformity in their points of view. But that is all in the past, and we are left only with a residue of conflicting nomenclature that nobody can change now and that as long as it is understandable makes little difference.

With the discovery of angiotonin, there was high hope that at last a vital link in the mechanism of at least renal hypertension had been found. Despite the current pessimism, I still think it has!

We all had the bad luck to have angiotonin turn out to be a polypeptide instead of some easily measurable aromatic pressor amine. This has prevented the elaboration of methods for its determination and thus blocked progress immeasurably. But with all these difficulties, the facts, circumstantial though they may be, strongly link angiotonin with the presence of certain types of hypertension. This evidence may briefly be schematized.

1. The reactants for the production of angiotonin are constantly present in the body and are liberated into the blood stream under a variety of physiological and pathological circumstances.

2. Changes in the circulatory dynamics within the kidneys cause both hypertension and possibly the liberation of renin.

3. When infused into animals or men, angiotonin produces a hypertension which has almost every hemodynamic observed in both ex-

perimental renal and human essential hypertension, differing only in detail.

This is important evidence, but it is not conclusive. Much testimony weighs against the genetic relationship of angiotonin and arterial hypertension. The chief points are:

1. Neither renin nor angiotonin has been demonstrated satisfactorily in increased amounts in the peripheral arterial blood of hypertensives, or even in normal amounts, for that matter. This is a problem we simply cannot answer at present because of lack of methods. Many ways have been suggested to get out of this dilemma, such as that angiotonin is taken up by the vascular musculature as soon as it is formed, but it is no use. We must face the problem, and I fear that, barring luck, until more is known of the chemistry of angiotonin, not very much can be expected in the way of progress.

2. Repeated injections of renin into hypertensive rabbits produces tachyphylaxis, but the blood pressure does not necessarily fall, as Taggart and Drury (20) first pointed out. Even in experimental renal hypertensive dogs, tachyphylaxis is not accompanied by a fall in blood pressure.

The problem of why tachyphylaxis to renin occurs is a vexed one. Doubtless it can occur as a result of the exhaustion of the substrate, but this does not seem the usual cause, since administration of purified substrate or fresh blood does not overcome it. In part, it is due to the activity of the autonomic nervous system, since dorsolumbar sympathectomy or the administration of tetraethylammonium chloride restores the response in some cases wholly and in others partially (Fig. 1). But there are still other factors which have as yet eluded us.

3. The arterial pressure is immediately reduced to normal levels in hypertensive rabbits by the destruction of the spinal cord in brief experiments, although such pithed animals show no parallel depression in response to injected renin (Dock, 21). The operation in dogs yields similar results, but after complete recovery, the arterial pressure again rises to hypertensive levels (Glenn, Child, and Page, 22).

4. The removal of both kidneys in hypertensive dogs does not necessarily reduce the blood pressure to normal, as many investigators have shown, whereas bilateral adrenalectomy will do so.

While there are several partial explanations of these facts which oppose the renin-angiotonin concept, none of them has a satisfactory factual basis. The testimony is simply not all in, on either side; hence the unwisdom of compelling a decision at this time.

To know the chemical constitution of angiotonin would be extraor-

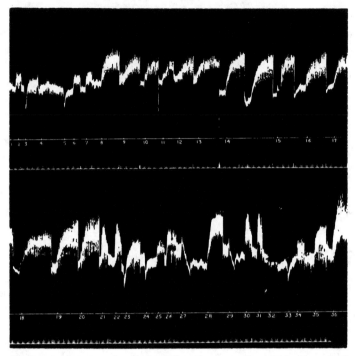

FIGURE 1. An example of the failure in some dogs with the spinal cord destroyed from C_6 caudad to develop tachyphylaxis from the repeated injection of renin. TEAC also somewhat enhanced the renin response. This is an example of the participation of the nervous system in the response to renin.

dinarily useful as giving a more rational approach to the problem. The evidence from physico-chemical investigation strongly suggests that it is a polypeptide with an isoelectric point at pH 6.8, and a molecular weight of about 2700, calculated from the diffusion constant. On the basis of paper chromatographic analysis, Edman (23) found a variety of amino acids in hydrolyzed angiotonin solutions— histidine 28%, alanine, 3.8%, proline, 5%, tyrosine < 2%, aspartic acid, 4.5%, glutamic acid, 5%, etc. Helmer (24) has recently shown that angiotonin can be separated by paper columns from components giving a positive ninhydrin reaction. Free histidine is readily removed.

To gather some notion of the configuration of the angiotonin molecule is extremely difficult, since it has not been got crystalline or pure and becomes increasingly labile with purification. The problem was approached by Plentl and Page (25), using the system of enzyme analysis of Bergmann and Fruton. This is based upon the fact that the rate at which proteolytic enzymes act upon a substrate of known structure is dependent upon the nature of the substrate and the enzyme. Comparing the rates for different enzymes such as pepsin, chymotrypsin, carboxypeptidase, and trypsin gives, from analogy with known substrates, some idea of what the various peptide linkages in unknown substrates are.

Subjecting angiotonin to enzymatic digestion with the four crystalline enzymes and measuring the rate and hydrogen ion optima allowed us to draw certain tentative conclusions, which are embodied in the following "working" structure for angiotonin. It is pictured as a tetrapeptide, but might well be a greater or lesser one.

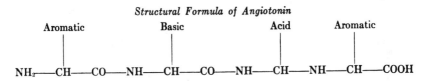

Structural Formula of Angiotonin

I do not propose to go further into the reasoning behind this tentative proposed structure, except to say that while some of the basic structure is doubtless as here conceived, many vital parts must have been omitted or wrongly portrayed. At any rate, it is a start and, I think, not a poor one.

The formation of angiotonin *in vitro* gives a few helpful clues to its nature. The evidence, largely circumstantial, suggested that renin was the enzyme which acted on a substrate contained in the blood to produce angiotonin. This was given substantial support by a kinetic analysis in which it was shown that the reaction was of the first order (Plentl and Page, 26), which is the order characterizing many enzymatic reactions. The system, however, is complicated by the presence in kidney and other tissue extracts of an enzyme or enzymes, discovered by Braun-Menendez, Fasciolo, Leloir, and Muñoz (27), which destroys angiotonin. Helmer, Kohlstaedt, and I (28) found at least 2 angiotonin-destroying enzymes. The one from muscle, liver, and intestinal mucosa showed maximum activity between pH 7 and pH 8, contrasting with that from kidney, in which activity was greatest at pH 4.0.

There now seems to be little doubt that the reaction between angiotonin and angiotonase is an enzymatic one and monomolecular (Plentl and Page, 25). What appear to be satisfactory methods for its determination have been developed by Braun-Menendez and his group and have been employed in this country especially by Dexter (29).

The enzyme or enzymes which destroy angiotonin do not appear from the work of Croxatto to belong to either the amino oxidases or phenol oxidases, but rather to the proteolytic group, more specifically to the aminopeptidases.

It is not clear what the precise part played by angiotonase in the inactivation of circulating angiotonin is. The distribution of the enzymes found by Fasciolo, Leloir, Muñoz, and Braun-Menendez (30) was not what might have been expected. Intestinal mucosa, for example, has a far greater concentration (1200–1600 units) than liver (80 units) or plasma (1–4 units). Red blood cells normally contain larger amounts. It is possible that the high angiotonase concentration in the intestine merely represents the presence in the unpurified extract of many proteolytic enzymes which will destroy angiotonin. If angiotonin is destroyed in the blood by angiotonase, it is surprising that the concentration is not greater.

In acute experiments most organs other than the kidney do not appear to be able to destroy angiotonin rapidly. On the basis of experiments in which a marked temporary increase in the response to angiotonin was observed after nonshocking hemorrhage in dogs, Sapirstein, Reed, and Ernest Page (31) concluded that blood is the major site of angiotonin destruction, with intact red cells contributing little or nothing. They recognize this as only suggestive evidence and by no means established.

I have a strong suspicion that the substance we have so confidently been calling hypertensinase or angiotonase is in fact only a mixture of enzymes which have the one property in common of destroying angiotonin and that this mixture depends on the tissue from which the extract is derived. It would surely be much simpler to think in terms of only one enzyme, but I have presented enough testimony to give one little confidence in this simple view.

Plant cells also contain angiotonin-destroying enzymes, as Croxatto, Croxatto, Manriquez, and Valuezuela (32) showed in 1942, when from yeast they separated enzymes which inactivate angiotonin and pepsitensin. Just what relationship these enzymes have to their animal counterparts that inactivate angiotonin is not known. Wheat bran is also a good source of angiotonases. Using such extracts, Gollan, Richardson, and Goldblatt (33) were able by the intravenous injection of large amounts to reduce the pressor response to angiotonin and abolish that to renin. In one hypertensive dog, the infusion of angiotonases lowered the arterial pressure to normal and reduced but did not abolish the angiotonin response. Inactivated enzymes were not hypotensive. After the return of the plasma angiotonase to normal, the arterial pressure rose to hypertensive levels. Clearly this would be strong evidence in favor of the view that angiotonin is the true mediator of renal hypertension if the evidence had not been drawn from a single experiment in a single dog and if the amounts of angiotonase administered had not been so enormous. At the same time it may be used as evidence against the view that essential hypertension or the toxemia of pregnancy is so mediated, for in these diseases the angiotonase content of the blood is not significantly changed (29, 34). This is an important area of endeavor; hence it cannot be treated lightly lest we be badly misled. I have said enough to indicate to you that in my opinion the groundwork has not as yet been satisfactorily laid; hence arguments based on it as to the participation of angiotonin in the genesis of various types of clinical arterial hypertension may well be faulty.

The conception of the simple enzymatic destruction in the blood stream of the mediator of hypertension is an appealing one, and has appealed to many investigators, all or most of whom, so far, have come away from the problem unconvinced of its validity. We had a try 10 years ago to determine whether the hypotensive action of kidney extracts is due to their ability to destroy angiotonin. A comparison showed, however, that the relationship between the two is questionable, even though they may follow each other during various precipitations, and further, that when the angiotonase fractions were deliberately concentrated, the hypotensive action was not enhanced in direct proportion. We have therefore never believed that the hypotensive action of kidney extract is directly due to its angiotonase content (35).

Pepsitensin. In 1942 the Croxattos (36) made the important observation that when pepsin is allowed to act on renin-substrate, a pressor substance is formed which they have called pepsitensin. One would not suppose from the name that this substance is almost identical with hypertensin or angiotonin. Consistency has never worried us in this field. Actually, physiological studies have disclosed no difference between the two substances (Fig. 2).

The reaction proceeds rapidly only at a quite strongly acid pH and hardly at all above 7.0. Helmer and Page (37) prepared it with crystalline pepsin, since there was some doubt about the enzymes used by the Croxattos, and were able to confirm their findings completely with the pure enzyme. According to Alonso (38) pepsitensin may be obtained alone by acid hydrolysis.

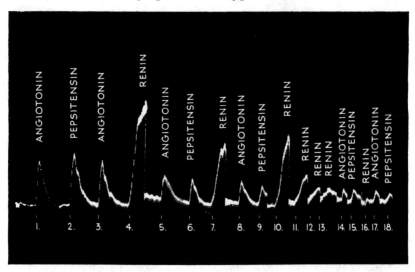

FIGURE 2. A comparison of the pressor effects of renin, angiotonin, and pepsitensin in a pithed cat. The gradual development of refractoriness is evident.

Certain chemical properties differentiate pepsitensin from angiotonin. Plentl and Page (14) showed that renin and renal pepsinase are not homospecific enzymes, it being therefore doubtful that the end products of their action would be identical. The rate of hydrolysis by crystalline pepsin was distinctly different, angiotonin being inactivated much more rapidly than pepsitensin. Further, with pepsitensin as a substrate, two hydrogen ion optima were observed, one at pH 5.5 and the other below 3.5, while only one optimum could be demonstrated for angiotonin. They concluded that angiotonin and pepsitensin are not identical and differ probably in the number, rather than in the nature, of the amino acid residues of which they are composed.

Braun-Menendez et al. (39) showed a further chemical difference in that red blood cell angiotonase rapidly destroys angiotonin but not pepsitensin. There is also a difference in the substrates, since alcohol-precipitated renin-substrate is not attacked by renin but pepsin is still able to liberate pepsitensin. Further, the molecular grouping causing the pressor action is probably identical since treatment of the substrate with renin causes it to lose its capacity to form pepsitensin when incubated with pepsin.

Certain physiological properties of angiotonin. I have so often presented the physiological properties of angiotonin both before audiences and in print, I am sure you will be relieved that I shall not trouble you with them again. The table on the next page gives the similarities between the action of angiotonin and the hemodynamic changes in patients with essential hypertension. While there is near identity in most of the comparisons, this could well be fortuitous. Until the quantitation of angiotonin in the blood is accomplished, this sort of testimony will carry no conviction. Hence my view that the next important step will come from painstaking chemical studies on the nature of angiotonin.

There is, however, another aspect of the action of renin and angiotonin that has an element of novelty—an aspect I should like briefly to discuss. It concerns the responsiveness of the blood vessels to these substances. The ability of the vasculature to respond is quite as important as the stimulating agent!

First, let us examine certain changes which result in an increased responsiveness to renin and angiotonin. I may say that the two usually, but not always, change simultaneously. The destruction of the nervous system by pithing or spinal cord section at C_6 very materially increases the responsiveness to angiotonin as well as to many other vasoactive agents. Under other circumstances, section of the brain at various levels may reduce the responsiveness to renin as von Euler and Sjöstrand (40) convincingly showed. We have found this also (42).

Total lumbodorsal sympathectomy produces almost the same increase as pithing. Autonomic ganglionic blockade with tetraethylammonium chloride also is highly effective. The removal of the inhibitory action of the sympathetic nervous system thus seems to heighten the response to the pressor action of angiotonin and renin.

The removal of both kidneys followed by a period of a day or two also significantly increases the responsiveness, especially to renin and angiotonin. This has been denied by some investigators, but we feel certain from a large number of experiments that it is true. Indeed, the heightened responsiveness is in some cases almost limited to renin and angiotonin.

Animal preparations can be made in which nephrectomy, cord destruction, and a small amount of TEAC have increased the responsiveness by from 6 to 10 times. An example of augmentation with angiotonin by TEAC is given in Figure 3.

Changes in the animal which reduce the responsiveness are several. The simplest and quickest is the breathing of 30 per cent CO_2 by the animal under curare. Within a few minutes the angiotonin response

TABLE 1. A Comparison between Certain Features of Experimental Renal Hypertension, Human Essential Hypertension, and Hypertension Induced by Angiotonin

	Experimental Hypertension	Human Essential Hypertension	Angiotonin-Induced Hypertension
Heart			
Hypertrophy	Left ventricular	Left ventricular	. . .
Force	Increased	Increased	Increased
Work efficiency	Increased	Increased	Increased
Output	Normal or reduced	Normal or reduced	Normal or reduced
Coronary sclerosis	Not found	Common	Not known
Rate	Normal	Normal	Normal or slowed
Pulmonary arterial pressure	Normal	Normal	Increased in acute experiments
Venous pressure	Normal	Normal	Often elevated in acute experiments
Kidneys			
Thickening of the arteries	Common	Common	Not known
Early morphological changes	None	None	Not known
Maximal ability to concentrate	Reduced early	Reduced early	Not known
Glomerular filtration	Maintained	Maintained	Maintained
Blood flow	Normal or reduced	Normal or reduced	Reduced in acute experiments
Filtration fraction	Elevated	Elevated	Elevated
Diodrast Tm	Slowly reduced	Slowly reduced	Slightly reduced
Unilateral renal disease	Sometimes cured by nephrectomy	Sometimes cured by nephrectomy	. . .
Salt metabolism	Possibly retained	Retained	Increased excretion
Liver			
Alpha$_2$ globulin production	Slightly increased	Slightly increased	Not known
Eyegrounds			
Arteriolar constriction	Present	Present	Present
Arteriolar sclerosis	Present	Present	Not known
Hemorrhages, exudates	Present	Present	Not known
Papilledema	Present	Present	Not known
Retinal detachment	Present	Present	Not known
Central Nervous System	No evident change	Many somatic expressions of hyperactivity in some patients. Need be none.	None
Sympathectomy	No change in blood pressure	May reduce blood pressure	Increases pressor response
Adrenalectomy	Reduces arterial pressure	Reduces pressure	Reduces response only terminally
Hypophysectomy	Reduces arterial pressure moderately	Possibly reduces pressure	No marked reduction in responsiveness
Pancreatectomy	No effect on pressure	Not known	No effect on responsiveness
Gonadectomy	No effect on pressure	No effect	No effect on responsiveness

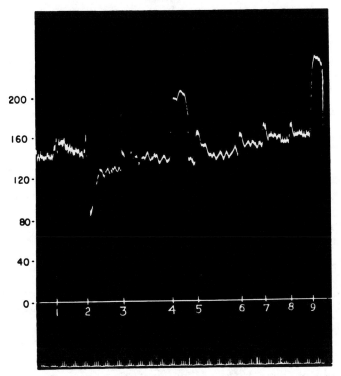

FIGURE 3. Augmentation of angiotonin (144). 1, Angiotonin; 2–3, tetraethylammonium chloride, 5 mg. per kg. of body weight; 4, angiotonin; 5–8, tetraethylammonium chloride; 9, angiotonin. This is an example of augmentation that might have significance in the renal hypertensive state.

disappears and returns on discontinuance of the CO_2. But if the lumbo-dorsal autonomic ganglia have been removed before CO_2 treatment, the response is not lost. The stimulation of the ganglia by the CO_2 thus in some fashion induces refractoriness of the blood vessels to angiotonin and to a variety of other pressor-depressor agents as well.

The removal of the liver is a second way to reduce or abolish the response to angiotonin (41). Within an hour after the operation the response may begin to decrease, and after several hours may disappear altogether. It may be gone before the blood pressure has begun its terminal descent, but its disappearance almost always heralds exitus. The renin responses after hepatectomy disappear well before those to angiotonin.

As Braun-Menendez has so well shown, removing the kidneys before removing the liver prevents the animal from being flooded with endogenous renin resulting from the operative procedures. The dog becomes tachyphylactic to its own renin. Thus part of the initial refractoriness of hepatectomized animals is due to endogenously produced renin tachyphylaxis. But this is probably not the most important cause of the refractoriness. Even if the kidneys have been removed and only angiotonin has been used as a test drug so as not to produce tachyphylaxis, still refractoriness occurs. There can be little doubt that the loss of the liver removes the source of something necessary for the responsiveness of the blood vessels, quite aside from renin-substrate, or causes the failure of the removal of something from the blood which blocks vascular reactivity to pressor-depressor substances.

A third way to reduce responsiveness is to throw the animal into shock, no matter by what method. This is a very reliable way and illustrates our belief that a loss of responsiveness is one of the important preludes to vascular collapse, a view not shared, I may say, by some physiologists (43). The correction of the blood volume and the restoration of the cardiac output and normal venous pressure do not necessarily lead to recovery in either animals or men who have been in shock. If at the same time vascular responsiveness returns, the chances of recovery are vastly enhanced. I am convinced that it is not a matter of secondary importance whether the blood vessels and the heart respond normally to humoral agents.

There are other ways of reducing vascular reactivity, such as the administration of intoxicating doses of a mixture of BAL and Benadryl, but for the most part these are a scientific tour de force and are used to demonstrate that refractoriness may precede by some time the fall in the arterial pressure and the final failure of the circulation.

These examples will, I hope, suffice to show that the responsiveness of the cardiovascular substrate on which humoral agents must act may determine the degree of hypertension quite as much as the amount of the agents producing the stimulation. This is a problem which is just beginning to receive attention in hypertensive patients and animals and will, I think, yield vital information on the nature of these diseases.

A Concept of the Mechanism of Renal Hypertension and of Renal-Adrenal Relationships in the Rat

At some time during the investigations of complex phenomena it is useful to formulate unifying concepts to provide a more orderly pattern for future experimental work. Masson, Corcoran, and I are now proposing such a pattern, which I can give only in the barest outline, without citing the not inconsiderable supporting evidence gathered in many cases by the investigators assembled at this symposium. The charts which follow show the proposed sequence of events which may occur.

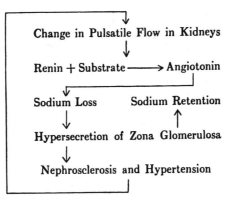

The concept begins with the recognition of the similarity between the vascular lesions in renal and in desoxycorticosterone hypertension (46, 47). Next it was noted by Deane and Masson that experimental renal hypertension, as well as the injection of renin, results in hypertrophy of the adrenal zona glomerulosa. This zone is the presumed source of desoxycorticoids. In rats it is relatively irresponsive to adrenocorticotrophin but responds especially to changes in the Na/K ratio of the body fluids (Laramore and Grollman, 48).

As Dr. Pickering and his group have clearly shown (49), renin and angiotonin cause a sodium loss, while desoxycorticosterone and, presumably, the glomerulosal desoxycorticoids cause sodium retention. But both renin and desoxycorticosterone raise the blood pressure. The glomerulosal hypertrophy caused by renin and renal hypertension is then possibly a response to the loss of sodium. The resulting increase in the glomerulosal desoxycorticoids would increase renin secretion and arterial pressure as a result of the vascular lesions which are known to result, at least under certain circumstances, from desoxycorticosterone acetate. Thus a vicious circle could become established. The sodium loss becomes balanced by the sodium retention due to an increased secretion of the glomerulosal desoxycorticoids.

Perhaps the greatest usefulness of this rather fanciful hypothesis is that it demands the demonstration of the hypersecretion of desoxycorticoids from the zona glomerulosa. As you know, many investigators do not believe that desoxycorticoids exist in any but the smallest amounts in the adrenal cortex. Much of present-day theory depends on this demonstration.

While I have discussed at some length the renin-angiotonin system, I should not like it thought that we believe this mechanism wholly responsible for even some types of hypertension. As some of you know, we (Page and Corcoran, 41) have proposed what is called the "mosaic theory of hypertension" (Fig. 4). This theory attempts to fit into the

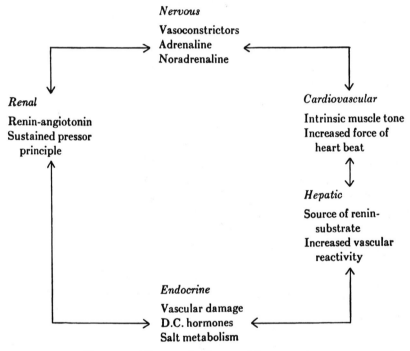

FIGURE 4. The mosaic theory of hypertension.

protean clinical picture of hypertension the many known mechanisms which elevate the blood pressure. These mechanisms are divided into (1) the nervous, (2) the endocrine, (3) the cardiovascular, and (4) the humoral (renal) panels, all of which contribute more or less, and in constantly changing interplay, to the maintenance of hypertension. Thus we come full circle around to our starting point, where it was submitted that the analysis of the problem of clinical and experimental hypertension would ultimately depend on the ability to measure the amount and kind of participation of each of the organs which contribute to the composite state called hypertension. Whether this theory proves ultimately the true one is not at the moment of importance. It is important, however, that it is one which can be subjected to direct and immediate experimentation. There is nothing ephemeral about it, and I think even its severest critics would grant that, barring some entirely unforeseen disclosure, it encompasses what seems for some time to be the knowable.

It must be evident that as I close I have not mentioned many of the important aspects of the renin-angiotonin pressor system. This has been no recital of all that has been published, but rather a brief disclosure of some aspects which at the moment interest me most. For this I have no apology; for is it not the purpose of this sort of gathering rather to talk among friends than lecture as to ignoramuses? You are all aware that since the discovery of angiotonin a host of other substances, more or less well defined, have appeared as contenders for the dubious honor of causing hypertension—the sustained pressor principle of Helmer and Kohlstaedt, the pharentosin of Schroeder, the VDM and VEM of Shorr and Zweifach, an angiotonin-like substance investigated by Gollan, Richardson, and Goldblatt, and so on. It is good that people's minds are so actively engaged in this vital problem. It is also most welcome, for 20 years ago the investigators of the humoral mechanisms in hypertension in this country numbered one or at most two. Only the most pessimistic would believe that time and the increased number of investigators will not in the foreseeable future bring about an understanding of at least some of these humoral systems, systems that may be at the bottom of the problem of arterial hypertension.

Questions and Discussion

DR. MAURICE B. VISSCHER: I understand that Dr. Leland Clark wishes to present several slides bearing on the renin-angiotonin pressor system and chemical studies which he, Dr. Frank Gollan, and Catherine Winkler are busy with at The Fels Research Institute at Antioch College, Yellow Springs, Ohio.

DR. LELAND C. CLARK: In order to save time, I'll turn my attention directly to the material on the slides.

The fact that renin has the characteristics of a proteolytic enzyme and that the renin-substrate, hypertensinogen, is an alpha globulin has led to the belief that hypertensin must be a polypeptide. And, indeed, crude or purified hypertensin preparations have many chemical properties common to polypeptides, among others that they are dialyzable and can be inactivated by proteolytic enzymes. Even the purest preparation obtained so far* yielded 11 amino acids on hydrolysis.

In preparing hypertensin by the usual methods, we have confirmed Dexter's observation that dialyzed preparations are much purer than those obtained by heat coagulation or alcohol precipitation.† These facts indicated that heat coagulation at an acid pH or precipitation of proteins by organic solvents tends to split off small molecular nitrogenous products, which are then carried over into the hypertensin preparation. We reasoned, therefore, that if we were rapidly to dialyze renin and plasma until the dialysate were free of detectable total nitrogen and free alpha amino nitrogen, then incubate for one day at 3° C.—a temperature which only slows down the activity of renin‡ but inactivates hypertensinase§—and then ultrafilter the mixture,

---

*P. Edman: Arch. f. Kemi, Minerologi o. Geolgi 22:1–50, 1945.

†L. Dexter, F. W. Haynes, and W. C. Bridges: J. Clin. Investigation 24:62–68, 1945.

‡C. Bean: Am. J. Physiol. 136:731, 1942.

§L. A. Sapirstein, R. K. Reed, and F. D. Southard: J. Lab. & Clin. Med. 29:633, 1944.

68

we should obtain a product that would contain only the ultrafiltrable alpha amino nitrogen from the newly formed hypertensin.

The non-protein nitrogen content and the ninhydrin positive alpha amino nitrogen of the ultrafiltrates of dialyzed renin, dialyzed plasma, and the resulting hypertensin were equally low in all three samples, but the expected increase of nitrogen in the hypertensin preparation did not materialize. These findings, however, could conceivably be attributed to possible volume changes during the process of ultra-filtration by pressure in a special ultrafilter devised in this laboratory. The ascending one-dimensional paper chromatogram (85 per cent phenol)[*] of the ultrafiltrates of dialyzed renin, dialyzed plasma, and their yield of hypertensin (0.03 mg. N per 30 mm. Hg rise in blood pressure in a chloralosed cat) confirmed the previous observation since no *new* ninhydrin spots appeared on the strip on which hypertensin was partitioned (see Figure 1). Thus all the ninhydrin-positive substances of the hypertensin preparation could be accounted for in quality and quantity as ultrafiltrable nitrogenous impurities contained in the renin and plasma. At this point the following interpretations seem justified: either that (1) hypertensin is not a polypeptide or (2) hypertensin is a ninhydrin-negative polypeptide or (3) the nin-hydrin reaction is not sensitive enough for the demonstration of any existing free alpha amino groups in an amount of hypertensin which gives an appreciable rise in the blood pressure.

Upon hydrolysis of these ultrafiltrates of dialyzed renin, dialyzed plasma, and hypertensin, further insight into the origin of ninhydrin-positive split products of hypertensin was gained. The ultrafiltered hypertensin was split by hydrolysis[†] and repartitioned to give 10 well separated spots (see Figure 1) instead of the previous 4, which were identical in size and rate of migration with those obtained from the hydrolyzed renin ultrafiltrate. The hydrolyzed plasma ultrafiltrate contributed only 5 ninhydrin-positive compounds to this hypertensin preparation. At this juncture, then, the conclusion can be drawn that an ultrafiltered preparation of hypertensin contains the same type and amount of amino acids as the ultrafiltrate of its mother substances. In other words, we are forced to conclude that all the amino acids in this hypertensin preparation were carried along during the purifica-tion procedure as impurities and that amino acids are not associated with hypertensin activity. This further strengthens our previous con-clusion that hypertensin is not polypeptide in nature or that an active

[*] H. Bull, J. W. Hahn, and V. H. Baptist: J. Am. Chem. Soc. 71:550, 1949.
[†] R. Consden, A. H. Gordon, and A. J. P. Martin: Biochem. J. 41:590, 1947.

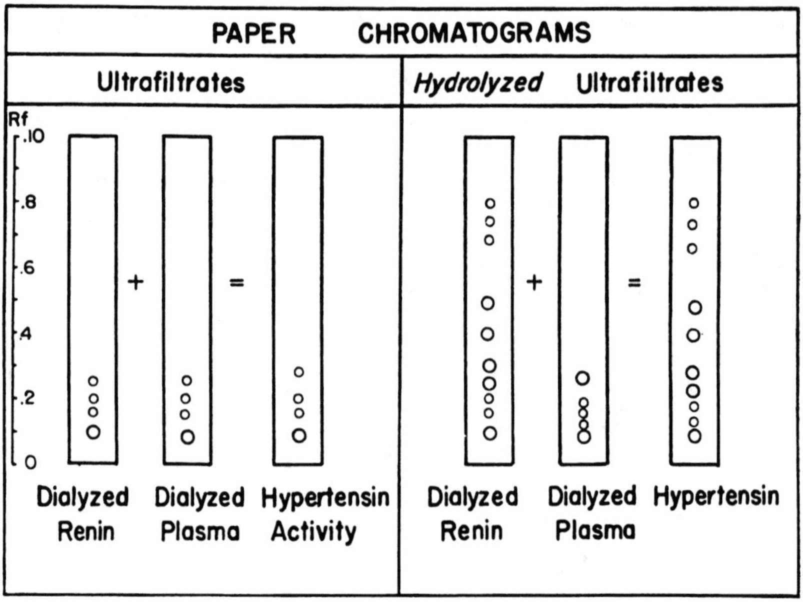

FIGURE 1

preparation may contain less than the 5-microgram amount necessary to obtain a clearly positive ninhydrin test. Similar results upon paper chromatographing were obtained for solutions which were found to have no vasoconstrictor activity due to inactivation of renin by prolonged dialysis.*

Because of the considerable variation in the sensitivity of the ninhydrin reaction to various amino acids on paper, together with the fact that the spot tests on paper are at best only semiquantitative,† the experiments were extended to include starch chromatography‡ with spectrophotometric analysis of the eluted fractions.§ On a standardized starch column, using 15 per cent water in butanol as a developing solvent and collecting consecutive 5-cc. effluent samples, we found that the first amino acid to appear is leucine, beginning in the 24th fraction. All of the pressor activity, however, was confined to the first 10 samples, which contained no alpha amino nitrogen detectable by the spectrophotometric ninhydrin reaction (see Figure 2).

Another series of experiments was concerned with the distribution between immiscible solvents. It was found that the partition of hyper-

*Y. J. Katz and H. Goldblatt: J. Exper. Med. 78:67–74, 1948.
†J. J. Pratt and J. L. Auclair: Science 108:213–214, 1948.
‡W. H. Stein and S. Moore: J. Biol. Chem. 176:337–365, 1948.
§S. Moore and W. H. Stein: J. Biol. Chem. 178:367–388, 1948.

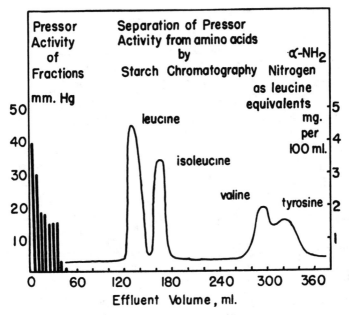

Figure 2

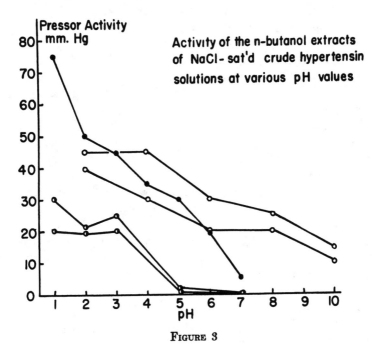

Figure 3

71

tensin between n-butanol and saturated sodium chloride solution was directly dependent upon the pH. When the aqueous layer was alkaline, no hypertensin was found in the butanol layer, but as the acidity increased, increasing amounts of hypertensin passed into the butanol (see Figure 3). At pH 1, hypertensin was quantitatively extracted from a salt-saturated crude aqueous solution. Such butanol solutions were adjusted to 15 per cent water and used directly for starch chromatography. This simple step results in a significant purification and incidentally excludes the possibility of hypertensin's being a basic amine. It seems to us that such an extraction procedure lends itself ideally to the detection of small amounts of hypertensin in large volumes of plasma. Indeed, it was possible to recover quantitatively a known amount of hypertensin from 300 cc. of beef plasma. The method has proved to be a definite improvement over a previously reported, relatively crude one* in the demonstration of hypertensin in the systemic blood of dogs with experimental renal hypertension.

Considering the complete dissociation of vasoconstrictor activity and alpha amino nitrogen as tested by such sensitive methods as the ninhydrin reaction in paper partition and starch chromatography, and considering the known lability of hypertensin to dilute alkali and oxygen and its unusual stability in acid, we believe that the accepted view of the polypeptide nature of hypertensin becomes nearly untenable.

DR. OSCAR M. HELMER (INDIANAPOLIS): As mentioned in Dr. Page's discussion, I have recently reported on the purification of angiotonin by means of paper chromatography.† I found that angiotonin solutions containing 10 to 20 units per cc. did not give a ninhydrin reaction. Secretin, a polypeptide, has been shown by E. Hammarsten not to give a ninhydrin reaction. On this basis the failure to give a ninhydrin reaction does not necessarily indicate that angiotonin is not a polypeptide.

DR. CLARK: It is very gratifying to know that you have also found purified angiotonin to be ninhydrin negative. Dr. Helmer, have you hydrolyzed your preparation?

DR. HELMER: No, I have not hydrolyzed the angiotonin separated by chromatography yet because I wanted first to be sure of its purity and it was assumed that we should find amino acids. Everyone seems to have this prejudice. As soon as more purified material is on hand, it will be hydrolyzed.

* F. Gollan, E. Richardson, and H. Goldblatt: J. Exper. Med. 88:389–400, 1948.
† O. M. Helmer: Proc. Soc. Exper. Biol. & Med. 74:642, 1950.

DR. EPHRAIM SHORR: These interesting experiments of Dr. Pickering raise a question which he may perhaps be able to answer. He has shown that the continuous intravenous administration of renin to the rabbit leads to a prompt and sustained elevation in the blood pressure. However, in the dog rendered hypertensive by the Goldblatt clamp, there may be a delay, varying from a few days to a week or more, before any appreciable rise in the blood pressure occurs. This is undoubtedly due, in part, to the degree to which the renal arteries are constricted by the setting of the clamp; but there is good reason to believe that this is not the whole story. Let us take, for example, the case of the dog which does not develop any significant rise in the blood pressure for a week after renal artery constriction. Despite the absence of immediate hypertension after clamping, it would appear from the work of the South American school and of Dr. Goldblatt that the renal vein blood of such an animal contains excessive amounts of renin almost from the moment of clamping.

Why should such an animal, then, exhibit a delayed response to the hypertensive effects of renin? Is it possible that compensatory peripheral vascular adjustments of the organism to the release of renin are able, temporarily, to overcome its pressor effect and that only when these compensatory mechanisms fail does hypertension develop?

These questions have a bearing on the participation in hypertension of other vasotropic humoral factors, such as VEM and VDM, whose effect on the blood pressure would be exerted in a chronic rather than an acute fashion.

In evaluating the role of humoral agents in hypertension, it will be wise to guard against the oversimplification of what must be a complex and subtle homeostatic system.

DR. PICKERING: Answering Dr. Shorr's question, I have experienced rather the opposite from renal artery constriction. If you cut out one kidney and constrict the renal artery of the other, the hypertension begins certainly within a few hours of the operation; before that time the animal is imperfectly recovered from the anesthesia, and we have not taken records of pressure. It is true that the onset of hypertension may be delayed for many days when one renal artery is constricted, but here you get atrophy of one kidney and hypertrophy of the other, and it is difficult to know exactly what you are doing; it is not a clean experiment. With renin infusions in the doses used, the arterial pressure began to rise within a few minutes of the entry of renin into the vein and reached its peak for that dose from a half to one hour after the starting of the infusion.

There are two minor points I might add concerning the infusions. I told you that at first we failed, that our animals became sick and died. We eventually found by analysis that something was going on in the burette and producing a product which killed the animals. The product was bacteria, chiefly coliform bacilli, and after we had introduced strict aseptic methods with bacteriological control for sterility, we had no further trouble. Secondly, about dosage: We found that the dose of renin producing hypertension of the same order as that in rabbits with hypertension of the same duration from renal artery constriction was 4 units per hour. We had previously found that the average renin content of the kidney of animals with Goldblatt hypertension in the first week was 32 units. If this hypertension is solely due to the release of renin, the whole amount in the kidney would need to be discharged about once every 8 hours, a not unreasonable suggestion.

DR. PAGE: Dr. Visscher, I have the greatest faith in my ability to complicate the matter further. During my speech I behaved as though the blood vessels on which the renin and angiotonin acted were constant in their response. Of course they are not, though we hate to admit it. In pharmacological testing, one is forced to make the assumption of probable constancy and attempt to rule out any changes in the responsiveness by large numbers of tests.

For the past 10 years we have been busy with the problem of what factors control vascular responsiveness. I need not remind you experts that these changes in reactivity may be very great, even converting depressor to pressor responses and vice versa. For instance, hepatectomy causes after a few hours the response to both pressor and depressor drugs, with the notable exception of TEAC, practically to disappear. On the other hand, nephrectomy heightens the responsiveness, especially to angiotonin. Denervation or the administration of TEAC may elicit exquisite supersensitivity.

If all these forces responsible for vascular reactivity remained constant, it would simplify things. But they change, and in no obvious pattern. No wonder the determination of "standard" responses under different experimental conditions is difficult and requires large numbers of experiments to yield significant results. But it seems to me quite as important to understand the components which make up the total response of the blood vessels as it is to understand the component stimuli which cause the response. Arterial hypertension is not due alone to an increased stimulation but possibly to an increased stimulation plus a change in the response to the vessels on which the stimuli are acting. It is this problem which we are trying to clarify.

A second problem which has always interested us in this connection is the mechanisms that control renin secretion. The obvious reason there has been no definitive advance in the knowledge of the subject is that satisfying methods for the determination of renin are not available. I think few of you will doubt that renin must be fed into the circulation in an orderly fashion, not in the disorderly quanta of the investigator. The amount fed in must bear some relation to other events in the body. In short, conditions of equilibrium must exist, and most of the components of the equilibrium system are either unknown to us or not considered in our thinking. Until they are, I fear our chaotic thinking will continue its gay and festive course.

. . . . *by* EPHRAIM SHORR

The Participation of Hepatorenal Factors in Experimental Renal Hypertension

I SHOULD like to preface my discussion with a brief statement of the major premise upon which our approach to the study of hypertension has been predicated. This is as follows: to the extent to which any concept of hypertension fails to provide for the participation of the terminal vascular bed, to that extent will it prove inadequate as an explanation of the genesis and evolution of the hypertensive syndrome.

The exclusion of the capillary bed from consideration in the dynamics of hypertension was justifiable only as long as the bed was thought to be composed of inert endothelial vessels which served merely for the passive transfer of blood from artery to vein, without taking an active part in this process. Since the fundamental contribution of Zweifach and Chambers (1) to the structure and behavior of the capillary bed, this latter concept has become untenable. These investigators have clearly shown that the capillary bed in tissues such as mesentery, skin, and muscle consists of a number of distinct structural elements. Certain of these have contractile properties and other functional characteristics by virtue of which they exert a profound and direct influence on the exchange of fluid between the blood and the extravascular spaces. There is, furthermore, a high degree of integration between the activity of the capillary bed and that of the terminal arterioles more directly and acutely concerned with the regulation of the blood pressure. Thus changes within the capillary bed proper are accompanied by readjustments in the arterioles proximal to it; conversely, constriction and dilatation of the terminal arterioles elicit appropriate responses in the capillary bed distal to them. Such an

NOTE. This paper is based on studies conducted with Drs. Benjamin W. Zweifach, Abraham Mazur, Silvio Baez, and Robert F. Furchgott, under grants from the National Institutes of Health, U.S. Public Health Service, the Josiah Macy, Jr., Foundation, the New York Heart Association, Eli Lilly and Company, and the Postley Hypertension Fund.

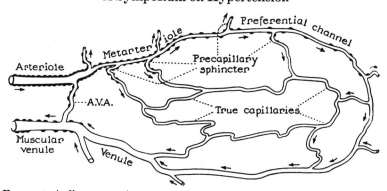

FIGURE 1. A diagrammatic representation of the architecture of the capillary bed. (Reprinted from B. W. Zweifach: Transactions of the Third Conference on Factors Regulating Blood Pressure, Josiah Macy, Jr., Foundation, New York, 1949.)

integration is obviously essential to achieve the homeostatic goal for which the circulation is fundamentally designed, namely, the maintenance of the constancy of the cellular environment. Indeed, in this broader sense, the remainder of the circulatory system may be regarded as subservient to the capillary bed, since only in the latter is there any communication between the blood and extracellular fluids.

Figure 1 presents in diagrammatic form the architecture of the capillary bed as revealed by the studies of Zweifach and Chambers. With minor modifications, the essential elements of this structure have been recognized in all the major tissues of the body. The terminal arteriole gives rise to a central preferential or thoroughfare channel, the metarteriole. This vessel is surrounded by smooth muscle cells for a considerable portion of its length, and represents the most direct route from the arterial to the venous circulation. It gives off numerous muscular offshoots, the precapillary sphincters, which because of their strategic location directly control the flow of blood entering the so-called "true" capillaries. The latter arise from the precapillary sphincters and are non-contractile endothelial vessels which join with one another to form collecting venules into which the muscular preferential channels, the metarterioles, also empty their blood.

A prominent feature of the muscular units of the capillary bed is the periodic activity termed "vasomotion," manifested by alternating periods of constriction and dilatation of the metarterioles and precapillary sphincters. These muscular units also exhibit variations in reactivity which are recognizable experimentally by alterations in the sensitivity of their constrictor response to the local application of

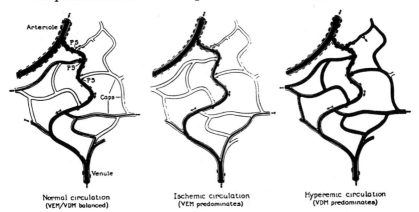

FIGURE 2. A diagrammatic representation of the capillary bed in different states of activity. (Reproduced, by permission of the copyright owner, from E. Shorr, B. W. Zweifach, R. F. Furchgott, and S. Baez: Tr. A. Am. Physicians 60:28–51, 1947.)

epinephrine or norepinephrine. Another feature which distinguishes this portion of the vascular tree from the larger blood vessels is its extreme sensitivity to blood-borne factors. Indeed, the activity of the capillary bed appears to be exclusively regulated by humoral principles of local or systemic origin, without the direct participation of the sympathetic nervous system which controls the larger blood vessels. The terminal arterioles, which lie between the larger blood vessels and the capillary bed, are physiologically intermediate in that they respond both to blood-borne agents and to systemic influences via the sympathetic nervous system (2).

In Figure 2, the phases of vasomotion are illustrated as seen in the mesenteric capillary bed. In the normal resting state there is an intermittent opening and closing of the precapillary sphincters, blood flowing now through one, now through another endothelial capillary. The central figure depicts a situation which results from the predominance of the constrictor phase of vasomotion. As a result of generalized precapillary sphincteric constriction, there is capillary ischemia, the blood flow being confined exclusively to preferential channels. This situation prevails during the hyperreactive phase of experimental shock when there is a predominance in the blood stream of the renal vasoexcitor, VEM (3). The third figure in the diagram is illustrative of the hyperemic capillary bed which results from the suppression of vasomotion and the accentuation of the dilator phase in the precapillary sphincters. This circumstance is characterized by an over-all blood flow through

the entire capillary bed and is observed in the mesenteric vessels dui-
ing the hyporeactive phase of experimental shock when the hepatic
vasodepressor, VDM, predominates in the blood stream (3).

The consequences of each of these situations for fluid exchange between the capillaries and the tissue spaces are illustrated in Figure 3.
The vertical vessels in the diagram represent the muscular metarteriole
which gives rise to a precapillary offshoot, the precapillary sphincter,
the extension of which is the true endothelial capillary. The stippled

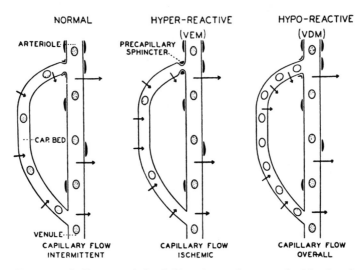

FIGURE 3. A diagram of the fluid exchange between the blood and
the tissues. The number of stippled cells in the side branch indicates the number of open capillary channels. The arrows indicate
the preponderance of the fluid movement, the length of the arrow
giving an approximation of the magnitude of the fluid movement
in comparison to that of the other capillary vessels. (Reprinted
from B. W. Zweifach: Transactions of the Third Conference on
Factors Regulating Blood Pressure, Josiah Macy, Jr., Foundation,
New York, 1949.)

cells within these vessels are meant to represent the number of open
capillaries through which blood is flowing at any one time. The arrows
are indicative of the direction and extent of fluid exchange between
the blood and the extracellular spaces. The normal pattern is representative of the state of fluid equilibrium in a resting tissue. During
the hyperreactive state, when the constrictor phase predominates in
the precapillary sphincters, the number of capillaries through which
blood is actively flowing is reduced; the hydrostatic pressure within the

capillaries is diminished relative to the osmotic pressure because of the resistance imposed by the contracted sphincters. The predominance of osmotic forces favors inward filtration, hemodilution, and tissue dehydration. The reverse situation is seen during the hyporeactive phase associated with VDM predominance, during which there is an over-all capillary flow because of generalized sphincteric dilatation. Hydrostatic pressure can now exert its predominance over osmotic pressure in a larger area of the capillary bed; outward filtration, hemoconcentration, and edema formation are favored by this situation.

It is evident that whenever either capillary ischemia or hyperemia are brought about by local or systemic humoral factors, a breakdown of homeostasis will occur unless appropriate compensatory readjustments take place in the arterioles proximal to the capillary bed. I have already referred to the experimental demonstration of such compensatory interreactions between capillaries and arterioles. It is our present hypothesis that any sustained changes of a chronic nature induced in the capillary bed by humoral factors such as those with which our studies have been concerned should, through the integrative action of arterioles and capillaries, lead to chronic changes in the systemic blood pressure. These considerations, which, I appreciate, have been dealt with all too briefly, have set the direction for our studies on hypertension. They have led to the disclosure of the existence of two hitherto undescribed vasoactive humoral principles, with opposite effects on the behavior of the capillary bed, of such a character as to suggest that they constitute one of the homeostatic systems for the regulation of the peripheral circulation. These studies have furthermore revealed specific alterations in these humoral factors in experimental renal and essential hypertension.

The vasoactive principles were detected by a bio-assay method, developed by Zweifach and Chambers, based on microscopic observations of the exteriorized mesenteric capillary bed of the anesthetized rat (4). This test involves the measurement of the reactivity of the muscular components of the capillary bed, specifically the precapillary sphincters, utilizing as an index their constrictor response to the topical application of epinephrine. After the determination of the threshold concentration of epinephrine to which the precapillary sphincters respond by a perceptible constriction and pronounced slowing of the blood flow through the corresponding capillary, the test sample is injected into the tail vein of the rat. The presence of a vasoexcitor principle is manifested by the development of a period of increased sensitivity to the constrictor effects of topical epinephrine. Vasodepressor activity is recognized from the depression in epinephrine reactivity following intravenous administration.

These oppositely acting factors were found to originate in specific organs under specific metabolic conditions. Thus the hepatic vasodepressor, which we have termed VDM and have since identified as ferritin (5), was found to originate chiefly in the liver and to arise normally only under anaerobic conditions, to judge from in vitro studies (3). Under aerobic conditions, none appeared; and indeed, the exposure of VDM to normal liver slices under these conditions rendered it physiologically inert. The kidney proved to be the sole source of VEM; and the same pattern of anaerobic formation and aerobic inactivation held for this renal vasoexcitor principle. (See Table 1.)

TABLE 1. The Formation and Inactivation of VEM and VDM (Ferritin) by the Normal Liver and Kidney

	In Oxygen	In Nitrogen
Hepatic vasodepressor— VDM (ferritin)		
VDM formation	0	+
VDM inactivation	+	0
Renal vasoexcitor—VEM		
VEM formation	0	+
VEM inactivation	+	0

We are actively engaged in the isolation and purification of these vasoactive principles and of the systems which regulate their metabolism. VDM has been identified as the iron-containing protein ferritin, which in crystalline form gives a positive vasodepressor effect with as little as 0.0005 micrograms injected into a 125-gram rat. The vascular activity of ferritin has been found to be related to the state of its thiol groups. Agents that combine with or oxidize its sulfhydryl groups to the disulfide form abolish the vasoactivity of ferritin (6). Activity can be restored by chemical agents that reduce the disulfide to the sulfhydryl form. This reduction can be accomplished by naturally occurring substances such as glutathione, cysteine, and ascorbic acid. This finding gains additional significance from our observation that the normal liver cell accomplishes the activation and inactivation of ferritin by affecting the same groups in the same manner. In the normal aerobic liver, ferritin is present almost entirely in the disulfide or inactive form. When the liver is exposed to anaerobic conditions, there is a progressive reduction to the sulfhydryl form, with a corresponding increase in vasoactivity. The inactivation of reduced SH-ferritin by aerobic incubation with normal liver slices is associated with the oxidation of the sulfhydryl groups to the disulfide.

The crystallization of ferritin made it possible to develop antisera to ferritins of various species by the injection of heterologous ferritin into rabbits. The combined use of antiferritin sera and the rat test permitted us to establish, by a specific immunochemical procedure, the identity of the vasodepressor in hypertensive bloods as ferritin. These antiferritin sera enabled us to fractionate bloods and other biological fluids in which the activity of ferritin, as measured by the rat test, might be masked by the simultaneous presence of the oppositely acting VEM. Indeed, the development of these procedures has proved of great value and actually essential for the elucidation of the role of these factors in the hypertensive syndrome.

In view of its importance, this fractionation procedure will be briefly described. When ferritin and VEM exist together, the response of the test rat is a resultant of the relative concentrations of each factor. Thus a neutral reaction can be obtained in the rat test when both factors are absent or when both factors are present in titers which are mutually antagonistic. When such a mixture is incubated with antiserum to ferritin, all ferritin vasoactivity is abolished and any VEM activity can exert its effect in the test rat. Conversely, any VEM present can be inactivated by the incubation at 37.5° C. with normal kidney slices under aerobic conditions, any ferritin present being thereby unmasked (see Figure 4).

We are not yet in a position to provide much specific information about the chemical characteristics and properties of VEM. Our efforts at purification of this factor are still in an early stage. It would appear either to be of a protein nature or to have a protein prosthetic group. Pharmacological studies are correspondingly incomplete, but the evidence to date would tend to differentiate it from the renin-hypertensin system on the basis of the absence of the musculotropic properties characteristic of the latter system (7).

With this background we are in a position to turn to the studies which have disclosed specific and characteristic derangements in the VEM-VDM mechanisms during the genesis and evolution of the syndrome of experimental renal hypertension. In Figure 5, which is based on studies of the blood and tissues in experimental renal hypertension in the dog as induced by the application of Goldblatt clamps, these changes are represented in semidiagrammatic form. The upper portion of this figure depicts the changes in the blood pressure during the various stages of the syndrome: the more abrupt rise during the acute

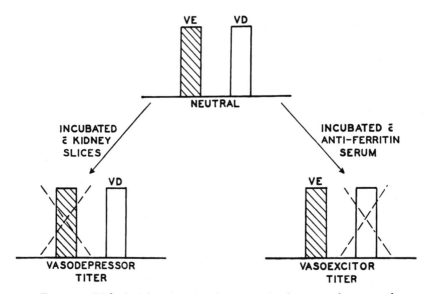

FIGURE 4. Biological fractionation for a vasotropic assay of untreated blood samples.

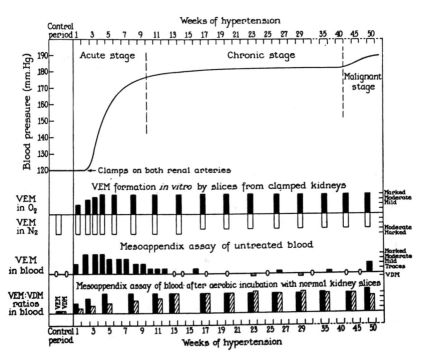

FIGURE 5. Metabolic and humoral alterations in hepatorenal vasotropic factors in renal hypertension.

stage, the leveling off during the chronic hypertensive phase, and the frequent terminal exacerbations in the malignant stage of the disease. The diagrams below present the parallel changes in the blood and tissues as they relate to VEM and VDM.

The application of the Goldblatt clamp, with a constriction of the renal artery sufficient to produce hypertension, results in a prompt derangement of the renal VEM metabolism, as a result of which the appearance of VEM, normally restricted to anaerobiosis, now takes place under aerobic conditions as well. Once this disturbance has set in, it persists throughout the course of the hypertensive syndrome. The significance of this defect stems from the fact that the kidney presumably has lost its intracellular homeostatic capacity to adjust VEM production in accord with local needs, and, in stress situations, with the peripheral circulatory needs of the organism as a whole; VEM production is continuous and unrestrained.

These changes are reflected in the bio-assays of unfractionated blood samples. VEM, normally undetectable in the blood, promptly appears after the application of the clamp and persists in considerable concentrations during the acute stage of hypertension. At about the time that the blood pressure attains the chronic hypertensive level, the VEM activity wanes and eventually disappears in the unfractionated blood. This phenomenon seemed at first glance analogous to the appearance of renin in the blood during the acute phase and its disappearance during the chronic stage of hypertension. However, as is indicated at the bottom of Figure 5, the actual situation is more complex. When blood samples were fractionated for VEM and VDM activity by the methods just described, it became evident that the neutral reaction of the test rat to the unfractionated blood in the chronic stage was the resultant of the presence of both VEM and VDM. It was then found that shortly after the appearance of VEM in the acute stage, VDM also appeared in the circulation, initially in low concentrations, thereafter in progressively increasing amounts until, with the transition to the chronic stage, the VEM and VDM titers reached a ratio in which they were physiologically equivalent as measured by the rat mesoappendix test. Thereafter, from time to time, there occurred a minor and intermittent predominance of one or the other factor.

In vitro studies of the VDM metabolism of the hypertensive liver disclosed the basis for the appearance of this factor in the blood. The hypertensive liver, as evident from *in vitro* studies, had undergone a shift in its metabolic pattern similar to that exhibited by the hypertensive kidney. Instead of forming VDM, as does the normal liver, only under anaerobic conditions, the hypertensive liver produces this vaso-depressor principle under both anaerobic and aerobic conditions. It was also found that in contrast to the normal liver, in which ferritin is present almost entirely in the inactive disulfide form, in the aerobic hypertensive liver about 15 to 25 per cent of ferritin is present in the active sulfhydryl form (8).

Hence we can conclude that the hypertensive kidney undergoes a characteristic alteration in the VEM metabolism as a result of which VEM formation occurs in oxygen as well as in nitrogen, hence continuously, and that this renal defect persists throughout the hypertensive syndrome. We can further conclude that the liver, in a manner that is still obscure, responds to this abnormal concentration of humoral VEM by an analogous shift in the VDM metabolism, which results in the appearance of VDM in oxygen as well as nitrogen. It is this shift in the VDM metabolism that leads to the appearance of increasing concentrations of humoral VDM until, at the chronic hypertensive stage, an equilibrium is reached with approximately equal titers of both VEM and VDM. Thereafter, and throughout the whole course of the syndrome, minor fluctuations in this equilibrium occur.

The fact that the presence of VEM in the blood in the hypertensive syndrome evokes the production of VDM by the liver would seem to add support to our concept that these vasoactive principles may constitute a homeostatic system for peripheral circulatory regulation.

As to the actual mechanisms involved in the production of these metabolic renal and liver derangements, it is perhaps relevant that a typical hypertensive pattern, as regards both VEM and VDM production, can be regularly produced in vitro. When a normal kidney, which forms VEM only in nitrogen, is exposed to nitrogen for a period of one hour and then restored to aerobic conditions, it acquires the typical hypertensive pattern, forming VEM equally well under both aerobic and anaerobic conditions (Table 2). The same procedure leads to a conversion of the normal hepatic VDM metabolism to the typical hypertensive type (Table 3). Hypoxia, which initially follows the constriction of the kidney by the Goldblatt clamp, could therefore account for the development of the defect in the renal VEM metabolism, but not for its persistence once the renal blood flow is restored with the development of hypertension. The persistence of this defect, therefore, has no present explanation. The sequence of the events which lead to the development of the hypertensive VDM pattern in the liver in vivo after the clamping of the kidney is also obscure.

In addition to the metabolic changes involving the VEM-VDM

TABLE 2. The Transformation of the Normal Renal VEM Metabolism
to the Hypertensive Type *in vitro*

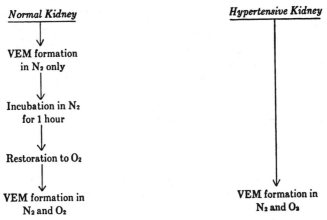

TABLE 3. The Transformation of the Normal Liver VDM Metabolism
to the Hypertensive Type *in vitro*

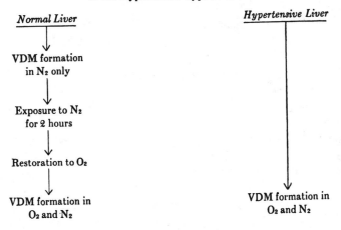

mechanisms in experimental renal hypertension, parallel alterations
have been noted in the behavior of the peripheral vascular bed which
is under the control of these humoral factors. During the acute stage
of renal hypertension in the rat, the mesenteric capillary bed becomes
more reactive, both to topical epinephrine and to the intravenous injection of VEM (9). The mesenteric capillary bed of the renal hypertensive dog is also hyperreactive to topical epinephrine during the
chronic stage of hypertension. Of particular interest is the striking
hyperplasia of the capillary bed of the mesentery in the renal hypertensive rat. This hyperplasia, which appears to involve largely the

true capillaries, has been noted as early as from 10 to 14 days after the wrapping of the kidneys and becomes progressively more marked with the progression of the syndrome (9). It is not limited to the rat but also occurs in the renal hypertensive dog. Of particular significance was the appearance of the same type of hyperplasia in the mesentery of a spontaneously hypertensive dog in our colony which exhibited, as well, all of the humoral VEM-VDM derangements and vascular hyperreactivity characteristic of the experimental renal hypertensive dog. It is unknown whether this capillary hyperplasia occurs in tissues other than the mesentery.

We are inclined to regard this capillary hyperplasia as of particular significance on several scores. In the first place, it is a structural and functional change in the specific components of the vascular tree upon which VEM and VDM exert their effects. In the second place, it represents an alteration of such a nature and magnitude as to affect the hemodynamic pattern in hypertension.

Let us, however, for the moment consider these humoral and vascular events in experimental renal hypertension on a purely descriptive level. Whatever their ultimate relation to the hypertensive syndrome, they provide a series of criteria for the evaluation of the variety of hypertensive states which can be produced experimentally. They should therefore permit the assessment of the relationship of any hypertensive state to the syndrome of experimental renal hypertension in animals and, as we shall see in my other paper, to essential hypertension in man.

I have assembled in Table 4 these criteria as they apply to the renal hypertensive rat and dog. I have included also one new criterion, the tetrazolium pattern of the renal tubule, which I shall discuss in detail in my second paper.

These criteria will serve as a basis for an assessment of the rela-

TABLE 4. Criteria for Evaluating the Hypertensive Syndrome

	Rat (Perineph.)	Dog (R. A. Clamp)
Aerobic formation of VEM by the kidney *in vivo*	...	+
Aerobic formation of VEM by the kidney *in vitro*	+	+
VEM in the blood during the acute stage	+	+
VEM and VDM in the blood during the chronic stage	+	+
Vascular hyperreactivity to epinephrine	+	+
Vascular hyperreactivity to VEM	+	...
Hyperplasia of the capillary bed	+	+
Renal histochemistry (tetrazolium pattern)	+	+

tion of the adrenal cortex to hypertension as it affects the VEM-VDM mechanisms and the capillary bed with which these systems are concerned.

From studies on adrenalectomized rats, dogs, and rabbits, it has become evident that an important relationship exists between the adrenal cortex and the renal VEM mechanisms. In the absence of the adrenal cortex, the kidney loses completely its capacity to form VEM. This function is maintained by DCA or adrenal cortical extract, but not by salt.

It then became of interest to see to what extent the VEM mechanisms and peripheral vascular reactivity might be impaired in the salt-maintained, adrenalectomized rat, subjected to the perinephric wrapping which induces hypertension in the rat with intact adrenals. The findings are given in Table 5. It is apparent that, together with the

TABLE 5. The Effect of Adrenalectomy on Perinephric Hypertension in the Rat

| | Bilateral Renal Capping | |
Criteria	Intact Adrenals	Adrenalectomy + NaCl
Blood pressure	160/220	100/135
Aerobic formation of VEM by the kidney *in vitro*	+	0
Anaerobic formation of VEM by the kidney *in vitro*	+	0
VEM in the blood during the acute stage	+	0
VEM and VDM in the blood during the chronic stage	+	0
Vascular hyperreactivity to epinephrine	+	0
Vascular hyperreactivity to VEM	+	0
Hyperplasia of the capillary bed	+	0

failure of the adrenalectomized rat so treated to develop hypertension, there is a complete absence of all of the changes in the VEM metabolism and of the vascular functional and structural changes which accompany perinephric hypertension in the intact animal (10).

It was further observed that dogs made hypertensive by Goldblatt clamps, adrenalectomized, and supported by adrenal cortical extract, developed the typical disturbances in the renal VEM mechanisms characteristic of hypertension.

It was now possible to apply the criteria described above to an evaluation of the extremely interesting type of hypertension produced by DCA. This type of hypertension bears directly on a very crucial question, namely, whether the adrenal cortical hormones are involved in the initiation of hypertension or whether the adrenal cortex should be considered merely an essential link in a chain of events initiated elsewhere and presumably in the kidney. DCA hypertension was induced in a series of rats according to the method of Selye. The findings with respect to the development of hypertension per se were confirmatory of Selye's observations, except for the lower incidence (20 to 25 per cent) of periarteritis nodosa in our strain of rats. However, the over-all pattern in DCA hypertension was in striking contrast to that seen in experimental renal hypertension. The differences are summarized in Table 6. Apart from the hypertension per se and the cardiac hypertrophy, none of the VEM disturbances or vascular changes characteristic of experimental renal hypertension were encountered, except in the small percentage of animals with extensive vascular damage including periarteritis nodosa. The photomicrograph (Figure 6) of the mesenteries of two rats, one with DCA

TABLE 6. A Comparison of DCA Hypertension with Experimental Renal and Essential Hypertension

	Rat (Perineph.)	Human (Essential)	Rat (DCA)*
Aerobic formation of VEM by the kidney *in vitro*	+	+	0
VEM in the blood during the acute stage	+	+	0
VEM and VDM in the blood during the chronic stage	+	+	0
Vascular hyperreactivity to epinephrine	+	+	0
Hyperplasia of the capillary bed	+	+	0
Renal histochemistry (tetrazolium pattern)	+	+	0

* From 15 to 20 per cent of DCA rats with severe hypertension show typical hypertensive metabolic lesions. This group is characterized by extensive vascular damage.

hypertension and one with perinephric hypertension, illustrates the absence of the type of mesenteric hyperplasia which regularly occurs with renal hypertension; the vascular pattern of the DCA rat is entirely normal. The absence of these humoral and vascular changes in uncomplicated DCA hypertension is strong evidence against the fundamental similarity of the DCA hypertension per se to experimental renal hypertension, and, as will be pointed out in my other paper, to human essential hypertension (11).

I have presented this afternoon the evidence for the participation of the vasotropic factors VEM and VDM in experimental renal hypertension. These factors appear in regular sequence in the blood of dogs and rats made hypertensive either by perinephric wrapping or renal artery constriction. The appearance of VEM and VDM in the blood

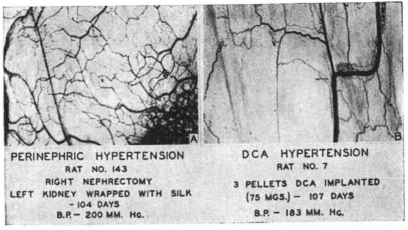

PERINEPHRIC HYPERTENSION
RAT NO. 143
RIGHT NEPHRECTOMY
LEFT KIDNEY WRAPPED WITH SILK
- 104 DAYS
B.P. - 200 MM. HG.

DCA HYPERTENSION
RAT NO. 7
3 PELLETS DCA IMPLANTED
(75 MGS.) - 107 DAYS
B.P. - 183 MM. HG.

FIGURE 6. Vascular hyperplasia in the mesentery.

has been shown to arise from metabolic derangements in the renal and hepatic mechanisms which regulate the metabolism of these factors. Similar derangements can be produced *in vitro* by a brief exposure of these tissues to hypoxia. These changes in the VEM and VDM metabolism are paralleled by alterations in the terminal vascular bed with whose regulation these principles are concerned. The changes are both structural and functional. There is pronounced hyperplasia of the capillary bed and an enhanced reactivity. The functional and structural characteristics of the terminal vascular bed have been discussed and their importance pointed out for circulatory homeostasis. The high degree of integration between the activity of the terminal vascular bed and the central blood vessels more directly responsible for the regulation of the blood pressure suggests that the altered condition of the capillary bed observed in experimental and renal hypertension and presumably dependent upon the altered VEM-VDM titers in the blood stream may be a contributing factor in the genesis and maintenance of experimental renal hypertension.

Questions and Discussion

DR. MARK NICKERSON: The vasotropic substances which Dr. Shorr and his co-workers have demonstrated provide us with an excellent new parameter in the study of hypertension. They are particularly important in studies such as the ones he has presented demonstrating the lack of similarity between the hypertension produced by DCA and human essential or renal hypertension.

However, one basic question comes to mind upon which I should like to have Dr. Shorr's opinion. That is, what is the role of these agents in the actual maintenance of the elevated blood pressure? As far as their studies go, and we have preliminary data of a similar nature, the primary activity of VEM appears to be in potentiating the response to epinephrine. It does not appear to prevent the blockade of responses to epinephrine by pharmacological agents. Yet in both experimental renal hypertension and human essential hypertension, agents which will completely block the effects of epinephrine and sympathetic nerve activity, with or without VEM, fail to reduce the pressure consistently.

DR. SHORR: Our studies have not as yet progressed to the stage of providing the data which would enable us to answer Dr. Nickerson's question about the exact role of VEM and VDM in the genesis and maintenance of hypertension. In my presentation I have briefly set forth the reasons for our view that any chronic changes in capillary behavior due to the continuous presence of high concentrations of these principles in the blood must inevitably lead to readjustments in the arterioles proximal to the capillary bed and hence to changes in the blood pressure. Beyond that, we are not prepared to go at present.

However, I should like to take advantage of this opportunity to clarify the relation of epinephrine to the action of VEM and VDM. In the first place, I want to emphasize the fact that the topical application of epinephrine to the rat mesoappendix should be regarded

94

merely as a useful method of assaying VEM and VDM. It should not be taken to mean that the action of these principles, when they occur in the circulation in shock or hypertension, is dependent on circulating epinephrine. Indeed, there are good reasons for feeling that this is not the case. It is much more likely that the effects of VEM and VDM on capillary vasomotion and reactivity are related to a locally produced sympathomimetic principle, such as sympathin. If this distinction between topical and circulating epinephrine is kept in mind, we should be able to avoid some of the confusion that has arisen in the evaluation of our observations on the relation of VEM and VDM to the function of the peripheral vascular bed.

With respect to the dibenamine blockade of epinephrine action, to which Dr. Nickerson is, I believe, referring, and its failure to lower the blood pressure consistently in both experimental renal and human essential hypertension, the implications of this phenomenon for the action of VEM have yet to be established. Our own preliminary observations show that it is possible to induce dibenamine blockade with epinephrine reversal, without altering the reactivity of the capillary vessels to topical epinephrine. Should this observation hold up in experiments now in progress, then it is evident that the dibenamine blockade of epinephrine cannot help us to assess the relation of VEM to hypertension.

DR. MAURICE B. VISSCHER: I should like to raise a question, Dr. Shorr. I take it, from your presentation, that your evidence indicates that after a period of some weeks the VEM and VDM activities reach approximate equality. Nevertheless, the blood pressure elevation remains. There is a fundamental physiological point in connection with the problem of hypertension which we should bear in mind. It seems quite obvious that the "barostat" in the body has its setting changed in essential hypertension in man, and in experimental renal hypertension in animals. Are we not paying too much attention to the effects of constrictor agents on the peripheral blood vessels and neglecting the actions on the central homeostatic mechanism?

I should like to have you comment first, if you will, on the question of the significance of your observed equalization of the VEM and the VDM over a period of time, with maintenance of the elevated blood pressure. Perhaps you would also care to comment on the more general physiological question of how hypertension can occur with an active "barostat" unless its "set" is changed.

DR. SHORR: I wish I had the information which would permit me to answer your question, which comes close to the core of the problem.

The sequence of events as far as the VEM-VDM system is concerned is as follows: During the acute stage of hypertension VEM predominates in the blood stream. However, even in that stage, VDM also appears early and in progressively increasing concentrations. When the blood pressure is stabilized at the chronic hypertensive levels, both these factors are present in amounts which counteract each other in the rat test so as to yield a neutral reaction. This new equilibrium at high concentrations of both VEM and VDM persists throughout the syndrome both in animals and in human essential hypertension. From time to time there are slight temporary shifts in this equilibrium, VEM gaining brief predominance at one time, VDM at another, as if there were a dynamic relationship between these two factors.

If we may regard these two principles as participants in the genesis and perpetuation of hypertension, why should not the blood pressure return to normal when this new equilibrium is reached? With our present knowledge, it is possible only to speculate rather than to provide answers.

In the first place, it may be pointed out that when we talk about a new equilibrium's being reached between VEM and VDM, the basis is the neutral reaction of the hypertensive blood injected into a normotensive rat on which the test is carried out. The blood may conceivably still exert a preponderant VEM effect in the hypertensive subject because of an increased vascular sensitivity to VEM which may have developed during the evolution of the syndrome. We know that the capillary bed of the hypertensive rat does become more sensitive to topical epinephrine and to VEM during the acute stage of hypertension, and that the capillary mesenteric vessels of the dog are hyperreactive to topical epinephrine all throughout the hypertensive syndrome. Thus changes may occur in the reactivity of the capillary bed in hypertension which render it more susceptible to the effects of VEM than in the normotensive state, so that what would be neutralizing concentrations of VEM and VDM for the normotensive would still represent VEM predominance for the hypertensive state. This possibility could be explored by using hypertensive instead of normotensive rats for the mesoappendix assay.

One might also regard the VEM-VDM equilibrium during the chronic stage of hypertension as a dynamic one, in which any fluctuations in the VEM-VDM ratio that would make for a higher or a lower blood pressure would call forth a compensatory change in the titer of the opposite factor, with a restoration of the previous equilibrium and blood pressure level. Thus, should a temporary predominance of VDM occur sufficient to lower the blood pressure, the kidney would respond with an increased production of VEM until the equilibrium was restored. How this might be brought about is still obscure, but it may possibly operate through a reduction in the renal blood flow and oxygen tension which would be favorable to an increased VEM formation. We do know, in the case of VDM, that the release of VEM in experimental renal hypertension does lead to a response on the part of the liver which results in VDM formation, and that the concentrations of VDM which are eventually attained in the blood stream are sufficient to set up the equilibrium between the two principles. This is the kind of behavior which could be anticipated from a homeostatic system.

I am inclined to look with favor on this concept of a dynamic equilibrium as the mechanism for maintaining the hypertensive level when both principles have come to equilibrium. When we clamp the kidney and VEM is produced, the higher the titers of VEM and the more rapid the rise in blood pressure, the more rapid is the production of VDM by the liver. However, in the present state of our knowledge we should be going further than the facts justify if we were to offer this as more than a working hypothesis.

• • • • • • • • • • • • • by EDUARDO BRAUN-MENENDEZ

Blood Volume and Extracellular Fluid Volume in Experimental Hypertension

THE importance of the circulating blood volume and especially of the extracellular fluid volume as a possible factor in the causation of hypertension has not received enough consideration. We were led to study this problem by the results obtained in rats after bilateral nephrectomy.

Hypertension after Bilateral Nephrectomy

The effect of bilateral nephrectomy on the arterial pressure has been the object of numerous investigations. Some authors observed a rise in the blood pressure, as Mosler did (1912) in 11 of 13 rabbits after total nephrectomy, while most of the others, like Backman (1916), Cash (1926), Hartwich (1930), Harrison et al. (1936), Goldblatt (1937), Dicker (1937), Houssay and Taquini (1938), Verney and Vogt (1938), Blalock and Levy (1937), Winternitz et al. (1940), could not confirm those results.

Jeffers et al. (1940) found that removal of three of the four kidneys in a pair of parabiotic rats resulted in hypertension in the nephrecto-mized animal. Grollman and Rule (1943) found in 2 pairs of para-biotic rats that the removal of the kidneys in one animal sufficed to induce hypertension. When these experiments were repeated by us (von Euler and Braun-Menendez, 1948), a definite rise in the blood pressure was found only in 5 out of 17 pairs (Fig. 1). We then modi-fied the procedure by joining three rats in parabiosis, one bilaterally nephrectomized between two normals. In all 6 trios prepared, definite hypertension was observed in the nephrectomized animal, occurring 2 to 4 days after the removal of the kidneys (Fig. 2).

These results led us to investigate more systematically the blood pressure of single rats after total nephrectomy (Braun-Menendez and von Euler, 1947). A total of 39 normal adult rats were nephrectomized,

98

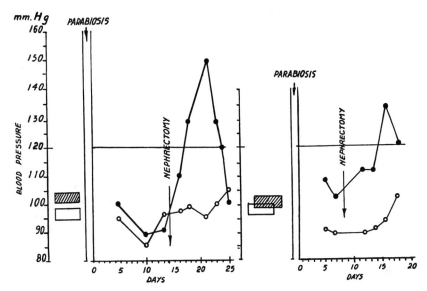

FIGURE 1. The blood pressure of rats in parabiosis. After 7–15 days of parabiosis total nephrectomy was performed in one member (indicated by the line
with solid dots) of the pair.

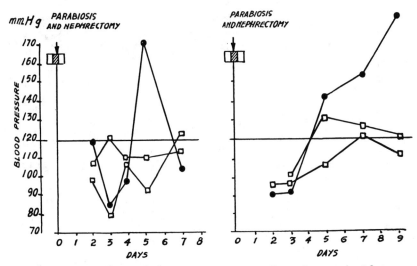

FIGURE 2. Three rats joined in parabiosis, one totally nephrectomized between
two normals. The blood pressure of the nephrectomized animal (indicated by
the line with solid dots) increased to hypertensive levels.

99

A Symposium on Hypertension

TABLE 1. The Blood Pressure in Normal Rats (mm. Hg) 1–4 Days
after Total Nephrectomy
(Braun-Menendez and von Euler, 1947)

First Day	Second Day	Third Day	Fourth Day
80	120	104	
94	144	90	
	92	130	
90	80	124	
118	80	106 *	200
112	116	148	
96	100	136	
104–128	116–116	104	124
100–104	108	96 *–126	108
96–100	112	148	
92	80	140 *–138	
100–90	128		
116	128		
110	92 *	140	

* Indicates peritoneal washing.

and the blood pressure determined daily until death occurred. A definite rise was observed in 13 rats (33 per cent) (Table 1). In all these
the blood urea was high. In 14 animals a solution of Ringer with 0.5
per cent gelatine was allowed to flow through the peritoneal cavity
at a rate of 1 ml. per minute during 1–3 hours, the animal being anesthetized with nembutal (30 mg/kg) or ether.

From Table 1 it is evident that the rise in the blood pressure mostly
occurs during the second or third day after nephrectomy and also
that peritoneal dialysis does not lower the pressure but may increase
it. In some cases there were indications of an improvement in the
general condition of the rat after washing, though the blood urea
showed only a slight fall.

To explain these results, it was tentatively assumed that the absence of renal function determined the accumulation in the blood of
some hypertensive substance of extrarenal origin and that the hypothetic hypertensive substance did not always manifest its action because of the accumulation in the organism of the nephrectomized rats
of other substances of antagonistic or toxic effects. In favor of this
explanation the following arguments could be adduced: (1) Apparently peritoneal dialysis had a beneficial action on the hypertension of
totally nephrectomized rats. The dialysis probably acted by eliminating more rapidly urea and other substances of low molecular weight,
leaving in the organism an excess of the assumed pressor principle.
(2) In the case of parabiosis a similar action could be involved:

through the parabiotic communication the depressor or toxic substances passed more easily than the pressor substances from the nephrectomized to the normal animal. This could explain also why in the parabiotic trios, where the communicating surface is greater, the hypertension was constantly present in the nephrectomized rat.

For circumstantial reasons we did not pursue the investigation of the hypothetic pressor substance, but we made determinations of the urea in the blood in order to see if some relation could be found between the concentration of this substance and hypertension. In 11 totally nephrectomized rats the blood urea concentration 48 hours after nephrectomy averaged 247 mg. per cent. No significant correlation could be found between the blood urea concentration and hypertension. However, hypertension was more often observed in rats with relatively low values of urea.

Peritoneal dialysis during 60 minutes with Tyrode solution did not cause a significant decrease in the blood urea; but, on the other hand, the control animals to which no peritoneal washing was given increased their blood urea concentration about 40–50 mg. per cent in the same interval. The parabiotic rats with hypertension had a definitely lower blood urea concentration than the single totally nephrectomized rats (112–161 mg. per cent 3 to 9 days after nephrectomy).

Our attention was drawn to the apparent relation between an increase in weight and hypertension. After the extirpation of both kidneys our rats were left in the same cage as the controls and had free access to drinking water and food. Not a single case of hypertension was found among those nephrectomized rats whose weight increased less than 15 gm. in the first 48 hours. On the contrary, hypertension was frequent when the increase in weight exceeded 15 gm. (Braun-Menendez and Covián, 1948).

The accumulation of fluid in the organism could be readily appreciated by simply making an incision in the skin: the subcutaneous tissues were edematous and ingurgitated. We thus decided to measure the blood volume (Evans blue) and the extracellular fluid volume (thiocyanate) in normal and totally nephrectomized rats and found both values definitely increased in the latter (Table 2).

In order to study the factors which caused the increase in the extracellular fluid volume, we arranged the following experiment. After total nephrectomy the rats were separated into 3 groups. The rats of Group 3 were kept in total fast, those of Group 2 were allowed to drink water *ad libitum* but received no food, and those of Group 1 were given daily by stomach tube a saline solution in amounts equiva-

TABLE 2. The Blood Volume and Extracellular Fluid Volume in Normal and Totally
Nephrectomized Rats
(Braun-Menendez and Covián, 1948)

	No. of Rats	Weight in Grams	Hema-tocrit	Blood Volume (ml/100 cm²)	No. of Rats	Weight in Grams	Extracellular Fluid Volume (ml/100 cm²)
Normal 32		245	44	4.43 ± 0.08 *	21	243	15.8 ± 0.39
Totally nephrec-tomized ...25		246	33.5	4.8 ± 0.11	21	239	21 ± 0.48

*Standard deviation of the mean $= \sqrt{\dfrac{\Sigma\, d^2}{n(n-1)}}$

lent to 0.15 gm. of sodium chloride per 100 gm. of body weight and
were allowed to drink water *ad libitum* (Table 3).

Determination of the blood volume and the extracellular fluid volume made 48 hours after nephrectomy showed that the thiocyanate space was increased in the 3 groups even in those which fasted or drank water and in which either no increase or a decrease (6 per cent) in weight occurred. The increase in the extracellular fluid volume in Group 1, which received sodium chloride and water, is easily accounted for: the absorption of sodium chloride given by stomach tube requires a proportional intake of water, which is distributed in the tissue spaces and in the blood. An increase in weight, in the extracellular fluid volume, and in the blood volume follows.

In Group 2, which had free access to drinking water, the increase in the extracellular fluid volume can also be explained: electrolytes originated in the processes of endogenous metabolism accumulate in the organism because of the absence of renal function. The animals drank water (from 20 to 25 ml. in 48 hours), which was distributed in the intercellular spaces, with a resulting increase in the extracellular fluid volume. The blood volume, however, remained within normal limits.

On the other hand, the increase in the thiocyanate space in those rats which fasted and could drink no water and which lost approximately 6 per cent of their weight can only be explained by assuming (1) that the thiocyanate space does not represent in these cases the extracellular fluid volume, or (2) that the increase in extracellular fluid is due to a passage of water from the interior of the cells to the intercellular spaces.

The first alternative was considered the more probable since it has been pointed out that in certain abnormal conditions the thiocyanate

TABLE 3. The Extracellular Fluid Volume of Totally Nephrectomized Rats in Different Experimental Conditions (Braun-Menendez and Covián, 1948b)

	No. of Rats	$\triangle$ Weight in Grams	Blood Volume (ml/100 cm^2)	Extracellular Fluid Volume		Hemato-crit
				SCNNa (ml/100 cm^2)	Inulin (ml/100 cm^2)	
Total nephrectomy, 48 hours						
Group 1 (NaCl plus water) 10		+30	5.1	22.6	19.1	27
Group 2 (water) 8		+2	4.33	20.9	13.9	39
Group 3 (total fast) 9		−19	4.45	20.6	13	33
Total nephrectomy, 1 hour						
Controls 10		...	(4.43)*	16.2	11.5	(44)

*The numbers in parentheses correspond to normal values obtained in another series (Braun-Menendez and Covián, 1948a).

space may increase while the mannitol space remains unmodified (Tharp, 1948; Overman, 1946). To test this possibility, we determined simultaneously the inulin space. Inulin, as was shown by Kruhoffer (1946), is exclusively distributed in the extracellular space. Its volume of distribution is smaller than that of sodium thiocyanate because (1) it does not penetrate into the red blood cells and perhaps into other cells as does thiocyanate and (2) it diffuses more slowly than thiocyanate into poorly vascularized tissues, such as tendons.

Determinations made in recently nephrectomized control rats confirmed Kruhoffer's results in rabbits: the thiocyanate space equaled 33 per cent of the body weight while the inulin space equaled 23 per cent. The equilibration time was less than 60 minutes in the rat and did not vary significantly after 4 hours. In this control group of 10 recently nephrectomized rats the inulin space averaged 11.5 ml/100 cm^2 of body surface. As can be seen in Table 3, in Group 1, which received sodium chloride and water, the inulin space was markedly increased; in the other 2 groups the increase in the inulin space was significant but less marked. On the other hand, the thiocyanate volume increased more or less in equal proportion in the 3 groups. This means that the apparently great increase in the extracellular fluid volume as depicted by the thiocyanate space in Groups 2 and 3 is due, in part at least, to the passage of thiocyanate through the cellular membrane into the cells.

These experiments show (1) that 48 hours after bilateral nephrectomy there is a definite increase in the extracellular fluid volume (thiocyanate or inulin volume); (2) that a close correlation exists between the accumulation of water in the extracellular spaces and hypertension. The water accumulation manifested itself by an increase in the body weight, in the extracellular fluid volume (thiocyanate and inulin space), and in the blood volume and by a decrease in the hematocrit value.

The increase in the extracellular fluid volume and blood volume is perhaps not a sufficient factor per se for the causation of hypertension, since we know of many experimental and pathologic conditions in which the blood and extracellular fluid volumes are increased without any definite change in the blood pressure. But the results of these experiments and the fact that water intoxication in normal rats caused also transitory hypertension in 30 per cent of the cases (Braun-Menendez and Covián, 1948) indicate that the accumulation of water in the organism is one of the factors capable of producing hypertension in the rat.

These results may also throw light on the results obtained by other workers who have studied the course of the blood pressure after total nephrectomy in animals with experimental hypertension. Thus Ogden (1947) in rats and Pickering (1947) in rabbits observed that after bilateral nephrectomy the blood pressure fell more or less rapidly in animals with short-standing renal experimental hypertension, but in animals in which hypertension had been present for a relatively long period of time the blood pressure remained high until death supervened. In the interpretation of these experiments one must take into account the possibility that in animals with chronic hypertension there has occurred an increase in the blood volume and extracellular fluid volume which pre-exists that determined by total nephrectomy and favors the maintenance of hypertension. Moreover, as Braun-Menendez and Martínez (1949) have shown, in rats with chronic hypertension due to unilateral perinephritis a significant increase in the blood volume and the extracellular fluid exists.

In the experiments of Oppenheimer et al. (1948), in which peritoneal dialysis was instituted in order to prolong the life of hypertensive dogs after total nephrectomy, a high blood pressure was maintained until death occurred. It must be borne in mind that already Braun-Menendez and von Euler (1947) had pointed out that peritoneal lavage seemed to favor the appearance of hypertension in totally nephrectomized rats and that Grollman et al. (1949) observed an increase in the blood pressure in all their totally nephrectomized dogs maintained in life by means of peritoneal dialysis. It is quite possible that this procedure causes an even greater increase in the extracellular fluid volume.

More recently Friedman and Friedman (1949) and Hall and Hall (1950) have shown that the blood pressure of rats rendered hypertensive by treatment with desoxycorticosterone acetate continues to rise following total nephrectomy. Incidentally, they also confirmed our results (Braun-Menendez and von Euler, 1947) by showing that the blood pressure of the controls (totally nephrectomized rats receiving no treatment) also rises after nephrectomy. The fact that treatment with desoxycorticosterone causes a rise in the extracellular fluid volume, as will be shown later, may explain the higher degree and greater incidence of hypertension in DCA-treated animals.

Experimental Renal Hypertension

The blood volume. The blood volume of hypertensive dogs was determined by Freeman and Page (1937) and by Gibson and Robinson

(1938) using Evans blue dye (T 1824). No significant variations were found. The blood volume of rats made hypertensive by subtotal nephrectomy was studied by Beckwith and Chanutin (1941), who found an increase in the plasma volume but no change in the total blood volume, a result implying low hematocrit values. On the other hand, Griffith and Ingle (1940) in 7 out of 8 rats made hypertensive by the same method found an increase in the blood volume. In the absence of the posterior lobe of the pituitary only 1 of 5 hypertensive rats showed an increased blood volume. The authors suggest that in the presence of a marked continuous diuresis an increased blood volume is more difficult to maintain.

We have not been able to find in the literature any systematic study of the variations in the extracellular fluid volume in experimental hypertension. Having found a considerable increase in the blood volume and extracellular fluid volume in hypertensive totally nephrectomized rats (Braun-Menendez and Covián, 1948), we studied these volumes in our rats with chronic hypertension due to unilateral perinephritis. This procedure causes a rather moderate hypertension without symptoms of renal insufficiency: the renal clearance of inulin and diodrast remains within normal limits, as does the blood urea concentration (unpublished results). In these chronically hypertensive rats definite alterations in the water and salt metabolism have been described (Braun-Menendez, 1950).

TABLE 4. The Blood Volume and Extracellular Fluid Volume (Thiocyanate Space) of Normotensive and Hypertensive Rats, Both with Unilateral Perinephritis, Fed a Standard Diet
(Braun-Menendez and Martínez, 1949)

	No. of Rats	Blood Volume * (ml/100 cm²)	No. of Rats	Extracellular Fluid Volume (ml/100 cm²)
Hypertensive 17		4.65 ± 0.08†	13	18.56 ± 0.45
Normotensive 14		4.20 ± 0.11	11	16.47 ± 0.35

* Body surface = 11.36 × body weight 0.66

†Probable error of the mean $= 0.6745 \sqrt{\dfrac{\Sigma\, d^2}{n\,(n-1)}}$

Our results (Table 4) show that in this type of experimental renal hypertension there exists an increase in the blood volume and in the extracellular fluid volume of about 7 and 12.5 per cent respectively, the latter being statistically significant. Eichelberger (1943) had observed in renal hypertensive dogs an increase in the extracellular fluid, with an abnormal distribution of electrolytes. She demonstrated an increased sodium chloride and a decreased potassium content in the muscle of the hypertensive as compared to the normal animal. Laramore and Grollman (1950) confirmed these findings in the rat.

The water and salt metabolism in experimental renal hypertension. Chanutin and Ferris (1932) observed polyuria, with urines of low specific gravity, in their rats made hypertensive by a reduction of the renal tissue. Oster and Martínez (1943) record an increased water intake and polyuria in rats made hypertensive by renal ischemia or cellophane. The relation water intake/urinary excretion, which was 2.5 in normal rats, averaged 1.9 in hypertensive rats, and the urine specific gravity was 1044 in normal and 1027 in hypertensive rats. These authors also observed the interesting fact that if drinking water is replaced by an 0.8 per cent sodium chloride solution, in normal rats the increase in the fluid intake averages 55 per cent, while hypertensive rats double their fluid intake and edema supervenes. Abrams *et al.* (1949) found that hypertensive rats offered different salt solutions take less sodium chloride and sodium bicarbonate than the normal controls.

We have made several studies of rats made hypertensive by wrapping the left kidney in a gauze soaked in collodion, the right kidney being left intact (Table 5). We found first that the water intake in

TABLE 5. The Intake and Output of Water in 4 Groups of Rats during 24 Hours

	No. of Rats	Water Intake (ml/100 gm/ 24 hr)	Urine (ml/100 gm/ 24 hr)	$\dfrac{\text{Urine}}{\text{Water}} \times 100$	Non-Renal Excretion (ml/100 gm/ 24 hr)
Normal controls	6	11.5	3.3	29%	8.2
Normotensive rats with unilateral perinephritis	.19	9.18	2.56	28	6.62
Hypertensive rats with unilateral perinephritis	.13	14.9	6.53	44	8.37
Hypertensive rats with bilateral perinephritis	.. 2	19.35	11.2	58	8.15

24 hours was greater in hypertensive rats with unilateral perinephritis than in the normotensive controls and even greater in rats made hypertensive by bilateral perinephritis. The latter had malignant hypertension with evident signs of renal insufficiency (depression of renal clearances, increased blood urea concentration, etc.); on the other hand, the rats with unilateral perinephritis had no evident signs of renal insufficiency. The greater water intake is accompanied by a

greater diuresis, the amount of water eliminated by other routes (the lungs, skin, digestive system) remaining constant. In fact, the amount of water ingested that is not excreted by the kidneys is more or less equal in the 4 groups, while the percentage of water ingested that is eliminated by the kidneys increases from 28 and 29 per cent in the two control groups to 44 per cent in the hypertensive rats with unilateral perinephritis and 58 per cent in those with bilateral perinephritis.

In another series of experiments we administered by stomach tube an 0.8 per cent solution of sodium chloride in amounts corresponding to 5 per cent of the body weight. The urine of 3 periods was collected: from 0 to 3 hours, from 3 to 9, and from 9 to 24 hours, the animals (4 rats for each group) having been deprived of food and water. The urine volume and the amount of chlorides excreted were measured in each period and expressed as a percentage of the water and sodium chloride administered. During the first 3 hours no significant differences could be detected; but in the 2d and 3d periods it could be seen that the hypertensive rats eliminated a greater percentage of water and of sodium chloride than the controls, with the result that at the end of 24 hours normal rats had excreted 55 and 61 per cent of the ingested water and about 80 per cent of the sodium chloride, while the hypertensive rats excreted more than 70 per cent of the water and about 100 per cent of the salt administered (Figs. 3 and 4).

This phenomenon can be related to the aversion for sodium that hypertensive rats show when exposed to different salt solutions (Abrams *et al.*, 1949).

If considerable amounts of sodium chloride are administered to hypertensive rats, they eliminate all of it in 24 hours, while normal

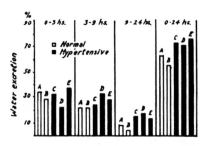 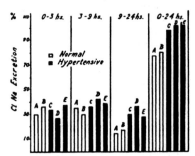

FIGURES 3 AND 4. The excretion of water and of sodium chloride (expressed as a percentage of the amount administered) in normal and hypertensive rats during the 24 hours following the administration of an 0.8 per cent solution of sodium chloride by stomach tube.

TABLE 6. The Volume of Urine and of Chloride Excreted by Rats during 24 Hours of Complete Fasting

	No. of Rats	Urine Volume (ml/100 gm/24 hr)	Urine Chloride	
			gm 0/00	mg/24 hr/100 gm
Hypertensive rats 6		1.87	3.2	5.95
Normal controls 8		0.65	10.2	6.65

rats retain about 20 per cent. This positive sodium balance has also been demonstrated in normal men (Stewart and Rourke, 1942). Furthermore, there are some indications of intolerance to great amounts of sodium chloride in hypertensive rats: some of them were in bad condition after the salt solution was given, and one died in 30 minutes with symptoms of acute pulmonary edema. It is worth re-membering that the administration of desoxycorticosterone to hyper-tensive dogs caused pulmonary edema and death in 2 of 5 animals (Rodbard and Freed, 1942).

Hypertensive rats also are more liable to dehydration than normal rats when deprived of drinking water (Table 6). In total fast they excrete in 24 hours a urine volume nearly 3 times as great as that of normal rats and eliminate a more or less equal amount of sodium chloride at a lower concentration (Braun-Menendez, 1950).

The mechanism of these alterations in the water and salt metabo-lism is not yet understood. Recently Ellis and Grollman (1949) have found an increased elimination of the antidiuretic principle in the urine of rats and dogs with experimental renal hypertension. If the increased renal excretion of the antidiuretic principle really means an increased production of the antidiuretic hormone by the posterior pituitary, it may be assumed that this increased production is a compensatory response to some endocrine or metabolic alterations, a response creating an increased water turnover. The experiments of Skahen and Green (1948) are in favor of this hypothesis. They found that the urinary elimination of the antidiuretic principle is proportional to the water turnover. When the fluid intake increases, following the administration of desoxycorticosterone or the substitution of water by an 0.8 per cent sodium chloride solution as a drinking fluid, the elimination of the antidiuretic principle also increases.

Some Experimental Conditions Causing an Increase in the Blood Volume and in the Extracellular Fluid Volume

Protein-rich diets. Many authors have studied the variations in the plasma proteins, hemoglobin, and blood volume produced by the administration of protein-poor diets. The results obtained are diverse; some authors have found an increase in the blood volume in malnourished rats (Chisolm, 1911), while others have found a decrease (Boycott and Chisolm, 1911) or no change (Scott and Barcroft, 1924). Metcoff *et al.* (1945) found in rats given 2 per cent casein in the diet a significant decrease in the circulating plasma volume after 7 days. On the other hand, Lippman (1948) in similar periods with a diet containing 3 per cent protein did not find a significant decrease in the plasma volume.

The effect of protein-rich diets on the blood volume has scarcely been studied. The only reference we have found is the work of Lippman (1948), who gives a diet with 77 per cent protein during 7 days to normal rats and finds an increase of about 10 per cent in the blood volume. We have studied the effect of the administration during several months of a diet containing 40 per cent protein and 4 per cent sodium chloride on the blood volume and extracellular fluid volume of rats in different experimental conditions (Table 7). The differences

TABLE 7. The Blood Volume and Extracellular Fluid Volume (Thiocyanate Space) of Rats Fed a Normal Diet and a Diet Containing 40 Per Cent Protein and 4 Per Cent NaCl

Experimental Condition	No. of Rats	Blood Volume (ml/100 cm²)	No. of Rats	Extracellular Fluid Volume (ml/100 cm²)
Standard diet				
Normotensive rats with unilateral perinephritis ...14		4.2 ± 0.11 *	11	16.47 ± 0.35
Pancreatectomized, normoglycemic rats 16		3.84 ± 0.15	19	16.45 ± 0.22
Protein- and salt-rich diet				
Normotensive rats with unilateral perinephritis ... 8		4.79 ± 0.13	9	19.1 ± 0.34
Pancreatectomized, normoglycemic rats 8		4.6 ± 0.16	9	22.1 ± 0.53

* Probable error of the mean $= 0.6745 \sqrt{\dfrac{\Sigma d^2}{n(n-1)}}$

between means in the 2 groups is statistically significant, the rats receiving the protein- and salt-rich diet showing an increase in the blood volume and extracellular fluid volume. The thiocyanate space is very much increased in pancreatectomized animals fed a protein-rich diet, but these male animals were probably in a prediabetic stage, having been operated on about 1 month before the volume determinations. In a small group of 4 normal rats fed the same diet during the same interval of time the average thiocyanate space was 19.7 ml/100 cm². The addition of 4 per cent sodium chloride to the diet has probably contributed to the increase in the blood volume and thiocyanate space. In normal persons the administration of considerable amounts of sodium chloride—from 20 to 30 gm. per day during 3 days (Grant and Reichsman, 1946) or 40 gm. in 48 hours (Lyons *et al.*, 1944)— caused a great increase in the plasma volume and extracellular fluid volume. Stewart and Rourke (1942) administered great amounts of saline solution to normal persons and obtained an increase of 80 per cent in the extracellular fluid.

The administration of desoxycorticosterone acetate. The administration of desoxycorticosterone is followed in normal persons by a slight increase in the blood volume and extracellular fluid (Perera *et al.*, 1944; Perera and Blood, 1947; Perera, 1948). Its effect is much more marked in Addison's disease. We have injected normal rats fed a standard diet and given water to drink with 2.5 mg. per day of DCA during 15 days. At the end of this period we found in the treated animals a definite increase in the blood volume (20 per cent) and in the extracellular fluid (13 per cent) when compared to the controls (Table 8). The administration of 1 mg. per day of desoxycorticosterone

TABLE 8. The Effect of Desoxycorticosterone Acetate (2.5 mg/day Per Rat during 15 Days) on the Blood Volume and Extracellular Fluid Volume (Thiocyanate Space)

	No. of Rats	Blood Volume (ml/100 cm²)	Extracellular Fluid Volume (ml/100 cm²)
DCA-treated 8		4.88	18.4
Normal controls 8		4.06	16.3

during 2 or more months to rats fed a protein- and salt-rich diet caused an even greater increase in the volume of extracellular fluid (Braun-Menendez and Martínez, 1949).

Gaudino and Levitt (1949) gave 30 mg. of desoxycorticosterone per day to dogs during 3 weeks. They observed a marked and immediate rise in the volume of extracellular fluid (inulin space), with a reduction in the intracellular fluid volume and a slight increase in the blood volume. Swingle *et al.* (1941) had also observed a moderate increase in the plasma volume in normal dogs injected with desoxycorticosterone.

Diabetes. Sunderman and Dohan (1941) observed in diabetic dogs

TABLE 9. The Blood Volume and Volume of Extracellular Fluid in Normoglycemic
Rats and Rats Made Diabetic by Subtotal Pancreatectomy

	No. of Rats	Blood Volume (ml/100 cm²)	No. of Rats	Extracellular Fluid Volume (ml/100 cm²)
Pancreatectomized, normoglycemic rats 16		3.84 ± 0.15 *	19	16.45 ± 0.22
Pancreatectomized, diabetic rats 15		4.72 ± 0.11	18	20.1 ± 0.24

$$* \text{Probable error of the mean} = 0.6745 \sqrt{\frac{\Sigma d^2}{n(n-1)}}$$

during ketosis an increase in the plasma volume (vital red) of about
30 per cent and in the volume of extracellular fluid (thiocyanate
space) of about 10 per cent. Sunderman (1943) also found that the
administration of glucose in diabetic patients is followed by an increase in the plasma water and that the administration of insulin produces a decrease in it.

We studied (Braun-Menendez and Martínez, 1949) the blood
volume and the volume of extracellular fluid in rats made diabetic by
subtotal pancreatectomy (Foglia, 1944). With this method diabetes
appears in the rat after a latent period of 1–3 months' duration and
follows a chronic course. As controls we took pancreatectomized rats
with normal blood sugar (Table 9). Most of the diabetic rats of
Table 9 had long-standing diabetes (4–11 months) and very high
blood sugar values (more than 300 mg. per cent). But even those in
which diabetes had appeared only recently (15–30 days) had high
values of blood volume and extracellular fluid volume. Compared to
the controls, the diabetic rats showed an increase in the extracellular
fluid and blood volume that is very marked (23 and 22 per cent respectively). The difference was so evident that when determinations
were made we could predict the existence or not of diabetes by the
values obtained (Fig. 5).

Experimental Conditions Which Modify the Incidence of
Renal Hypertension

In our laboratory we have adopted as a standard method of obtaining hypertension in rats the production of unilateral perinephritis,
the other kidney being left intact. With this procedure we obtain
only a low percentage (about 10 per cent) of hypertensive animals,
but on the other hand, it induces a chronic benign hypertension without evident symptoms of renal insufficiency.

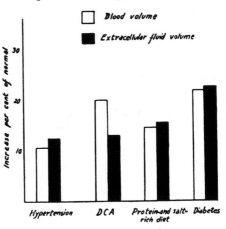

FIGURE 5. Changes in the extracellular fluid and blood volume
in rats with chronic benign hypertension, in diabetic rats, and in
rats given desoxycorticosterone
acetate or a protein- and
salt-rich diet.

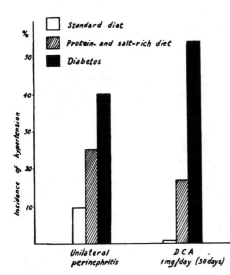

FIGURE 6. The incidence of hypertension in rats under different
experimental conditions.
(See text.)

The administration of a
protein- and salt-rich diet increases the percentage of hypertension in rats with unilateral perinephritis from 10
per cent (with the standard
diet) to 24 per cent (Fig. 6).
The association of diabetes
(subtotal pancreatectomy) increases the incidence to 41
per cent (Braun-Menendez
and Martínez, 1949).

These results acquire greater significance if we consider the frequency with which hypertension is observed in human diabetes. White
and Waskow (1948) observed hypertension in 55 per cent of their
patients who had been diabetic since childhood and for more than 20
years, and Millard and Root (1948) in from 46 to 77 per cent of their
patients. Hypertension in diabetic patients is usually accompanied
by renal lesions and in many cases also by ocular lesions, constituting
the Kimmelstiel and Wilson syndrome (1936).

In human diabetes arteriosclerotic lesions of various grades are
found in the great majority of patients. In rats with chronic diabetes

diffuse arteriosclerotic lesions were not found, but in 88 per cent of the cases histologic lesions of the renal glomerulus (Foglia *et al.*, 1948) and renal hypertrophy (Foglia, 1945) were observed. This renal lesion may be a factor in the increased incidence of hypertension found in our rats with unilateral perinephritis. But it is probably not the only factor. The protein-rich diet and the diabetes both may produce an increase in the intensity of the protein metabolism, a factor which may play a role in hypertension. But apart from this we have shown that both determine an increase in the blood volume and volume of extracellular fluid.

From these experiments we can conclude that some factors which are capable of increasing the frequency of hypertension after unilateral perinephritis also cause an increase in the blood volume and extracellular fluid. Is the latter a causal factor in arterial hypertension? I do not believe it can be per se, for if it is true that in hypertension due to bilateral nephrectomy or unilateral perinephritis, an increased volume of extracellular fluid is found, the inverse is not always true. In diabetes, for instance, we found in the rat a very marked increase in the blood and extracellular fluid volume, and spontaneous hypertension was only occasionally observed. But I believe the increased volumes can be an important cofactor or at least the manifestation of some causal factor in hypertension which we do not yet know.

The relation of these experiments to the problem of human hypertension is perhaps not immediately apparent. Determinations of the blood volume and volume of extracellular fluid have been made in hypertensive patients in basal conditions, and no abnormality has been found. However, this argument is only partially acceptable. The organism tends to maintain its homeostasis, but the new equilibrium may be unstable or may be obtained at the expense of some chronic abnormality. In the first stages of cardiac failure, everything is apparently normal under basal conditions, but an effort will reveal a decrease in the heart's reserve force. In the later stages the only abnormality may be a slight increase in the venous pressure or in the circulation time. In hypertension the renal clearances are sometimes normal: but they are perhaps normal because of the high level of the blood pressure and would not be so at a normal pressure. The same argument may be applied to the volume of extracellular fluid, which may be found normal in hypertensive patients in basal conditions but which is perhaps normal because of the increased blood pressure.

Furthermore, it would be interesting to compare the stability of this normality in hypertensive and normotensive persons. How does a tolerance test-infusion of sodium chloride solution or a diet rich in sodium chloride modify the blood pressure and the volume of extracellular fluid in normal and hypertensive patients?

Perera and his associates have made interesting studies in this respect. In a recent review Perera (1950) states that in his opinion "there is convincing evidence that the disorder [hypertensive vascular disease] is associated with a disturbance of salt and water metabolism." His experiments with the administration of sodium chloride or desoxycorticosterone show a definite difference between the pressor response of hypertensive and that of normotensive patients: the former are much more sensitive to the pressor action of DCA or NaCl. He also observed an increase in the volume of extracellular fluid and the blood volume following the administration of these substances, but he concludes that the "prompt rise in blood pressure in those [patients] with hypertension could not be ascribed to changes in salt and water retention *alone,* as there were comparable transitory changes in the normotensive group." To this conclusion I respond: (1) Perhaps it is true that changes in salt and water retention are not *alone* responsible for the increase in the blood pressure, but this does not exclude them as a causative factor. (2) The fact that similar changes in the normotensive group did not alter the blood pressure is not conclusive evidence. The administration of 5 gm. of sodium chloride per day to a normal person does not cause any manifestation, but the same dose of sodium chloride given to a patient with compensated cardiac failure may precipitate failure, with an increase in the venous pressure and body weight (Newman and Fishel, 1950).

There are in human pathology two other cases in which the volume of extracellular fluid and the blood pressure are rather closely related: Addison's disease and the toxemia of pregnancy.

For all these reasons I believe it would be most interesting to study hypertensive patients from the point of view of their salt and water metabolism and the variations in the volume and composition of their extracellular fluid. Perhaps these studies might throw more light on the difficult problem of the mechanism of arterial hypertension.

Questions and Discussion

DR. ARTHUR GROLLMAN: The studies of Dr. Braun-Menendez and his collaborators on the effects of bilateral nephrectomy in the rat are open to several criticisms which render invalid some of the conclusions which one might be tempted to draw from them. In his experiments with von Euler and with Covián, to which Dr. Braun-Menendez has referred, no effort was made to maintain the nephrectomized rats on an electrolyte-free diet. To do this is essential if one is to study the effects of nephrectomy uncomplicated by the edema and overload of the circulation which inevitably must follow the ingestion of salt by a nephrectomized animal. It is not surprising, therefore, that these authors observed an increase in the blood volume in their animals 2 days following nephrectomy. The increase in the blood pressure observed in such animals may be attributed, as Dr. Braun-Menendez has done, to this plethora of the circulation rather than to the absence of renal tissue. In my own experiments in the rat, I have, however, also noted an increase in the blood pressure following nephrectomy which is not dependent on the development of edema and an increased blood volume. However, this rise in pressure is evident only in animals which survive from 4 to 6 days following nephrectomy. Such long survival* is possible if one maintains the animals on an electrolyte-free diet following nephrectomy. If Dr. Braun-Menendez were to repeat his experiments under these conditions, I doubt if he would encounter the changes in the blood volume or the elevations in the blood pressure which he has described.

The starvation of animals following nephrectomy does not cause an overload of the organism with salt, but this procedure, likewise, leads to an undesirable state of affairs, since it intensifies the rate of endogenous protein catabolism and hence shortens the survival period following nephrectomy.

* Cf. Arthur Grollman and Béla Halpern: Proc. Soc. Exper. Biol. & Med., 71:394, 1949.

116

The facts just described are also applicable clinically. To maintain the patient with anuria it is necessary (1) to exclude potassium and other electrolytes from the diet (except in an amount lost by vomiting or diarrhea), (2) to administer an amount of water equal to that lost in the insensible perspiration and excreta, and (3) to feed the patient a salt-free diet with minimal protein but adequate caloric value to reduce endogenous protein catabolism to a minimum. Under such conditions anuric patients may be maintained in good condition for several weeks or more.

The failure to observe the above-described conditions accounts for the short survival reported by earlier observers of dogs following nephrectomy, their poor state during the brief period of their survival, and their failure to manifest a rise in blood pressure. In patients, likewise, the injudicious administration of saline or salt-containing foods leads to short survival, pulmonary edema, convulsive movements, and other manifestations erroneously attributed to "uremia."

DR. BRAUN-MENENDEZ: In our experiments, as I said, we only tried to demonstrate the relationship between the blood volume and extracellular fluid volume and the existence of hypertension.

I agree with Dr. Grollman that there may be other factors causing hypertension after total nephrectomy. But what I wish to emphasize here is that in our rats hypertension was correlated with an increased blood volume and extracellular fluid volume. Hypertension occurred only in those cases where an increase in body weight was present.

It is possible that if our rats had been given a potassium-free diet or subjected to other treatments, hypertension could have developed without any increase in the blood volume or extracellular fluid volume.

But in our experiments we have found a very close relationship between the increase in these fluid compartments and hypertension. Here we have these animals of Group 1, who were given food and saline solution by stomach tube and had free access to water. They gained weight and had a marked increase in their blood volume and thiocyanate or inulin space.

In Group 2, where only water was given and no food, there was a slight increase in weight and there was a very definite increase in the extracellular fluid volume. Now in these rats there was no hypertension, in spite of the increase in the thiocyanate space. This increase in the extracellular fluid volume is due probably to the passage of water from the intercellular space to the extracellular space.

The animals of Group 3, in total fast, lost weight. They also showed an increase in extracellular fluid volume when compared with the normal controls and had no hypertension. I believe these experiments show that a close correlation exists between the accumulation of water in the extracellular spaces and hypertension. The increase in the blood volume and extracellular fluid volume may be a co-factor in the genesis of hypertension.

· · · · · · · · · · · · · · · · · · *by* HANS SELYE

The Role of the Adrenal Cortex in the Pathogenesis of Experimental Hypertension

MANY of us have come a long distance in order to participate in this symposium and thus to pay homage to the three great scientists of the University of Minnesota whom we honor today. Dr. Pickering represents one of the prominent clinical research centers of England; Dr. Braun-Menendez has spoken about the important contributions made in South America by the Argentinian investigators, and I consider it indeed a great privilege to have been chosen to report upon pertinent studies performed by our group in Canada. The work of all of us has been greatly stimulated by the fundamental contributions made here at your University. Hence the opportunity on this occasion to discuss present-day views on hypertension and cardiovascular disease is most welcome.

Several other speakers on this symposium have referred to the probable participation of the adrenal cortex in the genesis of arterial hypertension in man. Our own observations are mainly based on animal experimentation and evolved from the concept of the general-adaptation-syndrome (G-A-S). The latter has given rise to a very extensive literature which I cannot discuss here in detail. Those interested in it are referred to my pertinent monograph *Stress,** which was completed only a few months ago. Suffice it here to give merely a diagrammatic outline of it, as an introduction to my remarks on hypertension as a disease of adaptation, since it is this concept that directed our attention to the role of the adrenal cortex in the pathogenesis of hypertensive disease.

The Concept of the General-Adaptation-Syndrome and the Diseases of Adaptation

In 1936, we demonstrated, by animal experimentation, that the organism responds in a stereotypical manner to a variety of widely

*Montreal, Acta Endocrinologica Inc., Medical Publishers.

different agents such as infections, intoxications, trauma, nervous strain, heat, cold, muscular fatigue, or X-irradiation. The specific actions of all these agents are quite different. Their only common feature is that they place the body under a situation of stress. Hence we concluded that the stereotypical response—which is superimposed upon all specific effects peculiar to the agent—represents a *reaction to stress as such*.

The first noticed manifestations of this stress-response were *adrenocortical enlargement*, with histological signs of hyperactivity; *thymicolymphatic involution*, with certain concomitant changes in the blood count; and *gastrointestinal ulcers*, often accompanied by other manifestations of damage or "shock." We were struck by the fact that while during this reaction all the organs of the body showed involutive or degenerative changes, the adrenal cortex actually seemed to flourish on stress. We suspected this adrenal response to play a useful part in a nonspecific adaptive reaction, which we visualized as a "call to arms" of the body's defense forces and which we named the "alarm-reaction."

Later investigations revealed that the alarm-reaction is merely the first stage of what is a much more prolonged *general-adaptation-syndrome*. (The syndrome itself comprises three distinct stages, namely: the *alarm-reaction*, in which adaptation has not yet been acquired; the *stage of resistance*, in which adaptation is optimal; and finally, the *stage of exhaustion*, in which the acquired adaptation is lost again.)

The experimental analysis of the mechanism of this syndrome was carried out as follows:

Animals were adrenalectomized and then exposed to stress. This showed us that in the absence of the adrenals stress can no longer cause thymico-lymphatic involution or characteristic blood-count changes.

When adrenalectomized animals were treated with the impure cortical extracts available at that time, it became evident that thymicolymphatic involution and blood-count changes could be produced by adrenal hormones even in the absence of the adrenals. The latter therefore were considered to be indirect results of stress mediated by corticoids.

On the other hand, the gastrointestinal ulcers and other manifestations of pure damage were actually more severe in adrenalectomized than in intact animals and could be lessened by treatment with cortical extracts. It was concluded that these lesions are not mediated by the adrenal and are combatted by an adequate cortical response to stress.

In 1937 we found that hypophysectomy prevents the adrenal response during the alarm-reaction and concluded that stress stimulates the cortex through ACTH.

Later, when pure cortical steroids became available, we could show that the administration of mineralo-corticoids (such as desoxycorticosterone) produces experimental replicas of the so-called hypertensive and rheumatic diseases, notably nephrosclerosis, hypertension, and vascular lesions (especially periarteritis nodosa and hyalin necrosis of the arterioles), as well as arthritic changes resembling, in acute experiments, those of rheumatic fever and after chronic treatment those of rheumatoid arthritis.

Yet even very high doses of mineralo-corticoids did not induce any significant thymico-lymphatic or blood-count changes.

Gluco-corticoids (such as cortisone), on the other hand, were highly potent in causing thymico-lymphatic involution and in eliciting the characteristic blood-count changes of the alarm-reaction. Furthermore, they tended to inhibit the hypertensive and rheumatic changes which can be elicited in animals by mineralo-corticoids. Thus, in many respects, the two types of corticoid hormones antagonize each other.

Inflammatory granulomas, especially those produced in the vicinity of joints by the local application of irritants, as well as certain allergic reactions, are also aggravated by mineralo- and prevented by gluco-corticoids.

We conclude that the pathogenicity of many systemic and local irritants depends largely upon the function of the hypophysis-adrenocortical system. The latter may either enhance or inhibit the body's defense reactions against such agents, and we think that derailments of this adaptive mechanism are the principal factor in the production of certain maladies, which we therefore consider to be essentially diseases of adaptation.

Experiments concerning the Role of the Adrenal Cortex in the Genesis of Hypertensive Disease

In discussing the role of the adrenal cortex in the various clinical hypertensive syndromes, it is well to remember a few rather fundamental facts:

1. Several types of clinical hypertension (hyperplasia of the adrenal cortex whether secondary to a basophil anterior lobe adenoma or "idiopathic," certain adreno-cortical tumors) are accompanied by an

increased corticoid elimination in the urine and can be considerably improved or cured by ablation of excess cortical tissue.

2. Various types of stressors cause an increased urinary elimination of corticoids, as established by accurate and specific bio-assay methods.

3. The excessive administration of synthetic (desoxycorticosterone) or naturally occurring corticoids (desoxocortisone or Reichstein's compound "S") has been shown to produce marked hypertension both in experimental animals and in man.

4. Adrenalectomy causes a decrease in the normal blood pressure and abolishes most types of experimental hypertension. The administration of mineralo-corticoids after adrenalectomy restores the blood pressure at least to the previously established level. Hence the participation of corticoids in the maintenance of hypertension may be regarded as definitely established. The question is only the importance of their role in this connection.

5. There is no evidence of a constant and marked increase in the total excretion of corticoids in the majority of patients suffering from hypertensive disease. It must be kept in mind, however, that the homeostasis of the blood pressure, like that of most other vitally important functions, is guaranteed by several alternative mechanisms. Hence a derangement of any one factor does not necessarily cause abnormal changes in the blood pressure under all conditions. The pressor effect of the corticoids themselves, for instance, is largely dependent upon metabolic factors (e.g., sodium). It is for this reason that the effect of corticoids upon the blood pressure can be profitably discussed only in conjunction with other factors capable of influencing the vasopressor system.

Exposure to nonspecific stressor agents is undoubtedly the most common cause of an increased corticoid production, and since this is accompanied by other manifestations of the G-A-S, we shall now consider cortical participation in vasopressor reactions in conjunction with the G-A-S as a whole.

In the G-A-S the manifestations of passive, nonspecific *damage* are intricately intermixed with those of active *defense*. This is an inherent characteristic of the stress, which elicits the G-A-S. In the biologic sense stress results from the interaction between damage and defense, just as in physics tension or pressure evolves from the interplay between a force and the resistance offered to it.

In addition to damage and defense, every stressor also produces certain *specific actions* (e.g., anesthetics act upon the nervous system, diuretics upon water metabolism, insulin upon the blood sugar), quite apart from its stressor effects. Hence the G-A-S never occurs in its pure form, but is always complicated by superimposed specific actions of the eliciting stressors. In contemplating any biologic response (e.g., a spontaneous disease, an intoxication, a psychosomatic reaction), it is usually quite difficult to identify individual manifestations as due respectively to damage from, defense against, or the specific actions of the provocative agent. Only nonspecific damage and defense are integral parts of the G-A-S, but the specific actions of the eliciting stressors modify the course of the resulting G-A-S (e.g., the glycemic curve will deviate from the characteristic pattern if insulin is used as the stressor agent; the neurologic manifestations will be atypical if the G-A-S is provoked by ether). In this sense they act as "conditioning factors." Certain circumstances, not directly related to the stress situation, are also prone to alter the course of the G-A-S. Among these heredity, pre-existent disease in certain organ systems, and diet are especially important.

The adjacent schematic drawing (see Figure 1) disregards the specific actions of stressors, since they are not part of the G-A-S. It attempts to depict only the main pathways through which nonspecific stress itself affects the organism and the manner in which such reactions are conditioned.

DEFENSE

The systemic defense measures, against both general and localized (topical) injuries, are coordinated through the hypothalamic vegetative centers and the hypophysis. The initial pathways through which stressors act upon these centers are not yet known. Probably either humoral or nervous impulses, coming from the site of direct injury, can induce the hypothalamus-hypophysis system to gear the body for defense. Subsequently both of the two great integrating mechanisms, the nervous and the endocrine system, are alerted.

The nervous defense mechanism. Nervous impulses descend from the hypothalamic vegetative centers, through the autonomic nerves, to the peripheral organs. The splanchnics induce the adrenal medulla to discharge adrenergic hormones (adrenaline and noradrenaline) into the blood. Other adrenergic nerves influence their target organs directly, through fibers, which in the final analysis again act through the liberation of adrenergic compounds, in this case at their endings in the effector organs themselves (blood vessels, glands, etc.). Presumably the discharge of adrenergic hormones into the circulation is most effective when they are needed throughout the body, while the

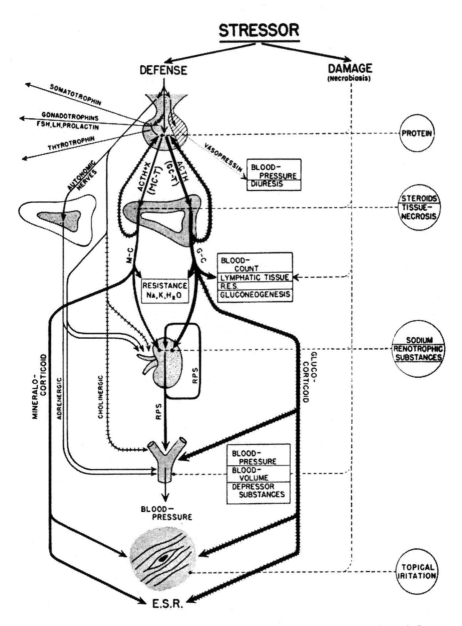

FIGURE 1. Interrelations during the G-A-S. (Reproduced, by permission of the copyright owner, from Selye: *Stress*, Montreal, Acta Endocrinologica Inc., 1950.)

sympathetic nerves are better suited to impart similar impulses selectively, to certain circumscribed territories. The most conspicuous results of such neuro-humoral discharges are changes in the contractility of smooth muscle. Owing to an adrenergic vasoconstriction, the peripheral resistance increases and the blood pressure rises. This hypertensive response may be further accentuated by an increased cardiac volume and the opening of the "renal shunt," which deviates blood from the cortical glomeruli to the juxtamedullary region of the kidney. This neurogenic activation of the "shunt" is comparable to that induced by mechanical interference with the arterial inflow (Goldblatt clamp, "endocrine kidney" operation) into the kidney; hence it augments the production of renal pressor substances (RPS). The latter also cause peripheral vasoconstriction; thus they further augment the peripheral resistance in the cardiovascular system, and hence the blood pressure rises (see below).

There is some evidence of a simultaneous cholinergic discharge during systemic stress. The concurrent activation of both agonists and antagonists occurs in many effector systems during the G-A-S. Presumably it helps to stabilize the target organs, in the face of very powerful stimuli which might otherwise cause excessive deviations from the norm. This concurrent tension of agonists and antagonists is somewhat reminiscent of the simultaneous contraction of flexor and extensor muscles, for instance, in a limb, to prepare it against possible displacement by a blow which may come from any direction. However, damage (shock) endangers life particularly through vasodepressor and hypotensive actions; hence the predominant response during the G-A-S is a defensive (prophylactic) vasoconstriction and hypertension.

The nervous system also participates in many other defensive reactions during the G-A-S—e.g., the regulation of water metabolism (through the hypophyseal stalk and posterior lobe), the blood sugar (through the hepatic branches of the sympathetic division), and the blood count (through splenic contraction); but for the sake of simplicity, these are not specifically indicated in our schematic drawing.

The hormonal defense mechanism. The principal endocrine response to stress is characterized by the so-called shift in anterior-lobe hormone production. This consists in a diminished secretion of somatotrophin, the gonadotrophins (FSH, LH, prolactin), and thyrotrophin —which are not essential for the maintenance of life during conditions of emergency—accompanied by an increase in the secretion of ACTH. Apparently the anterior lobe is unable to produce all its hormones at an optimal rate, if it is called upon to discharge extraordinarily large amounts of corticotrophin.

ACTH is a "gluco-corticotrophic" (G-CT) hormone. It induces the adrenal cortex to produce predominantly gluco-corticoids (G-C), e.g., "compound F," cortisone. The latter act upon the blood count (lymphopenia, eosinopenia, polymorphonuclear leucocytosis), the thymicolymphatic tissue (lympholysis), the reticulo-endothelial system (increased phagocytosis and antibody formation), and gluconeogenesis (the transformation of non-sugars into carbohydrates).

The gluco-corticoids presumably influence resistance in many additional ways, which have not yet been fully analyzed. Through all these actions such steroids help to maintain adrenalectomized animals, even during exposure to stress.

All the gluco-corticoids so far examined possess some mineralocorticoid activity (action upon the sodium, chloride, potassium, and water metabolism); thus they resemble the pure mineralo-corticoids, but the latter are much more potent in this respect and possess no gluco-corticoid action. Hence changes in the mineral and water metabolism, observed after the injection of ACTH, do not necessarily reflect the production of pure mineralo-corticoids by the adrenal.

The action of gluco-corticoids upon the kidney has not yet been extensively studied. However, preliminary investigations show that they cause marked hyperemia of the glomeruli and may render the latter permeable to proteins and even blood. Heavy overdosage with gluco-corticoids can produce severe hyalinization and disintegration of the glomeruli. This is followed by a rise in the blood pressure, presumably mediated through the RPS system. In this respect gluco-corticoids and mineralo-corticoids may mutually synergize each other.

The gluco-corticoids inhibit the production of arteriosclerotic changes (especially periarteritis and hyalinosis). In this respect they antagonize the effects of mineralo-corticoids.

The gluco-corticoids generally inhibit excessive proliferation of fibrous tissue, the formation of intercellular protein deposits (e.g., hyalinosis, collagen disease, allergies), and excessive granulomatous defense reactions against those local irritants which stimulate fibroplastic inflammatory reactions in mesenchymal tissue. They also tend to decrease the erythrocyte sedimentation rate (ESR), through their effect upon the blood-proteins. In all these respects they act as antagonists of the mineralo-corticoids.

The mechanism of the marked antiallergic and antihistaminergic actions of the gluco-corticoids has not yet been elucidated. It may depend upon the breakdown of the proteins which store histamine as a protein-histamine complex.

Many data suggest that under conditions of stress mineralo-corticoid production is likewise increased. Such a rise can also be elicited by certain impure, mineralo-corticotrophic (M-CT), anterior-pituitary extracts, for instance, lyophilized anterior-pituitary tissue (LAP). Threshold doses of LAP are further activated in this respect by the simultaneous administration of ACTH. Apparently the action of the latter can be qualitatively altered by some factor (X) present in crude pituitary extracts and LAP. This X factor appears to be a specific pituitary principle, as it has not been found to occur in similar preparations of other tissues (e.g., liver). The X factor is manifestly not ACTH, but it may be identical with one of the other, already known, hypophyseal hormones. It could also be a special hypophyseal principle, not hitherto identified. Be this as it may, it has now definitely been established that certain pituitary extracts produce a gluco-corticoid type, others a mineralo-corticoid type of reaction. Furthermore, in response to stress, the pituitary itself may discharge predominantly gluco-corticotrophic or mineralo-corticotrophic principles.

The mineralo-corticoids share with the gluco-corticoids the ability to increase the general resistance of adrenalectomized animals. They also cause severe lesions in the kidney, if large quantities of them are given over a long time. There are distention of the convoluted tubules, proliferation of the spiral segments, hyalinization of the glomeruli, proteinuria, hyaline-cast formation, and, eventually, nephrosclerosis.

It is highly probable that mineralo-corticoids increase RPS production especially through some direct functional effect upon the convoluted tubules. Even the subsequent morphologic changes in this part of the nephron precede the development of glomerular sclerosis. Eventually, however, the gradual constriction of the glomerular capillary bed acts somewhat like the Goldblatt clamp or the "endocrine kidney" operation and, simultaneously with the inhibition of glomerular filtration, increases the endocrine activity of the nephron. At the same time the inactivation of RPS is impeded, and a hormonally induced renal hypertension ensues.

Presumably both the stimulation of RPS formation and the inhibition of RPS destruction are thus induced by mineralo-corticoids. This affects the blood vessels. At first the resulting excess of RPS causes a functional vasoconstriction with an increase in the peripheral resistance and blood pressure. More prolonged overdosage with mineralo-corticoids results in arteriosclerotic changes (especially peri-arteritis nodosa and hyalinosis), with a consequent permanent increase in the peripheral resistance and blood pressure.

In this respect mineralo-corticoids and gluco-corticoids mutually antagonize each other, but since (at least at certain dose levels) their actions upon the kidney are synergistic, it depends upon the "conditioning" circumstances whether the administration of gluco-corticoids to animals overdosed with mineralo-corticoids increases or decreases the blood pressure. (Cf. also the conditioning effect of sodium and renotrophic substances, below.)

There is no definite evidence to prove that either type of corticoid has any direct vasopressor effect. The addition of corticoids to perfused vessel preparations does not cause them to contract. Nevertheless, mineralo-corticoids can augment the blood pressure even in the absence of the kidney, presumably by raising the blood volume through their effect on the mineral and water metabolism.

Both types of corticoids act back upon the anterior lobe and inhibit its ACTH production, through the so-called phenomenon of "compensatory atrophy." It is not yet known whether corticoids also impede the endogenous production of that X factor which renders ACTH mineralo-corticotrophic. However, that they do is very probable, since otherwise ACTH therapy would only aggravate conditions characterized by symptoms of mineralo-corticoid overdosage. If the production of the X factor is inhibited in the same manner as that of ordinary ACTH, then the therapeutic action of ACTH is readily explicable. In both instances the pituitary is exposed to an excess of gluco-corticoids. The latter are even more potent in eliciting the phenomenon of compensatory atrophy than are the mineralo-corticoids. Consequently, endogenous corticotrophic stimuli (including the X factor) are virtually eliminated, and the exogenously administered, predominantly gluco-corticotrophic, ACTH acts uninfluenced upon the adrenal cortex.

There is much to suggest that at least certain types of stress (e.g., emotional stimuli) can increase the production of the antidiuretic hormone, which is probably identical with vasopressin. This effect is undoubtedly mediated by nerve tracts descending from the hypothalamus to the posterior lobe, since (unlike the discharge of ACTH) it is abolished by transection of the hypophyseal stalk.

Vasopressin exerts important effects upon the blood pressure and diuresis; these may be superimposed upon the typical reaction pattern during the G-A-S. However, the role of vasopressin secretion during systemic stress has not yet been adequately investigated.

DAMAGE AND OTHER FACTORS CONDITIONING DEFENSE

As we have said before, many nonspecific actions of stressors merely represent manifestations of damage and are not mediated through either the humoral or the nervous defense systems outlined above. These changes appear to result from the necrobiosis of cells not sufficiently protected by the systemic defense mechanism. Thus tissue catabolism occurs under conditions of stress even in the absence of the pituitary, the adrenals, or the sympathetic nervous system. Although gluco-corticoids enhance catabolism, especially of readily dispensable proteins (e.g., that of the thymus, the lymph nodes, and connective tissue), extensive losses of body protein, fat, and carbohydrate can occur even after adrenalectomy.

Catabolites, thus produced, can condition the defensive chain-reaction of the G-A-S at various links. We have seen that protein tends to favor the mineralo-corticotrophic type of hypophyseal discharge, that sodium increases, while renotrophic steroids decrease, the sensitivity of the kidney to overdoses of mineralo-corticoids, that topical chemical irritation augments the fibroplastic and hyalinosis-producing action of mineralo-corticoids, and so forth. There is every reason to believe that endogenously liberated protein (or amino-acids), sodium, renotrophic steroids, and irritating metabolites, would influence such hormone actions in the same manner as these substances do when they are exogenously introduced into the body. The intensity and the quality of such "endogenous self-conditioning" of the G-A-S largely depend upon the body's reserve of these metabolites and the intensity with which they are discharged into the blood. Presumably this in turn is influenced by heredity, differences in species, previous exposure to stress, the nutritional state of the organism, etc.

We have seen that the specific actions of individual stressors may likewise act as conditioning factors. Thus agents causing intense renal damage can sensitize the body to the pressor effects of the G-A-S, somewhat in the same manner as partial nephrectomy does; pyrogens, histamine, and other stressors capable of causing severe vascular paralysis will selectively "decondition" the arterial tree to the pressor action of endogenous RPS; microbes, allergens, or local mechanical trauma can stimulate the tissues which come into direct contact with them (somewhat like the formalin or mustard in our "topical irritation arthritis" test) to the formation of a fibroplastic and hyalin-containing granuloma tissue.

Such conditioning factors affect the defense mechanism at different points and may either increase or decrease the efficacy of any one among its individual components. Hence it is evident that the essentially stereotypical defense-pattern of the G-A-S can manifest itself in widely different ways, depending upon such conditioning factors.

This is particularly important for the understanding of the diseases of adaptation. Unless conditioning factors could considerably alter the reaction-pattern to stress, it would be impossible to ascribe rheumatoid arthritis, periarteritis nodosa, allergies, certain types of diabetes, or hypertension to the same causative agent, namely, systemic stress. The concept *that such widely different maladies should result from the same cause* has often been considered to be quite contrary to accepted views concerning the causation of disease. Since this tenet is rather fundamental to our interpretation of the diseases of adaptation, it deserves special attention.

Let us point out first that such an assumption is not without precedent in medicine. For example, an excessive production of thyroid hormone may be associated with predominantly ophthalmic, metabolic, or cardiac derangements. Before the tuberculosis bacillus had been isolated, it would have been considered most improbable that such dissimilar conditions as Pott's disease, phthisis of the lungs, miliary tuberculosis, and the tuberculous lupus of the skin are all caused by the same pathogen; yet this is the case.

We have attempted to demonstrate that the polymorphism of the G-A-S symptomatology is due to two principal reasons. First, every stressor has specific actions, in addition to its stress-producing ability. The former modify the response caused by stress as such; hence the polymorphism of the G-A-S manifestations can be due to specific effects of the evocative stressors.

This type of conditioning may also be illustrated by an example taken from chemistry. All acids have many properties in common; yet the reactions of each member in this group are essentially different. The characteristics they share are due to their acidity; the properties which distinguish them are the specific reactions of the carriers of this acid function. In pharmacology the stressor effect is what the drugs have in common; their other properties endow them with "specific pharmacologic actions." Both in chemistry and in pharmacology the specific properties condition that nonspecific feature (acidity, stress) which the entire group shares. Hence no two acids—

and no two stressors—act exactly alike. This may help to illustrate conditioning by specific properties of the stressor.

We have seen, however, that even exposure to the same stressor agent may result in qualitatively different responses. Here the polymorphism of the G-A-S manifestations is due to selective conditioning, by factors extraneous to the stressor. This "peripheral conditioning" may occur at the various intermediate stations of the G-A-S or in the target organs themselves. We have compared this to the manifold effects one can obtain with the same electric current. During an emergency it may be necessary to supply more electricity for a community. This current will always be of the same quality, and it will always travel along the same pre-existent main channels. Yet, depending upon the kind of emergency and the special needs of each district, both its quality and quantity have to be regulated locally in the periphery. Thus the same current can be used to produce mechanical work, sound, light of any color, heat, or cold, and indeed it may be shut out completely from a locality where it would represent a fire hazard. Of course, the more we approach the periphery of such an electric circuit, the more subject it will be to conditioning—first, because the thin terminal wires can more easily be handled than the thick principal cables, and second, because interventions anywhere along the line, above such a peripheral point, would affect the latter.

Essentially the same is true of the G-A-S. The more we approach the periphery, the more often do we note deviations from the standard G-A-S pattern. All stressors cause an ACTH discharge, but this may or may not be accompanied by the production of the X factor, which is necessary for mineralo-corticotrophic action. Interference at a lower level may cause even more selective deviations from the typical stress response. Thus transection of the splanchnics may impede adrenaline discharge during the A-R, without interfering with any G-A-S manifestations except those resulting directly from hyper-adrenalinemia. The possibilities for conditioning become ever more selective as we approach the peripheral target organs, each of which can be individually protected or sensitized to the typical actions of the G-A-S.

Summary

Increased corticoid production undoubtedly plays an important part in the genesis of certain types of clinical hypertension (e.g., basophil adenomas of the anterior pituitary, adreno-cortical tumors).

Various stressor agents increase corticoid production in animals and man, as shown by demonstrably augmented corticoid elimination in the urine.

Mineralo-corticoids and certain corticotrophic pituitary extracts cause hypertension, with nephrosclerosis and hypertensive vascular lesions, in animals both on normal and particularly on high-sodium, high-protein diets.

The pressor and nephrotoxic effects of pituitary extracts and mineralo-corticoids can be prevented by dietary measures (metabolic "conditioning" factors).

Probably both the actual amount of corticoids secreted and the metabolic factors which determine their activity play an important part in the development of clinical hypertensive disease.

The degree to which corticoid secretion and corticoid-conditioning metabolic factors are involved in the development of the various types of clinical hypertension remains to be established.

• • • • • • • • • • • • *by* EDUARDO BRAUN-MENENDEZ

The Mechanism of Hypertension Due to Desoxycorticosterone

PROBABLY the first observation of the pressor effect of desoxy-corticosterone in animals was made by Kuhlman *et al.* (1939), who after injecting 25 mg. per day during 70 days into two dogs observed increases in the blood pressure of 45 and 20 mm. Hg respectively. This study was a consequence of the observation of Loeb *et al.* (1939), who called attention to the abnormal rise in pressure obtained in two Addisonian patients treated with desoxycorticosterone, a fact which was subsequently confirmed by many others. In 1940 Grollman *et al.* reported hypertension in rats treated with desoxycorticosterone, and Swingle *et al.* (1941) obtained transitory hypertension in normal and adrenalectomized dogs. Rodbard and Freed (1942) confirmed the pressor effect of desoxycorticosterone in dogs, and Mrazek *et al.* (1942) and Briskin *et al.* (1943) confirmed it in rats.

Selye (1942) showed that desoxycorticosterone causes nephrosclerosis and generalized tissue edema accompanied by cardiac hypertrophy in the chick, and Selye and Stone (1943) observed that high doses of sodium chloride added to the drinking water of chicks suffice to elicit these changes. Relatively small doses of desoxycorticosterone become toxic if given in conjunction with a solution of sodium chloride which by itself causes no abnormal symptoms. Then Selye and Hall (1943) and Selye *et al.* (1943) showed that in the rat chronic overdosage with desoxycorticosterone causes malignant nephrosclerosis with rapidly progressing hypertension. The production of both the renal changes and the hypertension was facilitated by the administration of a 1 per cent sodium chloride solution instead of ordinary tap water (Selye and Pentz, 1943). To obtain these effects desoxycorticosterone was administered daily by subcutaneous injection in rather large doses (5 to 10 mg.), but later the same results were obtained by single subcutaneous implants of one or two 20–40 mg. pellets (Selye *et al.*, 1945) from which sometimes less than 1 mg. per day was absorbed.

133

The Reaction of the Organism to the Chronic Administration
of Desoxycorticosterone

Before considering the possible mechanism of desoxycorticosterone-induced hypertension, we should review some of the reactions of the organism to the chronic administration of this steroid.

Electrolyte changes. Following the administration of desoxycorticosterone, there is a striking and rapid reduction in the renal excretion of sodium, chlorine, and water, accompanied by an increased renal excretion of potassium. The mechanism of these actions is not yet well understood, but it seems that the retention of sodium is mediated through the ability of the cells of the kidney tubules to reabsorb more or less sodium from the glomerular filtrate. According to the hypothesis of Wesson *et al.* (1948), a fixed percentage (about 87.5 per cent) of the filtered sodium is actively reabsorbed in the proximal tubules, and the rest is reabsorbed in the distal tubule, which has a maximal rate of reabsorption. The amount of sodium excreted would depend, according to this hypothesis, on the load of sodium offered to the distal tubules, which depends in great part on the rate of glomerular filtration. But many investigations show that this hypothesis cannot explain all the facts. In cardiac failure or hepatic cirrhosis, where sodium retention is known to occur, the rate of glomerular filtration may be normal (Farnsworth and Krakusin, 1948a, b). On the other hand the disappearance of edema during recompensation in cardiac patients may occur without changes in the glomerular filtration rate (Briggs *et al.*, 1948; Earle *et al.*, 1949; Kattus *et al.*, 1949).

An increase in the renal venous pressure increases the renal reabsorption of sodium (Blake *et al.*, 1949; Selkurt *et al.*, 1949); an increase in the blood pressure (Green *et al.*, 1949) or an increase in the sodium load (Selkurt and Post, 1949; Green and Farah, 1949) diminishes the tubular reabsorption of sodium. It seems, therefore, that the capacity of the tubules for reabsorbing sodium is subject to great variations, which depend on many physiological factors. Among these the antidiuretic hormone of the posterior pituitary probably decreases (Little *et al.*, 1947; Anslow *et al.*, 1948) and desoxycorticosterone increases the tubular reabsorptive capacity for sodium.

Changes in the blood volume and extracellular fluid volume. The retention of sodium following the administration of desoxycorticosterone is accompanied by an increase in the plasma volume and extracellular fluid in patients with Addison's disease as well as in normal subjects (Clinton and Thorn, 1943; Loeb, 1942; Perera *et al.*, 1944;

Perera and Blood, 1947), its effect being much more marked in the former.

Swingle *et al.* (1941) and Clinton *et al.* (1942) observed a moderate increase in the plasma volume in normal dogs injected with desoxycorticosterone, and we have seen (Table 1) an increase in the blood

TABLE 1. The Effect of Desoxycorticosterone Acetate (2.5 mg/day Per Rat during 15 Days) on the Blood Volume and Extracellular Fluid Volume (Thiocyanate Space)

	No. of Rats	Blood Volume (ml/100 cm^2)	Extracellular Fluid Volume (ml/100 cm^2)
DCA-treated	8	4.88	18.4
Normal controls	8	4.06	16.3

volume (20 per cent) and extracellular fluid volume (13 per cent) in rats to which 2.5 mg. of desoxycorticosterone per day were administered during 15 days (Braun-Menendez and Martínez, 1949b). Selye and Dosne (1941) also obtained in the intact rat a slight rise in the blood volume following the administration of desoxycorticosterone. Gaudino and Levitt (1949) gave 30 mg. of desoxycorticosterone per day to dogs during 3 weeks and observed a marked and immediate rise in the volume of extracellular fluid, with a reduction of the intracellular fluid and a slight increase in the blood volume.

Renal lesions. I have already reviewed the early work of Selye and his collaborators on the renal changes resulting from the administration of desoxycorticosterone and of desoxycorticosterone plus a sodium chloride drinking solution. Later on they demonstrated that in the absence of salt in the diet or the drinking fluid the administration of desoxycorticosterone is not followed by renal changes (Selye *et al.*, 1949). We have confirmed the latter results (Braun-Menendez and Prado, 1950) (Fig. 1). Some authors claim that renal hypertrophy and renal lesions can be observed in rats after the administration of desoxycorticosterone without any sodium implement (Friedman and Friedman, 1949; Green and Glover, 1948). But their rats were fed diets containing appreciable amounts of sodium chloride.

Cardiac hypertrophy. Following the administration of desoxycorticosterone in the presence of sodium chloride, cardiac hypertrophy has been observed by Selye and Stone (1943) in the chick and by many authors in the rat. The increased weight of the heart goes hand in hand with the increase in the blood pressure and is probably a consequence of the latter.

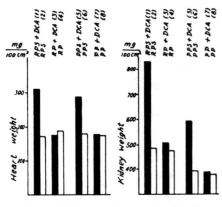

FIGURE 1. The heart and kidney weights in rats 7 weeks after the implantation of 40 mg. of desoxycorticosterone acetate. Rats were separated into 8 groups, and 4 types of diet were employed: RPS, rich in protein (40 per cent) and salt (4 per cent); RP, rich in protein without salt; PPS, poor in protein (13 per cent) and rich in salt (4 per cent); and PP, poor in protein. Of the two groups on each diet one received desoxycorticosterone and the other remained as control. As may be seen, desoxycorticosterone caused no renal or cardiac enlargement in the absence of salt in the diet.

FIGURE 2. The same experiment as in Figure 1. In the absence of salt in the diet and the drinking fluid, desoxycorticosterone caused no increase in the blood pressure.

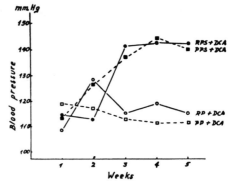

Hypertension. An analysis of the literature concerning the action of desoxycorticosterone on the blood pressure of the rat shows some contradictory results. But these contradictions may be explained if due consideration is given to the experimental conditions in each case. In our rats (Braun-Menendez and Prado, 1950) fed a sodium-poor diet and drinking tap water the implant of 40 mg. of desoxycorticosterone was not followed by a rise in the blood pressure in the course of 6–8 weeks (Fig. 2). On the other hand, the addition of 4 per cent sodium chloride to the diet was enough to cause hypertension in rats implanted with the same dose of desoxycorticosterone. The presence of sodium chloride in sufficient amounts in the diet or the drinking fluid is thus necessary for the pressor action of desoxycorticosterone to become manifest. Our experiments confirm the previous work of

Knowlton *et al.* (1947) and Selye *et al.* (1949). Some authors have obtained negative results, which can be attributed to one of the following causes: (1) The rats drank water (Braun-Menendez and Foglia, 1944; Gaudino, 1944; Leathem and Drill, 1943; Selye *et al.*, 1943) or very dilute sodium chloride solutions (Knowlton *et al.*, 1946). (2) The diet was very poor in salt (Braun-Menendez and Foglia, 1944; Gaudino, 1944). (3) Desoxycorticosterone was administered in low doses (Leathem and Drill, 1943) or during too short a time (Leathem and Drill, 1943; Gaudino, 1944). (4) Perhaps some strains of rats are less susceptible to the nephrosclerotic and pressor action of DCA (Friedman, 1949; Bechgaard and Bergstrand, 1949).

On the other hand, some authors claim that hypertension can be obtained by desoxycorticosterone without any additional sensitization (Friedman and Friedman, 1949), meaning that the administration of a 1 per cent sodium chloride solution as a drinking fluid or unilateral nephrectomy is not indispensable to obtain hypertension. Green and Glover (1948) also obtained hypertension following the administration of desoxycorticosterone to rats without the addition of salt to the diet or the drinking fluid. But in neither case was sodium chloride absent from the diet: the animals were fed Purina fox chow or other similar diets, which contain salt in appreciable quantities.

The action of desoxycorticosterone is in such a way related to the presence of sodium chloride (or, more properly speaking, to the presence of sodium) that it is difficult to decide whether sodium chloride sensitizes the animals to the action of desoxycorticosterone or whether desoxycorticosterone "potentiates the effect of subthreshold doses of sodium chloride," as Selye and Stone expressed it in 1943. The latter is true at least in the chick, where the administration of sodium chloride in high concentration (2 per cent as a drinking fluid) causes hypertension (Lenel *et al.*, 1948) and renal lesions (Selye, 1943), the latter being identical with those observed when subthreshold doses of sodium chloride (0.2 per cent), which in themselves are not toxic, are administered in conjunction with small doses of desoxycorticosterone (Selye and Stone, 1943). Sapirstein *et al.* (1950) administered during 6 weeks saline solutions (2 per cent) as a drinking fluid to rats. The animals developed arterial hypertension, which at autopsy was found to be associated with hypertrophy of the heart and kidneys, relative to body weight.

Disturbances in the water metabolism. Most authors affirm that the administration of desoxycorticosterone is followed by a diabetes insipidus-like syndrome with polydipsia and polyuria. Our results show that this action of desoxycorticosterone is also dependent on the presence of sodium chloride in the diet or the drinking fluid.

If a salt-free (or salt-poor) diet is administered together with tap water as a drinking fluid, the administration of desoxycorticosterone (the implant of 40 mg. of desoxycorticosterone or the daily subcutaneous injection of 2.5 mg.) does not cause any increase in the water intake or urine output (Fig. 3) (Braun-Menendez and Prado,

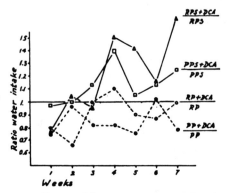

FIGURE 3. Same experiment as in Figure 1. The ratio of the water intake of the rats implanted with desoxycorticosterone and of the control rats is plotted against time. No increase in the water intake was produced by desoxycorticosterone in those groups that received no salt in the diet.

1950; Braun-Menendez, 1950). In the presence of sodium chloride in the diet (4 per cent sodium chloride) the administration of desoxycorticosterone is followed by a slight increase in the water intake. It is only when the only drinking fluid available is an 0.8 or a 1 per cent solution of sodium chloride that the intake and output of fluid are greatly increased by the administration of desoxycorticosterone.

An analysis of the literature showed that this observation had already been made by others, without any special emphasis having been given to it. The results obtained may be divided into two groups:

1. Those that show a "moderate" increase in the *water* intake following the administration of desoxycorticosterone (Carnes *et al.*, 1941; Selye *et al.*, 1945; Skahen and Green, 1948; Harned and Nelson, 1943; Winter and Selye, 1942; Corey and Britton, 1941; Green *et al.*, 1948). But none of these authors studied the action of desoxycorticosterone on the water intake of rats fed a sodium chloride-free diet. In every case the animals were fed standard diets (Purina fox chow, etc.), which contain sodium chloride in a proportion surely greater than 1 per cent.

2. Those showing that the action of desoxycorticosterone on the water intake depends on the amount of sodium chloride in the diet (Ragan *et al.*, 1943; Rice and Richter, 1943; Braun-Menendez and Prado, 1950; Braun-Menendez, 1950) and that in the absence of

sodium chloride in the diet desoxycorticosterone causes no increase in the water intake or urine output.

The majority of authors just mention the fact that the fluid exchange increases when desoxycorticosterone is administered to animals which drink a sodium chloride solution.

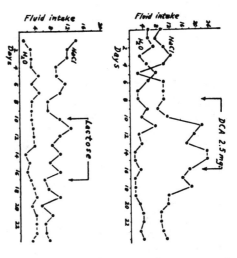

FIGURE 4. The effect of desoxycorticosterone administration on the fluid intake of rats given free access to tap water and a 1 per cent solution of sodium chloride.

We have studied recently the response to desoxycorticosterone of rats which were allowed to regulate their own salt intake (Fig. 4). When given access to a 1 per cent sodium chloride solution in a container separate from the one used for their drinking tap water, the animals into which desoxycorticosterone was injected in daily doses of 2.5 mg. increased their daily intake of salt solution several times and decreased the intake of tap water. The increased appetite for sodium chloride solution became manifest the 2d or 3d day after the initiation of the injections and persisted 2 or 3 days after the end of the injection period. Rice and Richter (1943) obtained more or less similar results.

This is indeed an unexpected response. We have seen that renal lesions, renal hypertrophy, and hypertension appear only when desoxycorticosterone is given in conjunction with sodium chloride in the diet or drinking fluid (Braun-Menendez and Prado, 1950). According to Richter's ideas, specific appetite is for rats a defense mechanism: the appetite increases for those substances that are more favorable for their subsistence (NaCl in adrenal insufficiency, $CaCl_2$ in parathyroid insufficiency, etc.) and decreases for those that are detrimental to the organism. As an example of the latter situation,

Abrams and his associates (1949) found that rats made hypertensive by perinephritis have a decreased appetite for sodium: hypertensive rats having access to different salt solutions drank less sodium chloride and sodium bicarbonate solutions than the normal controls. One would expect that allowed to choose between tap water and sodium chloride, the rats to which desoxycorticosterone had been administered would reject the saline solution, as on the election of the drinking fluid would depend the presence or absence of subsequent renal lesions and hypertension.

An explanation of the anomalous increased appetite for sodium chloride following the administration of desoxycorticosterone might be found in the loss of potassium caused by the steroid. Perhaps the rats took more sodium because no other cation was available to compensate the loss of potassium. To test this hypothesis, we arranged an experiment in which the rats had access to 3 graduated water bottles: one contained a 0.17 M. solution of sodium chloride, the second contained a 0.17 M. solution of potassium chloride, and the third distilled water. The administration of desoxycorticosterone (2.5 mg. per rat per day during 8 days) caused a marked increase in the intake of sodium chloride solution and no significant change in the intake of water or potassium chloride solution.

We then made another experiment in which each group of rats had access to various salt solutions (Fig. 5). To one of these groups we

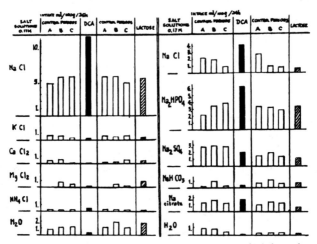

FIGURE 5. The effect of desoxycorticosterone administration during 10 days on the spontaneous intake of different salt solutions.

gave 0.17 M. solutions of NaCl, KCl, CaCl₂, MgCl₂, NH₄Cl and water; to the other we gave 0.17 M. solutions of Na₂HPO₄, Na₂SO₄, NaHCO₃, NaCl, Na citrate and water. The administration of desoxycorticosterone (2.5 mg. per rat per day) during 10 days caused in the former group a very marked increased intake of sodium chloride solution (from 9 ml. per rat per day in the control period to 20.6 ml. per rat per day) and of ammonium chloride solution (from 0.17 per rat per day to 0.77 ml. per rat per day), while the intake of water and magnesium chloride decreased from 1.8 to 0.7 and from 0.9 to 0.27 ml. respectively. In the second group the intake of sodium chloride and of sodium phosphate both increased significantly, with the particularity that as the injection period progressed the rats seemed to drink the sodium chloride solution in preference to the sodium phosphate.

The Mechanism of the Action of Desoxycorticosterone

The role of sodium. We have already pointed out that in the absence of sodium chloride the administration of desoxycorticosterone is not followed by renal lesions or hypertension or an increased intake of water. For these changes to appear, salt must be given in the diet or the drinking fluid. The sodium ion is the one responsible for the action of salt, as has been shown by Selye *et al.* (1949), Friedman *et al.* (1948), and others. We also know that desoxycorticosterone causes a retention of sodium in the organism, probably owing to the increased tubular reabsorption of this cation.

The first point to be considered is whether sodium sensitizes the organism to the action of desoxycorticosterone or, on the contrary, this steroid sensitizes the organism to the action of sodium. This question has not yet been solved, although, as we have already pointed out, the second proposition has some evidence in its favor. In fact, the administration of sodium chloride alone in high doses causes renal lesions and arterial hypertension in the chick and the administration of desoxycorticosterone together with subthreshold doses of sodium chloride causes the same effect as sodium chloride alone. In rats the administration of desoxycorticosterone even in great doses does not cause alteration in the water turnover, renal morphology, or blood pressure if sodium chloride is absent from the diet. On the other hand, Sapirstein *et al.* (1950) have obtained hypertension and renal hypertrophy in the rat after administering during 6 weeks a 2 per cent sodium chloride solution as a drinking fluid.

Why sodium chloride in high doses should produce renal lesions and how it does so are still unknown.

The relation between hypertension and renal lesions. The hypertension which follows upon the administration of desoxycorticosterone plus salt is always accompanied by renal lesions. One can thus almost affirm that the kidney plays an active role in this type of arterial hypertension. The evidence in favor of this point of view derives from the following facts: (1) When desoxycorticosterone is administered in conjunction with sodium salts, both renal changes and hypertension follow. If salt is withdrawn, desoxycorticosterone causes no renal lesions and no rise in the blood pressure. (2) Friedman and Friedman (1949) found a "remarkable parallel" between alterations in the blood pressure and an increase in the kidney weight. An elevation of the blood pressure even at the earliest date studied was always accompanied by an increase in the kidney weight. (3) Studies on the persistence of hypertension after the cessation of treatment with desoxycorticosterone show that hypertension may become permanent in from about 50 to 60 per cent of animals (Prado, 1950). This type of hypertension could be compared to metahypophyseal diabetes (Houssay, 1942), a permanent diabetes due to pancreatic lesions produced by the temporary administration of anterior pituitary extracts.

Before considering the mechanism by which the kidneys participate in the desoxycorticosterone-induced hypertension, we must discuss some experimental findings which may seem contradictory.

1. Friedman *et al.* (1948) studied renal function in rats to which desoxycorticosterone had been administered and noted that the rise in the blood pressure appeared to be independent of alterations in renal function as determined by the clearance of inulin and PAH; in other words, though desoxycorticosterone caused alterations in renal clearances, the blood pressure elevation seemed to occur well before the onset of renal interference. But they also recognized the presence of renal hypertrophy, which "indicated that some renal change had occurred." Later on Friedman and Friedman (1949), by correlating the renal functions with the kidney weight, concluded that since renal function was maintained only at the normal level despite the increase in the size of the kidney, it seemed reasonable to assume that this process is a compensatory hypertrophy. If the renal function tests are correlated with actual renal mass, the renal involvement becomes apparent. In other words, the previous finding that the rise in the blood pressure antedates the alterations of renal function loses its significance: normal renal function was maintained by an increase in the renal mass and, I would add, probably by the increase in the blood pressure.

2. The blood pressure that is increased following the administration of desoxycorticosterone can return to normal levels on interruption of the treatment with this steroid. This happens most easily and most rapidly when treatment has not been very prolonged. Friedman and Friedman (1949) withdrew the 75 mg. pellets of desoxycorticosterone 25, 37, and 51 days after the implant in intact rats. In all the hypertensive animals the blood pressure returned to normal in about 6 days. The duration of the hypertension before the interruption of the treatment was not more than 36 days. Prado (1950) removed the pellets 140 days after initiation of the treatment in rats, which had had hypertension of at least 120 days duration. Thirty-four days after the removal of the pellets the blood pressure was still elevated in all the animals. If the pellets were removed after shorter periods of hypertension, only a percentage of the rats remained hypertensive. In the rest, the blood pressure returned to normal levels in from 20 to 27 days. A thorough study of the residual hypertension has not yet been made. The fact that in some cases the elevated blood pressure can return to normal on cessation of the treatment can be taken as evidence against the participation of the kidney in the process. Nevertheless it seems reasonable to assume that the renal lesions caused by desoxycorticosterone can regress after withdrawal of the steroid or be compensated by hypertrophy of the non-damaged renal structures.

3. Why are the renal lesions caused by desoxycorticosterone and salt accompanied by hypertension, while more extensive renal lesions caused by a great number of other agents may not be accompanied by hypertension? A very typical case is offered by the experiments of Knowlton and his co-workers. Rats rendered nephritic by means of a rabbit anti-rat kidney serum did not develop hypertension, but when desoxycorticosterone was given in the dose of 2.5 mg. per day, striking hypertension resulted in every instance (Knowlton et al., 1946). The administration of the same dosage of desoxycorticosterone to nephritic animals receiving a diet with only 8 m. eq. Na per 100 gm. of diet did not cause hypertension (Knowlton et al., 1947). These authors point out that the renal changes were somewhat more pronounced in the rats receiving desoxycorticosterone plus cytotoxic serum, but the lesions caused by the serum were as extensive as those produced by desoxycorticosterone alone.

The interpretation of these facts constitutes a real problem, which we shall try to elucidate later.

The mechanism of the renal participation in renal hypertension. Assuming that the kidney plays an important role in the hypertension which follows upon the administration of desoxycorticosterone plus salt, what is the mechanism of its participation?

Many hypotheses have been put forward by those who have studied this problem.

1. The renin-hypertensin system may be involved, according to Selye. The injection of desoxycorticosterone would, according to this hypothesis, initiate the vicious circle of hypertension "by increasing the vasopressor (renin?) production by the kidney." Knowlton *et al.* (1946) also refer to this possibility. But to my knowledge nobody has yet studied the renin concentration in the blood or kidneys of animals rendered hypertensive by the administration of desoxycorticosterone.

The possibility that desoxycorticosterone might increase the efficiency of the reaction Renin + hypertensinogen → hypertensin was explored *in vitro* by Croxatto and Croxatto (1949) with negative results. The same authors also found that the acute administration of desoxycorticosterone did not increase in the rat the pressor response to hypertensin or adrenalin.

2. The possibility that the kidneys are concerned with the excretion and possible inactivation of desoxycorticosterone is suggested by Friedman and Friedman (1949). These authors extirpated the kidneys in both normal rats and rats treated with desoxycorticosterone. In the former they observed a rise in pressure in 3 of 9 animals, an observation almost superposable to that of Braun-Menendez and von Euler (1947). An even more marked rise was observed in all the desoxycorticosterone-treated animals after total nephrectomy. A similar observation was made by Hall and Hall (1949). I do not believe that these observations confirm the assumption of Friedman and Friedman (1949) or exclude the participation of the kidneys in desoxycorticosterone hypertension as claimed by Hall and Hall (1949). They merely show that the previous administration of desoxycorticosterone causes a change in the organism that favors the appearance of the hypertension which frequently follows total nephrectomy in non-treated animals. We shall presently come back to this subject.

VEM formation by the kidney is abolished by adrenalectomy, and this can be restored by desoxycorticosterone (Shorr, 1948). The vasopressor substance produced by the kidney following the administration of desoxycorticosterone is perhaps VEM rather than renin or both. This possibility has been tested by Zweifach and Shorr (1950), who were not able to find any increase in VEM, or changes in the reactivity of the terminal vascular bed, or modifications in the formation of VEM by the kidneys in rats made hypertensive by DCA administration.

The kidney may participate also in the desoxycorticosterone-induced hypertension by retaining sodium. And this leads us to the discussion of a possible extrarenal mechanism in the hypertension caused by desoxycorticosterone.

The participation of extrarenal mechanisms in desoxycorticosterone-induced hypertension. The retention of sodium and chloride and the excretion of potassium are a very striking action of desoxycorticosterone and have been demonstrated in rats, dogs, and men (Kuhlman et al., 1939; Harkness et al., 1942; Clinton et al., 1942; Loeb, 1942; etc.). The changes in the electrolyte metabolism due to the administration of desoxycorticosterone may be instrumental in the elevation of the blood pressure.

The retention of sodium is accompanied by an enhanced appetite for sodium and an increased ingestion of it (Braun-Menendez, 1950), by a marked and rapid increase in the extracellular fluid (Braun-Menendez and Martínez, 1949; Gaudino and Levitt, 1949), by a decrease in the intracellular fluid (Gaudino and Levitt, 1949), and by a slight increase in the blood volume (Swingle et al., 1941; Clinton et al., 1942; Braun-Menendez and Martínez, 1949; Gaudino and Levitt, 1949).

The explanation of all these changes is still completely hypothetical. DCA possibly initiates all of them by altering the cellular permeability for cations (Swingle, 1937): potassium leaves the cells and is excreted by the kidneys and is followed by the partial replacement of intracellular potassium by sodium. This change has been observed in the voluntary muscle (Buell and Turner, 1941; Miller and Darrow, 1941; Ferrebee et al., 1941) and also to a lesser extent in the cardiac muscle (Darrow and Miller, 1942). If no extra sodium chloride is given, all that happens is a shift of the fluid: a decrease in the intracellular fluid and a slight increase in the extracellular fluid. These changes are the reverse of those following sodium depletion in man (McCance, 1936) or the Darrow and Yannet experiment (1935). But if enough sodium is given in the diet or drinking fluid, renal lesions appear, the increase in the extracellular fluid is much more marked, and it is further increased by an enhanced appetite for sodium. The marked increase in the extracellular fluid is, I believe, a positive factor in the causation of hypertension. The evidence in favor of this point of view has been summarized in a previous presentation and will not be repeated here. But in desoxycorticosterone-induced hypertension the intervention of this factor seems evident.

When desoxycorticosterone is given in conjunction with a sodium-deficient diet, there is no significant increase in the extracellular fluid and no hypertension. On the other hand, all the factors which favor the retention of sodium in the organism, whether due to an increased ingestion or to a decreased excretion, facilitate the obtainment of hypertension. This happens in the following circumstances:

1. Unilateral nephrectomy (Selye, 1948), which in a way diminishes the capacity of the kidney for excreting sodium

2. The presence of renal lesions

   a. Toxic nephritis (Knowlton *et al.*, 1946)

   b. Experimental perinephritis (Braun-Menendez and Martínez, 1949)

   c. Experimental diabetes (Braun-Menendez and Martínez, 1949)

   d. Human essential hypertension (Perera and Blood, 1948)

3. The administration of sodium chloride or other sodium salts with the drinking fluid (Selye *et al.*, 1945; Selye and Stone, 1943, etc.)

Furthermore, the administration of great amounts of sodium chloride causes an increase in the extracellular fluid, and in the rat (Sapirstein *et al.*, 1950) and the chick (Lenel *et al.*, 1948) may cause hypertension.

Summarizing, the administration of desoxycorticosterone together with sodium salts causes hypertension accompanied by renal lesions and an increase in the extracellular fluid. Both these changes very probably play a role in the causation of hypertension.

Questions and Discussion

DR. MAURICE B. VISSCHER: We have been interested in the relationship of desoxycorticosterone and hypertension for some time in our laboratories. We have been troubled by several points. First, let me remind you that one of the characteristic things in essential hypertension is that it occurs without appreciable disorder of renal function in many, if not in most, instances.

We were interested in ascertaining whether hypertension could be produced in dogs and other animals by desoxycorticosterone, along with very large quantities of sodium chloride in animals with normal renal function.

Our most extensive studies have been done in the dog. I refer particularly to the work done in cooperation with Dr. Rodney B. Harvey.

Dogs were maintained for periods of a month with a daily administration of 25 mg. of desoxycorticosterone acetate and of between 75 and 125 gm. of sodium chloride. The dogs were fed the salt by stomach tube, along with the ground horse meat diet.

In none of these animals was there a maintained gain in body weight. In none of them was there an increase in the systolic or diastolic blood pressures as measured with the van Leersum loop by the cuff method or as measured directly by puncture.

We were, in other words, unable to obtain appreciable retention in these dogs of either salt or water over a long period of time. We had expected that we might have obtained salt and water retention with such large salt loads combined with high desoxycorticosterone dosage. We had also anticipated a production of hypertension. We have been disturbed by this set of observations because it seems to us that it should not be necessary to inactivate part of the renal mechanism in order to produce this effect in animals, but that it ought to be possible to push the administration of desoxycorticosterone and salt with a normal renal mechanism to the point where such effects occur, if

147

indeed the agents in question are of primary importance in the pathogenesis of hypertension.

I must say that we have not tested the effect specifically of our diet. I should not be at all surprised if the character of the remainder of the diet had determined what the results were and I rather surmise that the high potassium content of the horse meat may have had some protective effect. These observations cause me to raise a word of caution concerning the interpretation of the observations made on animals with renal impairment.

DR. ELEXIOUS T. BELL: I am puzzled by the structure of the endocrine kidney which Dr. Selye showed us. I understood him to say that he produced this by a modification of the Goldblatt technique. The kidneys which I have studied, which were prepared by the Goldblatt method, showed atrophy of the tubules when the constriction was too severe. They showed a structure quite different from Dr. Selye's endocrine kidney. I wonder if Dr. Goldblatt would comment on this.

DR. HARRY GOLDBLATT: I have seen sections of kidneys from Dr. Selye's rats and I myself have produced the so-called endocrine kidney by a reduction of the blood flow to a rat's kidney, even without tying the ureter. The typical picture of the endocrine kidney is the result of a combination of two processes, namely, atrophy and regeneration induced by ischemia. In the dog, the atrophy is usually the dominant change.

DR. SELYE: With reference to the problem raised by Dr. Braun-Menendez I should like to say that an increased production of renin may well play a role in the pressor responses obtained with DCA in animals.

The question of the resistance of dogs raised by Dr. Visscher is particularly important. It is our impression, on the basis of experiments carried out in our Institute, that adult dogs are much more resistant than young ones. In unilaterally nephrectomized young dogs kept on 1 per cent sodium chloride instead of drinking water, we have been able to produce renal changes as well as hypertension quite regularly, but adult animals are less responsive. In any event it is important to realize that a number of other species such as the fowl, mouse, cat, hamster, and guinea pig lend themselves very well to the production of nephrosclerosis and hypertension by DCA. Even in man this steroid has been proved to raise the blood pressure, and here—as in animals—pressor responses are much more readily obtained if there is a pre-existent condition of renal damage.

In reply to Dr. Goldblatt, I should like to say that the rat lends itself much better than other animals to the production of the "endocrine kidney." This may be due to the fact that the rat kidney has only one pyramid and hence is supplied by a very simple type of renal circulation. In animals having several renal pyramids the constriction of the main renal artery is very difficult to gauge exactly in such a manner as to give you the desired decrease in intrarenal blood pressure throughout the organ. It is as a result of this that infarcts form more readily in the dog than in the rat when this operation is performed.

• • • • • • • • • • • • • • • • • *by* MARK NICKERSON

Sympatho-Adrenal Factors in Hypertension

WHEN neurogenic factors in hypertension are discussed, the role of the sympatho-adrenal system is the center of attention. Somatic motor nerves may affect the blood pressure and peripheral blood flow by altering the skeletal muscle tone, and cholinergic portions of the autonomic system may produce similar effects by altering the smooth muscle tone (e.g., gastrointestinal tract) and by limited direct vasodilatation (e.g., blush area). However, these effects are insignificant in comparison with the results of the activation of the sympathoadrenal system, which includes most sympathetic nerve fibers and the adrenal medulla. This functional division of the nervous system differs from all others in that it stimulates effector cells by an adrenergic (epinephrine-like) chemical mediator. Whether this mediator is epinephrine, norepinephrine, or a mixture of the two is unimportant for the present discussion.

The sympatho-adrenal system and its afferent connections, particularly from the carotid sinus and aortic arch (Fig. 1), are continuously involved in the maintenance of circulatory homeostasis, whether it be at a normal or chronically elevated level of pressure. This control involves the heart, the large and particularly the small arteries, the capillaries, or at least the precapillary sphincters, and the veins.

Under normal conditions the afferent pathways carry tonic impulses which depress the activity of the vasomotor centers and consequently inhibit the sympatho-adrenal system. As a result, the section of the afferent fibers (moderator nerves) in animals (1, 2) and man (3) induces an immediate and persistent elevation of the blood pressure. In addition, the pressor activity of the sympatho-adrenal system may arise on a central basis, as in "diencephalic epilepsy" (4) or "diencephalic hypertension" (5), in tabes dorsalis (6), and in tumors of the fourth ventricle (7). In animals hypertension has been induced by electrical stimulation of or injury to the hypothalamus (8, 9), and by the stimulation of certain cortical areas (10). The pressor response

150

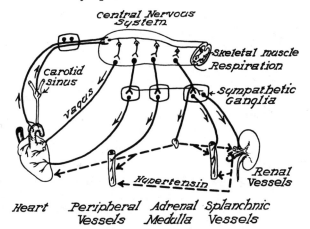

FIGURE 1. A diagrammatic representation of the nervous and humoral pathways involved in the maintenance of the systemic arterial pressure. The solid lines depict nervous pathways; the broken lines, humoral agents. (Reproduced, by permission of the copyright owner, from Nickerson: Am. J. Med. 8:343, 1949.)

to such cortical stimulation has been shown to be accompanied by a decrease in the renal blood flow, renal cortical ischemia (11), and a release of renin into the blood stream (12). Also, in both animals (13, 14) and man (15) hypertension may result from an increased intracranial pressure, at least in part because of the resultant cerebral ischemia (13, 15, 16). Studies on generalized cerebral ischemia indicate that it must be severe to evoke a pressor response after elimination of the carotid receptor areas (17, 18). However, little is known regarding the effects of localized areas of ischemia. An additional factor increasing the activity of the vasomotor centers and their sensitivity to reflex stimuli is a decreased pH of the blood such as may be induced by the accumulation of lactic acid or carbon dioxide (18, 19). This factor has received only limited attention.

Neurogenic renal vasoconstriction is not a major factor in most cases of neurogenic hypertension. Renal denervation induces little fall in pressure (20, 21), and prior nephrectomy fails to alter the acute pressor response to moderator nerve section (22). However, reflex renal vasoconstriction may produce a sustained hypertension after the sympathetic innervation of other body structures has been interrupted surgically (23, 24), and electrical stimulation of the sympathetic nerves to the kidney produces a similar effect (25).

A variety of clinical observations indicate that neurogenic factors in some way influence the development and course of essential hypertension. It has long been recognized that stressful situations may raise both the systolic and diastolic pressures (26, 27), an effect which may persist for varying periods after the termination of the external stimulus (28) and which may be associated with a considerable decrease in the renal blood flow (26). In addition, hypertensive people tend to have a characteristic type of personality. They usually exhibit important components of repressed antagonism and anxiety. They do not find emotional outlets in overt acts, but instead their emotions are expressed through an increased activity of the sympatho-adrenal system with a consequent increase in the blood pressure. The relief of psychic tension frequently produces salutary effects in these patients.

In spite of the multiple theoretical and empirical reasons for implicating the sympatho-adrenal system in the etiology of hypertension, it is clear that established human essential hypertension is not primarily neurogenic in nature. Table 1 illustrates the fact that the hemodynamic changes in neurogenic and essential hypertension are completely different. With the exception of the response to adrenergic blockade, the infusion of norepinephrine does produce a picture quite comparable to that observed in essential hypertension (29). However, the etiological significance of this similarity is questionable. Hypertension with these same characteristics may be induced by the infusion of any agent, e.g., various synthetic sympathomimetic amines or hypertensin, producing a generalized peripheral vasoconstriction which predominates over cardiac acceleration.

TABLE 1. Characteristics of Various Types of Hypertension

Mechanism / Indices	"Essential" Hypertension	Renal Hypertension	Neurogenic Hypertension	Epinephrine Infusion	Norepinephrine Infusion
Pulse Rate	N	N	↑	↑	N or ↓
Cardiac Output	N	N	↑	↑	N or ↓
Total Peripheral Resistance	↑	↑	N	↓	↑
Blood Flow in Extremities	N	N	↑	↑	↓
Blood Pressure Fluctuations	Marked Early Limited Late	Limited	Marked	Controlled	Controlled
Blood Pressure Response to Adren. Blockade	Variable Slight ↓ ?	Slight ↓ ?	↓ to Normal	↓ to Normal	↓ to Normal

N = Normal   ↑ = Increased   ↓ = Decreased

In spite of the obvious dissimilarity between human essential hypertension and neurogenic hypertension, a careful analysis of the latter is important as a basis for the intelligent recognition or exclusion of neurogenic factors in human hypertension.

One of the distinguishing characteristics of uncomplicated neurogenic hypertension is its dramatic response to sympathectomy and to chemical blockade of the sympatho-adrenal system. Paravertebral sympathectomy performed on animals with neurogenic hypertension results in an immediate reduction in the blood pressure to normal or to subnormal levels, with a gradual return to normotensive or slightly higher levels over a period of months or even years (20, 21, 24). In addition, moderator nerve section, hypothalamic stimulation, or increased intracranial pressure usually fails to increase the blood pressure in sympathectomized animals; if any rise is elicited, it is relatively slight and develops slowly (8, 21, 24, 30).

Dogs with neurogenic hypertension administered adequate doses of ergotamine, benzodioxanes, imidazolines, or Dibenamine consistently respond with a lowering of the blood pressure to the normal range (7, 8, 31, 32, 33, 34). A central inhibition of vasomotor activity as well as adrenergic blockade is undoubtedly involved in the response to ergotamine and to the benzodioxanes (35). However, the action of Dibenamine and its congeners is probably a specific inhibition of excitatory responses to adrenergic stimuli (35, 36, 37).

In contrast to neurogenic hypertension, the role of sympathoadrenal factors in experimental renal hypertension is obscure. The sequence of events by which the interference with renal hemodynamics leads to an elevation of the systemic blood pressure has been carefully studied and has been shown to operate independently of nervous mechanisms. However, studies involving the blockade of sympathetic pathways with spinal anesthetics and the induction of vasodilatation by inflammatory processes have demonstrated a component of dynamic renal vascular constriction in both experimental renal hypertension and essential hypertension (38, 39).

Sympathectomy does not prevent the development of renal hypertension and induces only slight and irregular reductions in pressure in renal hypertensive animals (40, 41, 42, 43). Similarly, a prolonged administration of adrenergic blocking agents induces only a limited and highly variable reduction in the systemic arterial pressure in animals with nephrogenic hypertension. This has been observed after the oral administration of yohimbine to dogs (44), the oral administration of Dibenamine to rats (45), and the intravenous administration of Dibenamine to dogs (46). In none of these studies involving the chronic administration of adrenergic blocking agents were the pressures consistently reduced to the normotensive range.

Single injections of 883F and 933F have little or no depressor action in either normal dogs or animals with chronic renal hypertension (31, 47). However, it has been reported that single injections of pentobarbital, yohimbine, and 883F, but not 933F, produce a greater depressor response in renal hypertensive rats which have had an elevated pressure for more than 2 months than in those with a shorter duration of hypertension (48, 49). On this basis it has been suggested that neurogenic factors are of importance in late, but not in early, renal hypertension (48, 49, 50). However, this effect of the duration of renal hypertension on the response to agents decreasing sympathoadrenal activity was not observed with the more effective adrenergic blocking agent Dibenamine in rats (45) or with Dibenamine and various anesthetics in dogs (51).

Other evidence which has been adduced to support the significance of neurogenic factors in renal hypertension is the observation that the arterial pressures of normal and renal hypertensive dogs and rabbits are reduced to essentially the same level after acute complete destruction of the central nervous system (52, 53). However, an interpretation of the results obtained with this drastic procedure is difficult. The elimination of the central connections of the sympathetics by cervical cord section in the region of C_7 reduces the pressures of early and late neurogenic hypertensive dogs even below those of normals. Under the same conditions the pressures of renal hypertensive animals are maintained significantly above those of normals (54). Other workers have observed a sharp fall in pressure when the spinal cord was destroyed below C_5 in renal hypertensive dogs, but the pressures returned to hypertensive levels as the acute effects of the operation wore off (55). In addition, chronic destruction of the spinal cord below C_5 does not prevent the subsequent development of a typical chronic renal hypertension (56). It appears that the less acute the trauma involved in the surgical elimination of the sympathetic nervous system in animals with nephrogenic hypertension, the less the effect of the procedure on the blood pressure. Indeed, it must be concluded that present evidence does not point to the development of a significant neurogenic component in the later stages of nephrogenic hypertension.

In general, human essential hypertension resembles renal hypertension more closely than it does neurogenic hypertension in its response to sympathectomy and adrenergic blockade. Although the reported results vary widely, 20 per cent would seem to be a reasonable estimate of the patients whose blood pressure is reduced to normal by either sympathectomy or chemical blockade.

The failure of adrenergic blockade consistently to reduce the pressure in essential hypertension cannot be explained on the basis that norepinephrine rather than epinephrine may be involved in the process (29). Dibenamine and its congeners block excitatory responses to epinephrine and norepinephrine to almost exactly the same extent (57). The failure of such agents consistently to lower the blood pressure in renal and essential hypertension appears effectively to rule out any sympathomimetic mediator as a primary etiological factor.

The observations discussed above indicate that sympatho-adrenal factors are of very limited significance in renal hypertension and that neurogenic hypertension, in which such factors are of primary importance, bears little resemblance to human essential hypertension. However, as mentioned above, a variety of clinical observations suggest that neurogenic factors in some way influence the development and course of essential hypertension. On the basis of present knowledge, the most reasonable postulate to reconcile the undoubted influence of the sympatho-adrenal system upon human essential hypertension with the fact that the established elevation of pressure is obviously not maintained primarily by neurogenic factors is to assume that the sympatho-adrenal system is involved primarily in the early stages of essential hypertension. It is possible that emotionally initiated sympatho-adrenal activity may cause repeated episodes of renal vasoconstriction, "ischemia," and hypertension which finally lead to the development of local changes capable of permanently altering the renal hemodynamics or renal metabolic activity. The experimental basis for such a conclusion is as yet incomplete, but certain points of evidence are of interest in this connection.

Many workers have noted a persistence of hypertension after the removal of a single "ischemic" kidney (58, 59, 60, 61). In addition, it has frequently been observed that hypertension induced by unilateral renal artery or parenchyma compression may induce structural changes in the vessels of the contralateral kidney in both man (62) and laboratory animals (59, 61, 63, 64). Indeed, it appears that vascular pathology in the contralateral kidney may so alter its hemodynamics or metabolic activity that it becomes capable of maintaining the hypertension after surgical removal of the kidney initially involved. This interpretation is strengthened by the observation that the persistence of hypertension is well correlated with the degree of vascular pathology in the unoperated kidney (61), and by the fact that releasing the renal artery constriction in unilaterally nephrectomized animals always causes the pressure to fall, although under comparable conditions, except for the presence of the other kidney, the pressure is frequently sustained after such release (65).

A similar sequence of renal vascular changes has not been demonstrated in connection with neurogenic hypertension. Indeed, the vascular pathology noted in cases of pheochromocytoma (66, 67, 68) and in animals with neurogenic hypertension from moderator nerve section (7), hypothalamic injury (9), or increased intracranial pressure (69) is less marked than in cases of renal or essential hypertension. However, highly suggestive evidence for the development of persistent hypertension on the basis of intermittent neurogenic vasoconstriction is found in observations on rats subjected to repeated audiogenic seizures (70, 71, 72). In these studies the blood pressures of young control and stimulated rats were found to be essentially the same, but it was noted that a large percentage of the experimental animals became hypertensive after they were 1 year of age. Hypertension was noted particularly among those animals which had consistently responded vigorously to the stimuli. It is of interest that these responses to auditory stimuli are characterized by a marked sympatho-adrenal discharge, including mydriasis, piloerection, etc. (73). Although the blood pressure was not determined during or immediately after the convulsive responses, it is reasonable to assume that a temporary elevation accompanied each reaction. Presumptive evidence for the occurrence of a similar process in human beings is found in the conversion of intermittent to persistent hypertension in some cases of pheochromocytoma and in the occasional persistence of hypertension after removal of the offending tumor (66, 68, 74).

It is quite possible that an etiological relationship exists between essential hypertension and neurogenic pressor episodes in man. Hypertensive persons have been shown repeatedly to have a more vigorous pressor response to psychic and physical stimuli than normotensives (75, 76), and it appears that subjects with even infrequent rises in pressure (76, 77, 78) or with a hyperactive cold-pressor response (79) are more prone than the average to develop hypertension in later life (cf. 80). The role of sympatho-adrenal factors in this sequence of events is indicated by the fact that the association of transient episodes of tachycardia with transient hypertension is particularly likely to presage the development of a sustained pressure elevation (78).

One may speculate that during the early stages of the development of hypertension the individual is subjected to repeated episodes of increased systemic pressure and renal vasoconstriction on a purely neurogenic (psychic) basis and that over a period of years he may secondarily develop organic renal vascular changes or functional alterations adequate to sustain a relatively stable hypertension. The mechanisms by which the kidney may perpetuate the hypertension as well as the questions of whether and to what extent non-neurogenic extrarenal factors may participate in the process are points beyond the scope of this paper. However, the sequence of events outlined above would explain the lability of early and the stability of late essential hypertension, the absence of organic vascular lesions in some, particularly early, cases, and the uniform bilateral distribution of renal vascular changes, as well as the observed correlation between psychic and sympatho-adrenal factors and the final development of a largely non-neurogenic hypertension.

Summary

Neurogenic hypertension differs markedly from human essential hypertension, both in its hemodynamic characteristics and in its response to sympathectomy and adrenergic blockade. In man, only hypertension due to pheochromocytoma, increased intracranial pressure, or other central nervous system pathology can be classified as primarily due to sympatho-adrenal factors.

However, a variety of clinical observations indicate that neurogenic factors are in some way related to the development and course of essential hypertension. Evidence is presented suggesting that neurogenic factors may be of importance in the early labile phases of essential hypertension and that the effects of this early sympatho-adrenal activity may lead to a persistent, self-perpetuated hypertension, perhaps nephrogenic, in later life.

Questions and Discussion

DR. WILLIAM KUBICEK (MINNEAPOLIS): We have been doing some experiments to try to elucidate the role of the sympathetic nervous system in hypertension.

The general attack on this problem was to produce sympathetic nerve hyperactivity by electrical stimulation and to determine the effects on the kidneys and systemic circulation.

We used well-trained dogs with a van Leersum carotid loop for blood pressure determinations. Bilateral unipolar electrodes were applied to either the renal arteries and associated nerves or to the splanchnic nerves below the diaphragm or the sympathetic nerves above the diaphragm. We measured the renal circulation by the clearance of para-aminohippurate to determine the renal plasma flow and creatinine for the glomerular filtration rate.

Initially, electrical stimulation produced either no change or a decrease in the renal circulation. After 48 hours or more of hypertension the renal circulation was found to be normal. In some experiments the renal blood flow was greatly reduced by damage to the renal artery. In these cases an elevation in the arterial blood pressure did not occur, which confirms the observations of other investigators that severe impairment of the renal circulation is not accompanied by hypertension. Stimulation accompanied by an elevated arterial blood pressure for as long as 45 days did not result in sustained hypertension following the cessation of stimulation. There is evidence that the carotid sinus aortic arch reflex can adapt to an elevated arterial blood pressure, as indicated by an increased pulse rate when the arterial blood fell toward normal upon the cessation of stimulation.

DR. MAURICE B. VISSCHER: Dr. Kubicek did not cover one point brought up earlier. I refer to the histology of the kidneys in the animals that had been subjected to up to 6 months of continuous stimulation in 2 or 3 periods.

There were no pathological changes of any consequence in the kidneys of any of the animals except those in which mechanical interference with the blood flow had occurred as a result of the placement of the lucite electrode block.

DR. ELEXIOUS T. BELL: I believe that emotional disturbances aggravate a pre-existing hypertension, but I wonder, Dr. Nickerson, whether the emotional instability of the hypertensive person is not an effect of the hypertensive state rather than the cause of it.

DR. NICKERSON: I will turn first to Dr. Bell's question. It is one which cannot be answered with any assurance at the present time. I think the best evidence, and it is far from conclusive, that a more or less "physiological" intermittent hypertension may predispose to persistent hypertension is found in the observations of Hines and his associates, which have been substantiated by Levy, White, and their co-workers in Boston and by others. These workers have shown that persons with transient rises in blood pressure and particularly those with an intermittent tachycardia indicating sympatho-adrenal hyperactivity are prone to develop a persistent hypertension. However, these studies only demonstrate a correlation. They admittedly do not prove a cause and effect relationship.

The ingenious experiments of Drs. Kubicek, Kottke, and Visscher have an objective similar to that of experiments now in progress in our own laboratory. They have produced prolonged, sympathetically-mediated renal vasoconstriction by electrical stimulation while we have attempted to do the same thing reflexly by section of the moderator nerves from the carotid sinuses and the aortic arch. As yet neither of us has succeeded in producing a hypertension which significantly outlasts the period of sympathetic hyperactivity. However, the duration and other features of these experiments are such that the present negative results certainly do not exclude the possibility of producing such a persistent hypertension.

I do not believe that the absence of pathological changes in the kidneys of animals subjected to prolonged periods of stimulation of the renal sympathetic nerve supply precludes the possibility of an elevated pressure per se producing alterations in kidney function or morphology. It is well known that in cases of hypertension due to unilateral mechanical renal artery constriction the secondary vascular changes occur in the opposite kidney. This is presumably due to the fact that the mechanical constriction protects the operated organ from the deleterious effects of the increased pressure. It is quite possible that the renal vasoconstriction induced by sympathetic nerve stimulation may perform a similar protective function.

The readjustment of pressure-regulating reflexes during a prolonged period of pressure elevation is an important and interesting factor in any study of hypertension. Prinzmetal and Wilson, Pickering, and many other workers have demonstrated that the peripheral vaso-motor tone is not significantly altered in essential and renal hyper-tension, although acute pressure elevations of a comparable magnitude may largely eliminate neurogenic vasoconstriction. The data which Dr. Kubicek has just presented indicate that an adjustment of the regulatory mechanisms to a new level may occur within 20 hours.

Finally, I believe that the data of Dr. Kubicek and his associates point to a necessary modification in our thinking about renal function tests. They have shown that when the sympathetic nerves to the kidneys are stimulated, the renal blood flow is decreased and the systemic arterial pressure is elevated, presumably a cause and effect relationship. However, during continued stimulation the renal circulation, as determined by conventional clearance methods, returns to normal, although the pressure remains elevated. This strongly suggests that the nerve stimulation has continued to evoke renal circulatory changes which are important to the maintenance of the hypertension but are not amenable to measurement by the techniques employed. These observations appear seriously to question the validity of excluding renal factors in cases of essential hypertension simply because the renal clearance values are normal.

· · · · · · · · · · · *by* EDUARDO BRAUN-MENENDEZ

Experimental Hypertension

THE title of this lecture is highly presumptuous. Nobody could possibly summarize in the relatively short space of an hour all of what we know and of what we do not know about experimental hypertension. Hypertension is today one of the deadliest enemies of mankind, and in the eagerness to fight with better arms this human disease, numerous research workers all over the world have tried to reproduce it in animals in order to obtain a better understanding of its mechanism. The mere enumeration of the different methods employed, of the type of hypertension obtained, and of the hypotheses formulated by the most outstanding investigators in this field would be surely boring and perhaps useless. As a lecturer I should try to avoid these two dangerous reefs. For this reason I will only make a general survey of the problem of experimental hypertension.

May I add that I am not particularly fitted for presenting an unbiased review of the subject. Perhaps I am too near the trees to see the forest. I know that every scientist must renew his efforts every day in order to look at the facts without prejudice. Claude Bernard said that you must hang up your overcoat and your hypotheses on entering the laboratory. I shall try to analyze the present situation without letting my own theories interfere, but I know in advance that I shall not be able to do so. Claude Bernard and my audience will excuse me: after all the lecture room is not the laboratory.

Experimental hypertension may be classified into three groups on the basis of the primary cause of the rise in the blood pressure: renal hypertension, neurogenic hypertension, and hormonal hypertension.

Experimental Renal Hypertension

Of all the methods devised to obtain experimental hypertension none reproduces more exactly human hypertension than Goldblatt's method. In 1934 Goldblatt and his co-workers produced chronic hypertension in the dog by partial compression of the renal artery with a metal clamp. This hypertension is not necessarily accompanied by renal excretory insufficiency; it is stable and associated with a normal heart rate and peripheral vasoconstriction. The epoch-making discovery of Goldblatt confirmed the relation of the kidney to hypertension, which had been envisioned by Bright and, after him, by many other workers. Ever since, all those who have studied clinical or experimental hypertension have had to reckon with this organ as a very important factor in the chain of events.

The present trend of the investigations related to the problem of renal experimental hypertension can best be shown by the exposition of the principal working hypotheses which try to explain its mechanism.

THE RENIN HYPOTHESIS

According to the renin hypothesis arterial hypertension is due to renal ischemia, which determines the liberation of renin into the blood, with the subsequent formation of hypertensin.

Houssay and Fasciolo (1937) showed that the ischemic kidney liberates into the blood a vasoconstrictor and pressor substance. Two years later Braun-Menendez, Fasciolo, Leloir, and Muñoz (1939, 1940) isolated from the renal venous blood of ischemic kidneys the substance responsible for this action and called it *hypertensin*. They also found that hypertensin could be formed *in vitro* by the interaction of *renin* (a protein found in extracts of renal cortex by Tigersted and von Bergmann, 1898) with *hypertensinogen*, which is a blood globulin. Simultaneously, from a different approach, Kohlstaedt *et al.* (1940), who were studying the vasoconstrictor action of crude preparations of renin, found that on purification renin lost its vasoconstrictor properties, which could be restored by mixing it with a fraction of plasma. Later Page and Helmer (1940) found that by this mixture a new vasoconstrictor and pressor substance was liberated, which they called *angiotonin*.

Hypertensin or angiotonin is a polypeptide which has a molecular weight of about 2.700 and which is thermostable and dialyzable, in contrast to its mother substances, renin and hypertensinogen, which are thermolabile and non-dialyzable.

It is generally accepted that renin is an enzyme which catalyzes the reaction Hypertensinogen $\rightarrow$ Hypertensin $+ X$. As hypertensin represents only a small fraction (about 1/100) of the hypertensinogen molecule, other products must be formed in the reaction.

Hypertensin is destroyed or inactivated presumably by the proteolytic action of enzymes present in the blood and extracts of organs. These enzymes or groups of enzymes are termed *hypertensinase*.

Leloir *et al.* in 1940 devised a method of estimating the renin in the blood. By means of this method, renin was found in the blood of dogs in the initial phase of renal hypertension (Dell'Oro and Braun-Menendez, 1942; Haynes and Dexter, 1947), in shock (Huidobro and Braun-Menendez, 1942), and in acute hemorrhagic hypotension (Huidobro and Braun-Menendez, 1942) and it was found in the blood of human beings during acute glomerulonephritis, the toxemia of pregnancy, and shock (Dexter and Haynes, 1944).

These findings, which I have presented in a very schematic and abridged form, seemed in 1942 to explain the pathogenesis of experimental renal hypertension, and many hoped that they would be ultimately applied to the cure of human hypertension. But the initial enthusiasm rapidly declined when the multiple therapeutic possibilities suggested by the renin-hypertensin system were tested and one after the other failed. The unfulfillment of these exaggerated hopes brought about unjustly the discredit of a hypothesis that has not yet been thoroughly studied in many of its fundamental aspects. Little is known about the formation of renin by the kidney, the cause and mechanism of its liberation, the mechanism of the action of hypertensin, and the factors which may increase or decrease its action.

The first blow to the renin-hypertensin theory of hypertension was the fact that renin could not be found, with the methods then available, in the blood of dogs with chronic renal hypertension.

Renin had been demonstrated in the renal venous blood and in the systemic blood of animals with renal hypertension during the acute phase of hypertension. It had been demonstrated during the first days following ischemia, especially when the constriction of the artery is extreme and when accompanied by signs of severe renal insufficiency. It had been detected in a few human beings during the acute phase of hypertension (acute glomerulonephritis, the toxemia of pregnancy). But in animals with chronic hypertension with or without renal insufficiency as well as in patients with essential or malignant hypertension, the results employing the method of Leloir *et al.* for detecting renin were uniformly negative (Braun-Menendez *et al.*, 1943; Dexter and Haynes, 1944).

A possible interpretation of these negative findings might be that the method of Leloir and his associates was not sensitive enough to detect minute amounts of renin in the blood. Fasciolo and Taquini developed in 1947 a method 200 times greater in sensitivity. The method is based on the same principle, e.g., the formation of hypertensin by the incubation of renin-containing blood with hypertensinogen in the absence of hypertensinase, but it differs in that the amount of hypertensin formed is estimated by its vasoconstrictor action on the perfused hind limbs of the toad instead of being tested by its pressor action on the dog or cat. With this fairly reliable method, no renin-like substance is found in the blood of nephrectomized animals, and quite small amounts of renin injected into the blood of these animals can be easily detected. On the other hand, small amounts of renin were found in dogs (Taquini and Fasciolo, 1947) and rats (Braun-Menendez et al., 1947) and in men (Taquini and Fasciolo, 1947) with normal blood pressure; but no increase in renin concentration could be detected in the blood of animals or subjects with chronic hypertension. According to these results and accepting this method of renin estimation as reliable, one should conclude that chronic renal experimental or human hypertension is not due to an increased concentration of renin in the blood. The results of Gollan et al. (1948) seem to contradict this affirmation, since they were able to find an increased formation of hypertensin in incubated blood from dogs with experimental renal hypertension.

But even if an increased concentration of renin is not present in the blood in chronic hypertensives, one cannot exclude the participation of renin in the process. Other possible ways by which renin might play a role in the pathogenesis should first be excluded. (1) The increased secretion of renin may cease when the blood pressure rises sufficiently to improve the circulatory conditions of the ischemic kidney. A new equilibrium would be reached at a higher level of the blood pressure. (2) In the hypertensive individual the organism may be sensitized to the pressor action of hypertensin. The fact that the injection of a given amount of hypertensin does not cause a greater rise in the blood pressure in hypertensive than in normal animals does not exclude this possibility: the initial blood pressure level is different, and I should be inclined to accept that for equal sensitivity, the higher the initial level the smaller should be the rise caused by the vasoconstrictor substance. (3) Renin could be adsorbed in the wall of the arterioles and produce its action by the formation of hypertensin in situ. This possibility has received some support from the recent work of Introzzi et al. (1949), who found renin in the heart and liver of shocked dogs. If previously nephrectomized, no renin was found in these tissues. (4) A fourth possibility which should be kept in mind, and which has not been sufficiently explored owing to technical difficulties, is that in chronic hypertension renin could act on hypertensinogen within the kidney, and hypertensin instead of renin be liberated into the renal venous blood. If this is the case, we must assume that the activity of renin within the kidney is enhanced by renal ischemia and that the concentration of hypertensin in the blood is increased.

Very little is known of the changes in the activity or concentration of renin in the kidneys. Some interesting work has been done by Taquini and Fasciolo (1949) in this respect. They have devised a method for the estimation of renin in small samples of renal tissue and studied the variation in the renin content of the renal cortex in different experimental conditions.

In order to localize the site where renin is stored or formed they took small pieces of tissue from the renal cortex in different species. Renin is mainly contained in the portion of the cortex which lies below the renal capsule to a depth of 2 mm. or more, a zone which in the dog is formed exclusively by convoluted tubules. These results show, as previously pointed out by Friedman and Kaplan (1942, 1943), that renin is formed in the tubules and that the juxtaglomerular apparatus appears not to be concerned with renin formation. The renin content of the kidney presents individual variations, but in the same animal is strikingly similar in both kidneys and in the same kidney in different regions. This may be an indication that the renin content of the kidney can be influenced by metabolic or hormonal factors.

Partial ischemia causes a 100 per cent increase in the renin content of the kidney in 15–30 minutes. Anoxia by the respiration of poor oxygen mixtures did not increase the renin content of the kidney. Complete ischemia causes also an increase when the renal pedicle is clamped. But no increase was found when the kidney was removed. Some experimental findings seem to show that stimulation of the renal nerves may cause an increase in the renin concentration within the kidney.

We have also confirmed in the rat the curious fact observed by Wakerlin in the dog that after unilateral nephrectomy the renin content of the remaining kidney is sometimes very low.

All these studies concerning the mechanism of the formation of renin within the kidney should be extended and perfected, as they open a new field of research.

To test the hypothesis that renin acts within the kidney and liberates hypertensin into the blood new methods should be devised for the estimation of hypertensin. The only methods at present are biological methods which measure the vasoconstrictor or pressor action of the mentioned substance. But biological methods have a tremendous disadvantage for the assay of vasoconstrictor or pressor substances in the blood, owing to the possible presence of other preformed substances or to the formation *in vitro* of new substances with similar action. Blood may contain adrenalin, noradrenalin, tyramin, pitressin, and perhaps other unknown vasoconstrictors; and serotonin, the serum vasoconstrictor, may be formed *in vitro*. If reliable chemical micro-methods were devised for the recognition of all these substances, this problem would be more easily solved. Perhaps the procedures used for the pharmocological determination of noradrenalin and adrenalin could be applied (Bülbring, 1949).

In the present state of knowledge our final judgment as to the role of the renin-hypertensin system in the pathogenesis of hypertension must be suspended.

OTHER PRESSOR SUBSTANCES

The renin-hypertensin system might not be the only pressor system which comes into play in renal experimental hypertension. From time to time new vasoactive substances are described in the blood of hypertensive animals, originating in the kidney or elsewhere.

1. According to Bing (1946) renal ischemia could cause a diminution in the activity of kidney amino-oxidases, thus bringing about the accumulation of pressor amines in the blood. This hypothesis has some interesting facts in its favor, but has not been further explored.

2. According to Shorr and his co-workers (1947, 1948), VEM (vasoexcitor material) formed in the cortical portion of the kidney in anaerobic conditions and VDM (vasodepressor material) of hepatic origin, which has been identified with ferritin, are the components of a homeostatic mechanism which participates in the regulation of the peripheral blood flow and the blood pressure. In the initial stages of hypertension in the dog and the rat they found an increase in VEM activity in the blood, but in the chronic phase of hypertension the reaction of the blood was neutral. However, by the use of procedures which permitted the specific inactivation of VEM or VDM an increased concentration of both substances was revealed in the blood of dogs and men with chronic hypertension.

The studies of Shorr, Zweifach, and their associates are very important, and I have always wondered why nobody has yet tried to repeat them. In spite of the enormous amount of work they have done, many problems have not been solved, and among these the most important to me is the concentration and fractionation of VEM in order to identify this principle and differentiate it from other known vasoactive substances.

3. An apparently new pressor principle of renal origin has been demonstrated in the blood of animals after prolonged periods of hypotension (Shipley and Helmer, 1947). This principle caused a sustained elevation in the blood pressure (of from 1 to 4 hours' duration) when injected intravenously into cats, dogs, or rats the kidneys of which had been removed 6–48 hours before. This principle is contained in renal extracts together with renin. Its differentiation from the latter has not yet been clearly achieved. Perhaps it is only renin plus something or minus something. I remember that in Houssay and Fasciolo's experiments in which an ischemic kidney from a hypertensive animal was grafted into the neck of a nephrectomized dog (for 24–48 hours) the rise in the blood pressure persisted, sometimes for a long time, after the graft was removed. Perhaps this was due to the presence of the sustained pressor principle. I think Drs. Shipley and Helmer are wise in postponing the baptism of this principle until we are quite sure that it is not disguised renin. After all, what we call renin is rather a complex protein.

4. Grollman (1946) believes that the kidney elaborates some humoral agent which regulates the blood pressure, the absence of which results in hypertension. The evidence in favor of this hypothesis seems to me inconclusive. But Grollman has the merit of having emphasized that hypertension may occur in the absence of any renal tissue in the organism.

5. Vasoconstrictor or pressor substances have lately been described in the blood of hypertensive patients by Schroeder et al. (1948) and by Croxatto and Muñoz (1949). These two unidentified substances are recent additions to a long list which was initiated some 25 years ago. The results obtained by different workers using a similar technique have often been contradictory, and in spite of the enormous amount of time and energy consumed in these investigations, we are still in a very uncertain position. Nevertheless, I am inclined to have faith in those who have obtained positive results, and I believe—though I recognize that this may be simply wishful thinking—that all we need is to find the appropriate technique and the vasoconstrictor agent responsible for hypertension will be displayed.

THE PARTICIPATION OF THE NERVOUS SYSTEM IN
NEPHROGENIC HYPERTENSION

In fact, experimental renal hypertension is accompanied by a generalized vasoconstriction, the mechanism of which is humoral and due with great probability to the presence of vasoconstrictor substances in the blood.

It has been demonstrated that this type of hypertension cannot be prevented or abolished by renal denervation (Page, 1935; Collins, 1936; Vallery-Radot et al., 1938), by excision of the splanchnic nerves (Goldblatt et al., 1937; Blalock and Levy, 1937), by resection of the lumbar sympathetic chain (Introzzi et al., 1938), by bilateral section of the anterior nerve roots from the 6th dorsal to the 2d lumbar inclusive (Goldblatt and Wartman, 1937), by complete resection of the paravertebral ganglions (Heymans et al., 1937; Alpert et al., 1937; Freeman and Page, 1937), or even by destruction of the spinal cord below the 5th cervical nerve (Glenn et al., 1938; Glenn and Lasher, 1938).

These results show that experimental renal hypertension is not caused by a nervous reflex arising in the kidney, but they do not exclude completely the participation of the nervous system.

The nervous mechanisms which regulate the blood pressure are still active in experimental renal hypertension as well as in human essential hypertension. The humoral agent of hypertension, whatever it may be, must exert its action against these powerful regulators or else influence the neural mechanisms in such a way as to set them at a new level of sensitivity (Heymans and Bouckaert, 1939; Dock, 1940).

No wonder, then, that procedures such as general anesthesia (Moss and Wakerlin, 1948), natural sleep (Kernodle et al., 1946), spinal anesthesia (Taylor et al., 1948), and pharmacological nervous block (Ogden et al., 1946; Moss and Wakerlin, 1948) should cause a drop in the blood pressure in hypertensive men or animals. It is noteworthy that the response of patients with essential hypertension to high spinal anesthesia is similar to that obtained in dogs with renal experimental hypertension (Taylor et al., 1948). This question I will not discuss further. The point I wish to make clear is that the nervous system is active in renal hypertension. There is no reason why all the vasoconstrictor nerves should become paralyzed because a humoral agent causes vasoconstriction and hypertension.

Ogden and his co-workers (1946) consider that in the rat appreciable differences exist between the early and late stages of experimental renal hypertension. In rats with short-standing hypertension the injection of sympathicolytic agents does not cause a great drop in the blood pressure, while in chronically hypertensive rats the blood pressure falls to normal levels. Ogden believes that early hypertension is dependent upon a disturbed kidney and may be caused by a renal humoral pressor mechanism; late hypertension responds to a neurogenic mechanism and could be denominated "neurohypertension of renal origin." That the nervous system is concerned in the maintenance of hypertension after the renal phase is completed has been inferred from the fact that this late hypertension is abolished by nembutal, yohimbine, and F 883 in rats. We repeated these experiments some years ago using the same and other drugs but were not able to confirm their results. What we have confirmed is the great individual variability of the responses to depressor drugs, a fact recently emphasized by Page and Taylor (1949).

But Ogden's hypothesis, though not firmly established, is a tentative explanation of a real fact: the existence of 2 apparently different stages in nephrogenic hypertension, a fact which has many other experimental observations in its favor and which has not yet received adequate explanation.

Experimental Neurogenic Hypertension

Hypertension can be produced experimentally in animals by the removal of the pressor regulator system (the aortic and carotid sinus nerves; for bibliography, see Braun-Menendez et al., 1946). This type of hypertension is accompanied by tachycardia and an increased cardiac output, is subject to great spontaneous variations, and is cured by total sympathectomy. Its characteristics are thus quite different from those of renal experimental hypertension and clinical essential hypertension.

Though this seems to be a purely nervous hypertension, humoral factors may also play a role. A vasoconstrictor substance has been found in the blood of rabbits and dogs made hypertensive by section of the pressor receptor nerves (for literature, see Braun-Menendez et al., 1946). It would be interesting to investigate with the new methods at our disposal the presence of adrenalin and noradrenalin in the blood of these animals.

There are other means of producing permanent hypertension of central origin: the intracisternal injection of a suspension of kaolin (Dixon and Heller, 1932; Heller, 1934; etc.) and the production of cerebral ischemia by ligation of the carotid, vertebral, and spinal arteries (Nowak and Walker, 1939; Fishback et al., 1943). Unfortunately these procedures give inconsistent results and have not permitted a thorough study of the hypertension produced.

A psychogenetic hypertension has been obtained by Farris et al. (1945) and by Yeakel and his collaborators (1948) by means of subjecting rats daily to intense explosive noises. These interesting studies should be continued since we have here a typical case of hypertension where the primary cause is a sensorial stimulus with psychical repercussion. But little is known yet of the mechanism which leads ultimately to hypertension. It may be through "stress" in the sense of Selye.

In all these types of neurogenic hypertension the kidney may be involved. In dogs with hypertension due to the removal of the pressor regulator nerves Grimson et al. (1939) and Grimson (1940) observed that the excision of the sympathetic chain produced only a partial fall in the blood pressure, provided the splanchnic innervation of the kidneys remained intact. The subsequent denervation of the kidneys produced a drop in the blood pressure to normal levels.

Braun (1933) and Braun and Samet (1934, 1935a, b) claim that renal denervation is capable of preventing or curing hypertension that is due to the intracisternal injection of a suspension of kaolin.

The demonstration by Trueta and his co-workers (1947) that the direct or reflex stimulation of the renal nerves produces a fundamental change in the renal circulation resulting in cortical ischemia, and the work of Kottke et al. (1945) showing that the continuous electrical stimulation of the renal pedicle is able to produce hypertension in dogs, suggest that the kidney may play a role in those types of hypertension that are apparently of purely nervous origin. The recent work of Introzzi and his co-workers (1949) and of Taquini and Fasciolo (1950) seems to show that the nervous system can also influence the formation of renin within the kidney. The stimulation of the renal pedicle increases the concentration of renin in the renal cortex. Further studies are needed to clarify this interesting fact.

Experimental Hormonal Hypertension

The adoption of the term "hormonal hypertension" by Prado and Dontigny (1948) to designate the hypertension which follows upon the administration of desoxycorticosterone, of pituitary extracts, and the exposure to noxious nonspecific agents seems to me fully justified. Hormonal factors may not only play a role in neurogenic or nephrogenic hypertension but they may also initiate changes leading to chronic hypertension. Under the term hormonal hypertension we shall review the possible influence on the blood pressure of other substances originated in the glands of internal secretion.

THE ADRENAL GLANDS

Adrenalin and noradrenalin. The secretion of adrenalin by the adrenal medulla plays no important role in the production or the maintenance of hypertension of renal origin. The removal of the adrenal medulla does not interfere with the hypertensive action of renal ischemia (Goldblatt *et al.*, 1934; Fasciolo, 1938; Page, 1938), and no increase in adrenalin secretion could be demonstrated in dogs made hypertensive by the constriction of the renal arteries (Rogoff *et al.*, 1938).

At one time Vaquez's theory (1904) that hypertension results from the increased secretion of adrenalin had many adherents. This theory was afterward abandoned in spite of the well-recognized fact that some tumors of the adrenal medulla are associated with attacks of paroxysmal hypertension. Recently, following the studies of von Euler, who identified sympathin with noradrenalin, new interest has arisen in this gland. Noradrenalin has been found to be present in the adrenal medulla (von Euler and Hamberg, 1949). In the normal gland, the relative amounts of adrenalin to noradrenalin were found to be about 4:1; in chromaffin tissue tumors the relation was inversed.

Goldenberg and his collaborators (1948) have shown that adrenalin is in man a vasodilator and cardiostimulating agent; injected into the blood of hypertensive subjects, it may cause a fall in the blood pressure. Noradrenalin, on the other hand, is a powerful vasoconstrictor and increases the peripheral resistance, causing an increase in the blood pressure, with little if any action upon the heart. Hypertensive subjects respond to the injection of noradrenalin with a greater rise in the blood pressure than normal subjects show. Goldenberg suggests that hypertension may be due to a disturbed equilibrium between the 2 sympathicomimetic substances: a relative increase of noradrenalin would overcome the action of its normal antagonist, adrenalin. As the only structural difference between the 2 substances is a methyl group, essential hypertension could possibly be regarded as due to a metabolic disturbance consisting of deficient transmethylation.

The adrenal cortex. The removal of the adrenals prevents the development or maintenance of hypertension of renal origin. In animals treated with cortical extracts it is possible to observe a certain degree of hypertension due to the substitution therapy which corrects, in part at least, the disturbance resulting from adrenalectomy. It is difficult to judge up to what point the changes depend upon a specific action of the adrenals as opposed to the general changes resulting from adrenal dysfunction.

The removal of the adrenals in normal animals causes a drop in the blood pressure to subnormal levels. The blood pressure is restored in these animals by the administration of sodium salts, by desoxycorticosterone, and also, in rats, by cortisone (for bibliography, see Gaudino, 1944).

When desoxycorticosterone became available for clinical use, its great activity on the regulation of the metabolism of electrolytes prompted its use in the treatment of patients with Addison's disease. It was soon found that desoxycorticosterone corrected not only the metabolic disturbances but also the hypotension of these patients. In 1939 Loeb and his co-workers called attention to the rise of the pressure to hypertensive levels in 2 Addisonian patients treated with this steroid, a fact which was subsequently confirmed by many other workers. Following Loeb's observation Kuhlman et al. (1939) injected 25 mg. of desoxycorticosterone per day during 70 days into 2 normal dogs and observed small rises in the blood pressure of 45 and 20 mm. Hg. This observation was repeated and confirmed by others in dogs and rats.

The contribution of Selye and his co-workers to the problem of hypertension due to desoxycorticosterone has been of fundamental importance. Selye (1942) first showed that the administration of sodium chloride to chicks caused renal lesions very similar to those found in human nephrosclerosis. The administration of desoxycorticosterone caused the same type of lesions in chicks fed a nontoxic dose of sodium chloride.

Then came from his laboratory a great number of experimental observations which have not only clarified many problems concerning the pathogenesis of hypertension but have also given us a new, simple, and efficient method of producing chronic experimental hypertension in the rat. The daily injection of massive doses of desoxycorticosterone (a method formerly used by Selye) has been replaced by the subcutaneous implantation of 1 or 2 desoxycorticosterone pellets (20–40 mg. per rat) into uninephrectomized rats fed an adequate diet and given a 1 per cent solution of sodium chloride as a drinking fluid. At the end of from 2 to 4 weeks hypertension appears in practically all the animals.

Unilateral nephrectomy is probably not indispensable, but the presence of sodium in the diet or its administration in the drinking fluid is a condition *sine qua non* for the production of renal lesions and hypertension (Braun-Menendez and Prado, 1950). The mechanism of this type of hypertension is still obscure, but many points of interest have been revealed.

1. It is well known that desoxycorticosterone causes a retention of sodium in the organism, probably owing to an increased renal tubular reabsorption of this cation. The first point to be considered is whether sodium sensitizes the organism to the action of desoxycorticosterone or whether, on the contrary, this steroid sensitizes the organism to the action of sodium. This question has not yet been solved, but I believe the latter proposition has some evidence in its favor. In fact, the administration of sodium chloride alone in high doses causes renal lesions and arterial hypertension in the chick, and the administration of desoxycorticosterone together with subthreshold doses of sodium chloride causes the same effect as sodium chloride alone. In rats the administration of desoxycorticosterone even in great doses does not cause alterations in the water turnover, renal morphology, or blood pressure if sodium chloride is absent from the diet. But if sodium chloride is given in sufficient amounts, the administration of very small amounts of desoxycorticosterone will be followed by an increase in the fluid turnover, by renal lesions, and by hypertension. Even more, Sapirstein *et al.* (1950) have obtained hypertension and renal hypertrophy in the rat by administering during 6 weeks a 2 per cent solution of sodium chloride as a drinking fluid.

2. Hypertension that follows upon the administration of desoxycorticosterone plus salt is always accompanied by renal lesions and renal hypertrophy. The mechanism by which the kidney participates in this hormonal hypertension may be an increase in the production and liberation of renin by the kidney, a possibility still unexplored. The participation of the VEM humoral system seems to be excluded by the results of Zweifach and Shorr (1950). But we must remember that one of the most striking effects of desoxycorticosterone is a retention of sodium due to an increased renal reabsorption of this electrolyte and a renal excretion of potassium. The changes in the electrolyte metabolism and the increased volume of extracellular fluid which follow upon the administration of this steroid may be instrumental both in the causation of renal lesions and in the elevation of the blood pressure.

Summarizing, hypertension induced by the administration of desoxycorticosterone appears to be a hormonally induced renal hypertension, caused by or associated with a disturbance in the water and salt metabolism, which also plays a part as a causative factor in the elevation of the blood pressure.

Desoxycorticosterone is not the only adrenal corticoid the administration of which can produce renal lesions and hypertension. Selye (1950) has obtained similar actions with 11-desoxycortisone, the compound S of Reichstein, which has been isolated from the adrenal cortex.

The hypertensive action of desoxycorticosterone was first discovered in patients with Addison's disease. In normal men desoxycorticosterone must be given during a relatively long period to produce an increase in the blood pressure over normal; on the other hand, patients with essential hypertension respond promptly to its administration by showing a definite rise in the blood pressure. As in the rat this steroid has no action if sodium is absent from the diet. In man as in the rat and the dog it causes a disturbance in the electrolyte metabolism and an increase in the extracellular fluid volume. The relation of the latter changes to the rise in blood pressure has not been definitely established; experimental observations in animals seem, however, to indicate that they play an important role.

The action of cortisone on the blood pressure has not yet been thoroughly studied. Administered to adrenalectomized rats, it promptly restores the decreased blood pressure to normal levels (Gaudino, 1944); in nephritic rats it may cause moderate hypertension; in nephritic adrenalectomized rats the rise in pressure is much greater (Knowlton *et al.*, 1949). It seems as if the presence of other adrenal steroids tends to diminish the pressor action of cortisone.

In normal man cortisone has no action on the blood pressure, but in patients with Addison's disease it causes an increase in it (Perera and collaborators, 1949).

THE HYPOPHYSIS

The removal of the *anterior lobe* of the hypophysis produces a fall in the blood pressure in normal dogs (Braun-Menendez, 1932) and rats (Braun-Menendez and Foglia, 1944). In the latter the normal level of the blood pressure can be restored partially by the administration of desoxycorticosterone and totally by the administration of adrenocorticotrophin (Anderson *et al.*, 1944; Braun-Menendez and Foglia, 1944).

In hypertensive animals also hypophysectomy causes a fall in the

blood pressure, which is due to adrenal hypofunction. Neither growth
hormone nor lactogenic hormone prevents the fall in the blood pressure which follows hypophysectomy, but adrenocorticotrophin restores the pressure to the former hypertensive levels (Anderson *et al.*,
1944; Braun-Menendez and Foglia, 1944).

The injection of crude extracts of the anterior lobe causes in the rat
renal changes (Selye, 1944) and hypertension (Prado *et al.*, 1947;
Dontigny *et al.*, 1948; Hay and Seguin, 1946; Masson *et al.*, 1949).
The production of hypertension is conditioned by the richness of the
diet in protein.

The pituitary principles that are responsible for renal changes and
hypertension have not yet been identified, but apparently they act
by stimulating the adrenal cortex, with increased production of
mineralo-corticoids of the desoxycorticosterone type. The mechanism
of hypertension would thus be similar to that induced by the administration of desoxycorticosterone. Together with the mineralo-
corticoids, the adrenals secrete other types of steroids which may have
an agonistic or antagonistic action to the former and thus complicate
the picture.

Pure adrenocorticotrophin has little or no action on the blood pressure of normal men, but may produce great rises accompanied by
severe symptoms in patients with essential hypertension (Perera,
1950) or nephritis (Sprague, 1950).

The removal of the *posterior lobe* of the hypophysis has no action
on the blood pressure of normal mammals or animals with renal hypertension. But pitressin, one of the active principles isolated from the
posterior lobe of the hypophysis, has a pressor and antidiuretic action.
It is adduced that this pressor action is too feeble in man and that its
skin-blanching and antidiuretic action would not fit into the clinical
aspect of human hypertension (Pickering, 1943). Nevertheless, it
probably plays a part in experimental and clinical hypertension. The
removal of the posterior pituitary lobe produces a decrease in the
blood pressure of toads (Orías, 1934). In rats and dogs with experimental hypertension and in hypertensive men Ellis and Grollman
(1949) have recently found an increased elimination of the antidiuretic
principle by the urine. This increased excretion of the antidiuretic
principle might be due to an increased production of the same by
the posterior lobe of the hypophysis, and the latter a reaction to some
endocrine or metabolic disturbance which increases the water turnover. This interpretation is supported by the findings of Skahen and
Green (1948) in rats. These authors found that the elimination of the

antidiuretic principle is proportional to the degree of fluid exchange. When fluid ingestion is increased following the administration of desoxycorticosterone or the substitution of water by saline in the drinking fluid, the excretion of antidiuretic substance in the urine is also increased.

OTHER ENDOCRINE GLANDS

Of the other endocrine glands, the gonads and the thyroid are apparently not essential for the maintenance of hypertension produced by constriction of the renal arteries. But the role of these glands and of the hormones secreted by them cannot be completely dismissed.

Testosterone does not cause an elevation of the blood pressure (Selye and Rowley, 1944; Blackman *et al.*, 1944; Page *et al.*, 1946; Sapeika, 1948), though Grollman *et al.* (1940) reported a rise in rats. Nevertheless, by its action on protein metabolism and by its renotrophic action, it may influence in some way or another the course of hypertension caused by other factors.

Estradiol seems to have a definite action on the blood pressure, although some results are contradictory (Grollman *et al.*, 1940; Sapeika, 1948; Page *et al.*, 1946; Page, 1948).

Progesterone does not cause hypertension in the rat (Selye *et al.*, 1945), nor does it raise the blood pressure in patients with Addison's disease. The lack of effect of progesterone is the more striking if one considers its structural resemblance to desoxycorticosterone.

The extirpation of the *thyroid* gland in the dog does not prevent or cure hypertension produced by constriction of the renal arteries (Glenn and Lasher, 1938; Katz *et al.*, 1939). Its effect on renal hypertension in the rat has not been studied. Through its action on the protein metabolism it is likely that the thyroid can exert some influence on the hypertensive effect of other factors. The work of Selye and his collaborators seems to support this point of view. In fact, the administration of thyroid powder increases the sensitivity of rats to the nephrosclerotic action of desoxycorticosterone and the anterior pituitary lobe (Selye *et al.*, 1945) and on the other hand the extirpation of the gland diminishes the sensitivity of these animals to the action of the named principles (Hall and Selye, 1945).

Metabolic Hypertension

I have reviewed in a very abridged form the three principle types of experimental hypertension: renal, nervous, and hormonal. This classification is, like all classifications, completely artificial and prompted only by our natural tendency to simplify the enormous complications of biological facts; thus we rest content for a short while until new facts oblige us to modify our previous classification.

I believe, nevertheless, that the time is ripe to present a new synthesis in the still obscure field of the mechanism of hypertension. We have seen the kidney become involved in all types of hypertension: in renal hypertension it is surely the culprit; in the other two it may be the victim, but I do not believe in its innocence: spontaneously or forcibly it has become part of the gang and a very important part too. One of its roles may be the elaboration and liberation of vasoconstrictor substances.

The other role is more complex, but perhaps as important as that just mentioned. The kidney is placed at the crux of a very complex set of mechanisms concerned with the regulation of body fluids and electrolyte interchanges. The latter suffer the direct influence of the metabolic processes of the body, which in turn are regulated by the glands of internal secretion, etc.

In this sense hypertension, even experimental hypertension, can be viewed as a metabolic disturbance initiated by different primary causes. This broader point of view can be criticized on the ground that it is too comprehensive. Nevertheless, in the present state of our knowledge on the subject, a more limited point of view—namely, that hypertension is exclusively due to the secretion of a pressor substance, to the exaggerated activity of the nervous system, or to the increased or decreased secretion of some hormone—is untenable. Whatever the initial or predominant cause of hypertension, a metabolic change occurs which participates in the pathogenesis of hypertension or may even take over the baton and become the conductor of the phenomenological orchestra.

When I refer to metabolic changes, I have in mind especially two of them: changes in the protein metabolism and disturbances in the water and electrolyte metabolism. But many others may come into play which have not yet received proper attention.

My present view of the pathogenesis of hypertension can be represented by a diagram (Fig. 1).

Let me close by quoting Professor Corner's words: "The collective thinking of mankind, forever struggling to understand this enormously detailed universe in which we find ourselves, inevitably takes comfort in diagrams. Faced with any unsorted array of facts or things, we begin automatically to sort and arrange them, and when they are too large or too subtle to be dealt with directly, we itemize their names

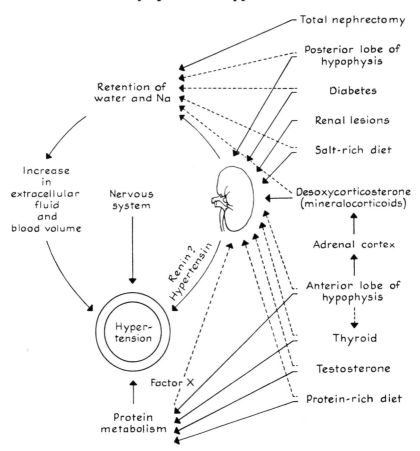

FIGURE 1. A diagrammatic view of the pathogenesis of hypertension.

on paper, draw lines between them, subordinate one to another, nominate their hierarchies and rest temporarily content, having achieved in some degree a better ordering of our restless thoughts."

But for this ordering to have any justification, it must have a dynamic consequence. Whenever a research worker makes a pause in his experiments in order to examine the work done and analyze his results, he may come to some conclusion about a definite problem, may discover some new relation or law, or, more often, may become disappointed by the futility of his efforts. But whatever the result of his survey, one unavoidable conclusion will come forth: more experiments are needed.

At the end of this lecture the conclusion which arises is the same:

we need further experiments to clarify the elusive problem of hypertension. And if I were given the privilege of delivering another similar lecture 50 years hence, I should certainly end in the same way; for while the more we seek, the more we know, it is also true that by extending our knowledge, we expand simultaneously the field of our curiosity.

· · · · · · · · · · · · · · · · · · *by* ELEXIOUS T. BELL

The Pathological Anatomy in
Primary Hypertension

THERE is no sharp separation between hypertension and normal blood pressure, but many observers agree that the upper limits of normal pressure are 150/90 mm. Hg in persons over 50 years of age and 140/90 mm. Hg in persons below the age of 40 years. Some investigators believe that the upper limit of normal systolic pressure is 140 mm. Hg. Repeated examinations are necessary to establish the diagnosis, since single high readings may be due to emotional disturbances. In the milder forms of hypertension the pressure may fall to normal levels after prolonged bed rest or during sleep, but it rises again when the patient resumes his usual activity. The reason that pressures of 150/90 mm. Hg or higher are regarded as abnormal is that persons with such pressures more frequently develop vascular diseases than normotensive persons.

Old people may show an elevation of the systolic but not of the diastolic pressure. This is not so serious as an elevation of the diastolic pressure; but a pressure such as 180/80 mm. Hg produces an increased strain on the arteries, since the average pressure is increased.

The majority of hypertensive persons over 50 years of age whose pressures do not exceed 170/90 mm. Hg never develop serious complications, but sometimes the pressure rises to more dangerous levels. In general, the danger of vascular complications and death increases directly with the height of the blood pressure. Women tolerate high blood pressure better than men. Although hypertension is more frequent in older women than in older men, the death ratios from hypertensive disease in persons over 50 years of age in our experience are 14.1 per cent for males and 11.9 per cent for females.

It is to be emphasized that about three fourths of the persons with primary hypertension, in the sense of a blood pressure of 150/90 mm.

183

Hg or higher, die of diseases unrelated to hypertension and that a majority of persons with mild hypertension have no symptoms.

In persons suffering from primary hypertension the principal alterations found in the body occur in the heart, the brain, the kidneys, and the arteries. The changes in the brain and kidneys are due entirely to arterial disease, and the damage to the heart is caused either by the load of the increased peripheral resistance or by coronary atherosclerosis. Basically, therefore, primary hypertension is a disease of the arteries and arterioles.

The Heart

The increased peripheral resistance almost invariably brings about hypertrophy of the left ventricle and increased weight of the heart. This is compensatory hypertrophy in response to increased work. It is not a primary disease of the heart. Heart failure is the most frequent cause of death in primary hypertension, but it is secondary to increased work or to coronary disease.

Myocardial failure. The heart responds to the increased peripheral resistance by hypertrophy of the left ventricle. It may remain compensated for years, but commonly the left ventricle begins to fail, causing congestion of the lungs, hypertrophy of the right ventricle, and finally general venous congestion. This is the most frequent form of death in primary hypertension. The weight of the heart is increased and its chambers are dilated. The weight that the heart attains before failure sets in depends in large measure upon its individual response, and cannot be correlated closely with the duration and intensity of the hypertension as one might expect. In the absence of primary renal disease and coarctation of the aorta, left ventricular hypertrophy is nearly always due to primary hypertension.

Coronary disease. Coronary disease occurs frequently in normotensive persons, but it is over twice as frequent in hypertensive persons as in normotensive. The increased intravascular pressure accelerates the aging process in the coronary arteries. In about 20 per cent of the deaths from primary hypertension, coronary disease is the major fatal complication. One or more of the large coronary arteries are markedly narrowed from atherosclerosis, and frequently thrombosis is found. There are scars in the myocardium, and fresh infarcts may be found.

The Brain

The effects of hypertension on the brain are intracranial hemorrhage and encephalomalacia.

Intracranial hemorrhage. About three fourths of the cases of spontaneous intracranial hemorrhage are associated with primary hypertension. The hemorrhage is due to rupture of a diseased artery in the substance of the brain.

Encephalomalacia. Encephalomalacia is infarction of the brain due to thrombosis or embolism of one of the arteries. In primary hypertension the lesion is a thrombus. Encephalomalacia is somewhat less frequent than hemorrhage in primary hypertension, but occurs more frequently than intracranial hemorrhage in normotensive persons.

A hypertensive person may have one or more strokes and die later of cardiac or renal complications.

Hypertensive encephalopathy is characterized by intense headache, convulsions, paralyses, and intellectual impairment. It is believed to be due to ischemia of the brain resulting from atherosclerosis.

The Kidneys

Approximately 12 per cent of the deaths from primary hypertension are due to renal failure resulting from disease of the small renal arteries and arterioles.

In order to determine the effects of hypertension on the renal vessels we must first study the aging process in these vessels in normotensive persons. The control group consisted of 741 persons of all ages who had no hypertensive symptoms of any kind and whose blood pressures were never higher than 140/90 mm. Hg. The hearts weighed less than 350 gm. in the females and less than 400 gm. in the males.

The small arteries. The incidence and the degree of intimal thickening in the small arteries of the control group with respect to age are

TABLE 1. The Incidence and the Degree of Intimal Disease in the Small Arteries of the Control Group with Respect to Age

Age in Years	No. of Cases	Percentage by Degree of Involvement			
		0	1	2	3
0–10 12		100	0	0	0
10–20 10		80	20	0	0
20–30 37		54	35.1	8.1	2.7
30–40 57		33.3	47.4	10.5	8.8
40–50 91		16.5	49.4	25.2	8.8
50–60 177		5.1	54.2	24.9	15.8
60–70 155		2.0	35.5	37.5	25.1
70–80 137		0.7	20.4	33.6	45.3
80+ 65		0	7.7	33.8	58.5
Over 50 534		2.4	34.5	31.8	31.3

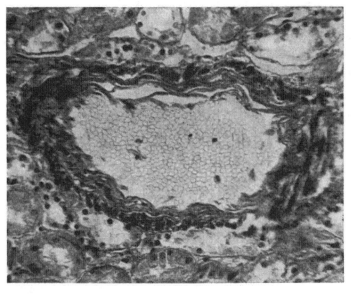

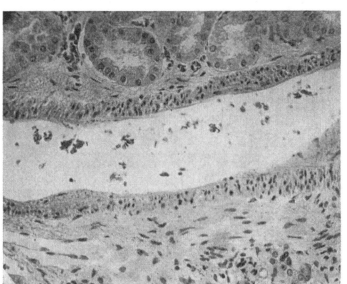

Figure 1 (left). Normal small renal artery. Figure 2 (right). Small renal artery showing Grade 1 intimal thickening. (Figures 2 through 8 are reproduced, by permission of the copyright owner, from E. T. Bell: Renal Diseases, ed. 2, Philadelphia, Lea & Febiger, 1950.)

186

shown in Table 1. A normal artery is shown in Figure 1, a Grade 1 intimal thickening in Figure 2, and a Grade 3 thickening in Figure 3. As the intima thickens, the media undergoes atrophy, and with a Grade 3 intimal thickening the muscular media has largely disappeared. In Table 1 it will be noted that the degree of intimal thickening increases progressively with age and that very few persons over 50 years of age have normal small renal arteries. The thickened intima

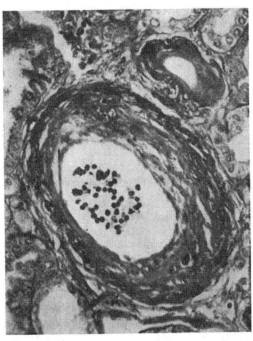

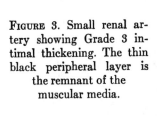

FIGURE 3. Small renal artery showing Grade 3 intimal thickening. The thin black peripheral layer is the remnant of the muscular media.

is composed largely of elastic tissue. Intimal thickening of these vessels is therefore an aging process and is commonly very severe in normotensive persons of advanced age.

In Table 2 there is shown a comparison between the intensity of intimal disease in the small arteries of the control group over 50 years of age and that of hypertensive persons. About 15 per cent of the hypertensives were less than 50 years of age. Grades 2 and 3 of intimal thickening were found in 63.1 per cent of the controls and in 80 per cent of the hypertensives. These data suggest that intimal thickening of the renal arteries of this caliber is an aging process which is somewhat accelerated by high blood pressure.

The arterioles. The wall of a normal arteriole is composed almost

Table 2. Intimal Disease of the Small Arteries in Hypertensive
Subjects and in a Group of Non-Hypertensive Controls

	No. of Cases	Percentage by Degree of Involvement			
		0	1	2	3
Controls over 50 years of age ..534		2.4	34.5	31.8	31.3
Myocardial 226		0.9	12.8	32.3	54.0
Cerebral 194		0	11.3	31.4	57.2
Coronary 80		1.2	16.2	40.0	42.5

Table 3. The Incidence and the Intensity of Arteriolosclerosis in the Control Group
with Respect to Age

Age in Years	No. of Cases	Percentage by Degree of Involvement					Total
		0	1p	1	2	3	1–3
0–10 12		100	0	0	0	0	0
10–20 10		100	0	0	0	0	0
20–30 37		91.9	5.4	2.7	0	0	2.7
30–40 57		86.0	10.5	0	1.8	1.8	3.6
40–50 91		81.3	11.0	6.6	0	1.1	7.7
50–60 177		79.1	13.0	6.2	1.7	0	7.9
60–70 155		78.0	12.9	7.1	1.9	0	9.0
70–80 137		62.0	19.7	13.8	2.2	2.2	18.2
80+ 65		61.5	9.2	20.0	6.1	3.0	29.1
Over 50 534		72.3	14.2	10.1	2.4	1.0	13.5

entirely of smooth muscle, and the intima consists of a single layer
of endothelial cells. In the older members of the control group there
was frequently a subendothelial deposit of a hyaline substance. This
is called arteriolosclerosis, and the intensity of the process is indicated
in Table 3 by the numerals 1, 2, and 3. The designation 1p in the table
indicates that hyaline was found only in an occasional arteriole, usually those originating from larger arteries. The numerals 1, 2, and 3 indicate that the majority of the arterioles are affected. Grades 1 and 2
of arteriolosclerosis are shown in Figure 4 and Grade 3 in Figure 5.

The incidence and intensity of arteriolosclerosis in the control group
with respect to age are shown in Table 3. Arteriolosclerosis is very rare
before the age of 40 years, but it increases from 7.7 per cent in the
fifth decade to 23.7 per cent after the seventh decade. In the entire
group over 50 years of age renal arteriolosclerosis was found in 13.5
per cent. The lesion was usually Grade 1, seldom Grade 3. It is apparent, therefore, that renal arteriolosclerosis is an age change which
may develop independently of hypertension.

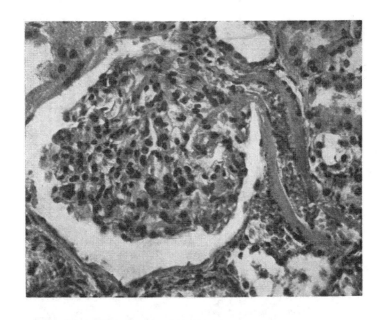

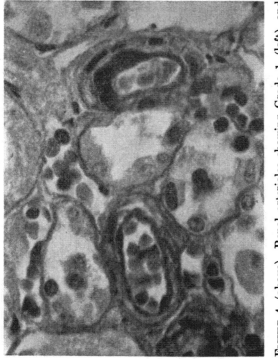

FIGURE 4 (above). Renal arterioles showing Grade 1 (left) and Grade 2 (right) hyaline arteriolosclerosis. FIGURE 5 (side). Afferent arteriole showing Grade 3 arteriolosclerosis.

The relation of arteriolosclerosis to disease of the small arteries. Arteriolosclerosis was never found in the control group except in association with a Grade 2 or 3 intimal thickening of the small arteries. But disease of the small arteries is very common in the absence of arteriolosclerosis. The disease seems to extend from the small arteries into the arterioles.

The relation of arteriolosclerosis to the level of the systolic blood pressure in persons over 50 years of age without hypertensive symptoms. From the figures in Table 4 it appears that arteriolosclerosis is

TABLE 4. The Relation of Arteriolosclerosis to the Level of the Systolic Pressure in Persons Over 50 Years of Age without Hypertensive Symptoms

Systolic Blood Pressure (mm. Hg)	No. of Cases	Percentage Showing Arteriolosclerosis Grades 1–3
90–129	410	12
130–139	164	19
140–149	70	24.3
150–159	76	21
160–169	70	24.3
170–179	49	22.4
180–210	48	20.8

TABLE 5. The Relation of Arteriolosclerosis to the Weight of the Heart in Non-Hypertensive Control Subjects Over 50 Years of Age

Weight of the Heart in Grams	No. of Cases	Percentage Showing Arteriolosclerosis Grades 1–3
Males 170–299 / Females 170–249	174	10.3
Males 300–349 / Females 250–299	181	14.9
Males 350–400 / Females 300–350	181	14.4

definitely less frequent in those with systolic pressures below 130 mm. Hg, but that there is no significant difference in its incidence in those with pressures above that level. This observation is difficult to interpret. Since these persons had no hypertensive symptoms, it may mean that their blood pressures were of the labile type and not persistently elevated.

The relation of arteriolosclerosis to the weight of the heart in the control group over 50 years of age. It may be seen in Table 5 that arteriolosclerosis is definitely less frequent in association with hearts weighing less than 300 gm. in males and 250 gm. in females than with larger hearts; but there is very little difference between its incidence in the second and third groups of the table.

It is clear that renal arteriolosclerosis of moderate intensity occurs frequently in older persons who had no symptoms of hypertensive disease and whose blood pressures and cardiac weights were within recognized normal limits. It is a primary disease of the arterioles which increases in frequency with age. The most important influence in the control group is the age of the individual. There can be no doubt that arteriolosclerosis may develop independently of hypertension.

It may be suggested that the older persons are the ones with the larger hearts and higher pressures, but a careful analysis shows that the size of the heart and the level of the blood pressure in this group are not related to age.

Scriba also found many normotensive subjects in the older age groups who had renal arteriolosclerosis.

The incidence of renal arteriolosclerosis in the different clinical forms of hypertensive disease. In Table 6 the incidence of arteriolo-

TABLE 6. The Incidence and the Degree of Renal Arteriolosclerosis among a Group of Non-Hypertensive Controls and in the Different Clinical Forms of Hypertensive Disease

	No. of Cases	Percentage by Degree of Arteriolosclerosis					
		0	1p	1	2	3	Total 1–3
Controls over 50 years of age 534		72.3	14.2	10.1	2.4	1.0	13.5
Myocardial 242		26.9	6.2	28.1	18.2	20.2	66.5
Cerebral 266		20.7	6.4	26.7	17.3	29.0	73.0
Coronary 80		32.5	12.5	30.0	12.5	12.5	55.0

sclerosis is shown in the myocardial, cerebral, and coronary forms of hypertensive disease. The renal form is not included, since by definition there is always a severe vascular disease. In all the cases shown in the table the patient was known to have had a high blood pressure, and death was due to hypertensive disease of the type indicated. The percentage with definite arteriolosclerosis (Grades 1–3) is smaller in the coronary than in the other forms. Nearly 25 per cent of all persons with typical clinical hypertensive disease of the non-renal types have normal renal arterioles (Grade 0), and about 7 per cent have only occasional hyaline deposits in the arterioles (Grade 1p).

Castleman and Smithwick examined biopsies from the kidneys of 100 hypertensive patients, the specimens being taken at the time of sympathectomy operations. Using the criteria of Moritz and Oldt (which includes prearterioles), they found no vascular disease in 7 patients, Grade 1 lesions in 21, Grade 2 in 25, Grade 3 in 33, and Grade 4 in 14. These observers believed that in a fairly high percentage the vascular lesions were an inadequate explanation of the hypertension.

It cannot be maintained that hypertension is always caused by renal arteriolosclerosis, since in about 25 per cent of the cases of hypertension without renal insufficiency the arterioles are entirely normal. If one includes the prearterioles, the percentage of involvement is higher, but there remain 17.5 per cent in which both arterioles and prearterioles are normal. Likewise hypertension cannot be attributed to disease of the small renal arteries, since this is almost invariably present in the normotensive controls over 50 years of age, and in about one third of them it is severe (Grade 3). Disease limited to the small arteries, when sufficiently severe to cause atrophy of the renal cortex, may, however, be associated with hypertension.

It has been demonstrated that clinical hypertension may develop in persons whose renal arterioles and prearterioles are normal and whose small arteries are no more severely affected than those of the normotensive controls.

In hypertension with renal insufficiency the blood pressure is commonly higher than in the other forms of hypertension, and the evidence seems convincing that the development of severe vascular renal lesions during the course of chronic hypertension may cause the blood pressure to rise to higher levels, and in exceptional cases of acute renal insufficiency the vascular lesions may initiate the hypertension.

To summarize the evidence presented above, it may be pointed out that mild renal arteriolosclerosis does not always cause hypertension, since it is found in about 13.5 per cent of normotensive older persons. It is also established that a fair percentage of subjects with typical clinical hypertensive disease do not have renal arteriolosclerosis; hence hypertension may develop in the absence of arteriolosclerosis.

Since renal arteriolosclerosis is much more severe and more frequent in hypertensive than in normotensive subjects, one must conclude that there is some causal connection between the condition of the arterioles and the level of the blood pressure. We may believe that primary hypertension is basically due to a spastic narrowing of the arterioles and not to organic changes in their walls, and that the persistent increase of intravascular pressure accelerates the aging process. According to this concept primary hypertension and renal arteriolosclerosis are independent in origin, but they intensify each other.

The relation of diabetes mellitus to renal arteriolosclerosis. In Table 7 the frequency and intensity of renal arteriolosclerosis in diabetic subjects is shown in relation to age. It appears that arteriolosclerosis is about as frequent in diabetics as in persons with primary hypertension. The tendency of diabetes to accelerate atherosclerosis is well known. It may be suggested that the high incidence of arteriolosclerosis is due to associated hypertension, but the arteriolar lesions are nearly as frequent in normotensive as in hypertensive diabetics.

The three known etiological influences in renal arteriolosclerosis are therefore age, hypertension, and diabetes mellitus.

Hypertension with renal insufficiency. In Table 8 the age distribution of the several clinical forms of hypertensive disease is shown.

TABLE 7. The Incidence and the Degree of Renal Arteriolosclerosis in Diabetic Subjects with Respect to Age and in a Group of Controls

Age in Years	No. of Cases	Percentage by Degree of Involvement				Total
		0	1	2	3	1–3
0–10	9	100	0	0	0	0
10–20	22	100	0	0	0	0
20–30	31	71.0	12.9	3.2	12.9	29.0
30–40	57	70.1	8.8	0.0	21.0	29.8
40–50	84	46.4	22.6	6.0	25.0	53.6
50–60 214		36.4	19.6	15.0	28.9	63.5
60–70 331		26.6	19.6	17.2	36.3	73.1
70–80 216		25.0	23.1	18.0	33.8	75.0
80–100	60	25.0	28.3	8.3	38.3	75.0
Over 50 821		28.6	21.3	16.2	33.9	71.4
Controls over 50 534		86.5	10.1	2.4	1.0	13.5

TABLE 8. The Distribution by Age Decade of the Different Clinical Forms of Hypertensive Disease (Age at Time of Death)

Group	No. of Cases	Percentage by Decade								
		1	2	3	4	5	6	7	8	9 & 10
Myocardial 338		0	0	0	1.2	13.0	21.9	30.8	26.6	6.5
Cerebral 315		0	0.6	1.0	2.2	13.6	22.2	29.2	24.1	7.0
Coronary 207		0	0	0.5	1.0	8.7	21.7	41.0	22.2	4.8
Renal										
Males 281		0	0.7	2.5	6.8	25.3	35.6	20.3	7.8	1.0
Females 173		0	2.3	4.6	20.8	26.6	16.8	15.6	10.4	2.9

Renal insufficiency develops early or late in about 12 per cent of persons with clinical symptoms of primary hypertension. In this table the number with renal insufficiency is much higher because the cases were selected from a much larger group of necropsies than were those with the other forms of hypertensive disease. It will be noted that in the earlier decades there is a higher percentage of the renal than of the other forms of hypertensive disease, and that this is particularly true of females. The total incidence of renal insufficiency is about the same in the two sexes, but in females 27.7 per cent of the cases occur before the age of 40 years, and 45.7 per cent after the age of 50, whereas in males 10 per cent occur before the age of 40 years and 64.7 per cent after the age of 50.

In the great majority of the renal group there is satisfactory evidence that hypertension was present a long time before the onset of renal insufficiency. The blood pressure is usually much higher in the presence of renal insufficiency, the systolic pressure being 200 mm. Hg or higher in 81 per cent of the group of 454 cases. The pressure tends to rise to higher levels as renal insufficiency increases.

In about one third of the cases the kidneys were small and contracted, the combined weight being less than 200 gm.; but in about 20 per cent there was no reduction in the size of the kidneys, the combined weight being 300 gm. or more. In the contracted kidneys, uremia is brought about by a slowly progressive occlusion of the small arteries and arterioles, whereas in the large kidneys it is due chiefly to acute occlusion of these vessels. On the clinical evidence we may distinguish a slowly developing uremia and an acute fulminating uremia.

1. Chronic uremia. This is more frequent than the acute form, and the kidneys are usually reduced in size. Microscopically there is extensive cortical atrophy due to severe intimal thickening of the small arteries and hyaline changes in the arterioles. Most of the glomeruli are hyaline (Fig. 6). The changes are similar to those often found in hypertension without renal insufficiency, but they are more severe and are associated with extensive cortical atrophy.

2. Acute uremia. The vascular changes characteristic of acute uremia are usually superimposed on those resulting from simple chronic hypertension. Three varieties of lesions are found.

a. Collagenous intimal thickening. This is found chiefly in the small arteries and prearterioles. The lumen of the vessel is greatly reduced in diameter by a very thick intima composed of loosely arranged collagenous fibers (Fig. 7).

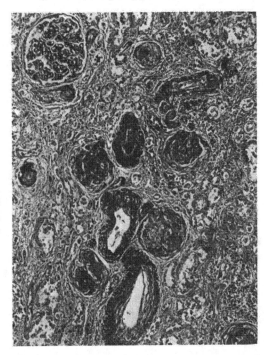

FIGURE 6. Hypertension with chronic uremia. Severe involvement of the small arteries, with hyaline arteriolosclerosis and many hyaline glomeruli.

b. Thrombonecrosis. This lesion is found chiefly in the arterioles. The lumen of the vessel is filled by a thrombus, and often the entire wall is necrotic (Fig. 8).

c. Focal glomerulitis. Frequently one finds occasional glomeruli associated with necrotic afferent arterioles in which the glomerular capillaries are filled with leucocytes. An epithelial crescent may be present (Fig. 8).

The changes characteristic of acute uremia are so different from the renal vascular lesions commonly found in other forms of hypertension that they are often interpreted as a special form of acute arteritis.

Summary

Primary hypertension is arbitrarily defined as a persistent blood pressure of unknown cause, 150/90 mm. Hg or higher in persons over 50 years of age and 140/90 mm. Hg or higher in persons less than 40 years of age.

Systolic hypertension with a normal diastolic pressure is not so serious as a high diastolic pressure, but it nevertheless produces an increase in the average intravascular pressure.

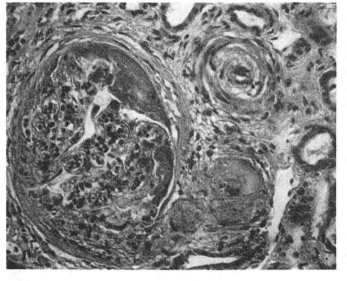

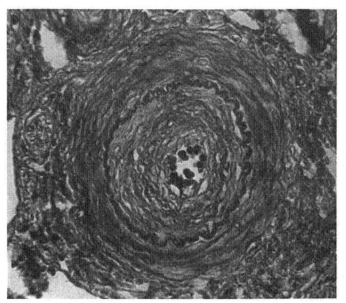

Figure 7 (left). Hypertension with acute uremia. Small artery showing severe collagenous intimal thickening. Figure 8 (right). Hypertension with acute uremia showing thrombonecrosis of the afferent arteriole and acute glomerulitis.

196

The majority of hypertensive persons over 50 years of age whose pressures do not exceed 170/90 mm. Hg, have no symptoms attributable to the high pressure, and there is no great increase in mortality from hypertensive complications in this group.

About three fourths of persons with hypertension, in the sense of having blood pressures of 150/90 mm. Hg or higher, die of diseases unrelated to the hypertensive state.

Although hypertension is more frequent in older women than in older men, the mortality from hypertensive complications is lower in females, and women with corresponding degrees of hypertension survive longer than men.

In the autopsies at the University of Minnesota, about 13 per cent of the deaths of persons over 50 years of age were assignable to some complication of primary hypertension.

The fatal complications of primary hypertension are myocardial failure, coronary atherosclerosis, intracranial hemorrhage, encephalomalacia, and renal insufficiency.

About 12 per cent of the deaths from primary hypertension are due to renal failure resulting from narrowing or closure of the small renal arteries and arterioles.

Intimal thickening of the small renal arteries is an age change found in some degree in practically all persons over 50 years of age. It increases in intensity with advancing age. In primary hypertension this lesion is somewhat more severe than in non-hypertensives of corresponding age.

In non-hypertensive controls renal arteriolosclerosis is rare before the age of 40 years, but it increases in frequency from 7.7 per cent in the fifth decade to 22.7 per cent after the seventh decade. The arteriolosclerosis is usually mild. Renal arteriolosclerosis is over five times as frequent in persons dead of primary hypertension as in non-hypertensive controls and is usually much more severe. About 25 per cent of persons dead of primary hypertension do not show renal arteriolosclerosis.

Primary hypertension and renal arteriolosclerosis are independent in origin, but they intensify each other.

The basic disturbance in primary hypertension is a spastic state of the arterioles, not an organic alteration.

In a majority of the cases of primary hypertension terminating in uremia the alterations in the small renal arteries and arterioles differ only in intensity from those occurring in the other forms of hypertensive disease; but in a fair percentage uremia is brought about rapidly by collagenous intimal thickening of the small vessels or by a necrotizing arteriolitis.

REFERENCE. E. T. Bell: Renal Diseases, ed. 2, Philadelphia, Lea & Febiger, 1950, pp. 391–395.

• • • • • • • • • • • • • *by* REGINALD H. SMITHWICK
and BENJAMIN CASTLEMAN

Some Observations on Renal Vascular Disease in Hypertensive Patients Based on Biopsy Material Obtained at Operation

THE observations of Richard Bright in 1827 (1) and in 1836 (2) called attention to the fact that diseased kidneys were at times associated with hypertrophied hearts. This important deduction resulted from the correlation of clinical evidence with gross pathological findings at autopsy. Thus it became established that kidney disease of one sort or another was evidenced clinically by dropsy and albuminuria and at autopsy by diseased kidneys and hypertrophied hearts.

The advent of the microscope permitted more detailed study of pathological material from patients dying of so-called Bright's disease or with hypertrophied hearts. The brilliant observations of Gull and Sutton in 1872 (3) led them to question the then current theory of the cause of hypertrophied hearts. As a result they suggested that cardiac hypertrophy might result from kidney disease but also could be present in the absence of kidney disease. Their careful study of the blood vessels from various organs of patients dying of Bright's disease led them to suggest that a widespread arterio-capillary fibrosis existed in which the blood vessels of the kidney might or might not participate. They also contested the then current concept of the nature of the pathological changes in the blood vessels and showed that in addition to medial hypertrophy, a hyaline fibroid degeneration also existed. With increasing refinement in the fixation and staining of tissues their observations have since been repeatedly confirmed.

By 1940 it had thus been firmly established that widespread vascular disease was invariably present in patients dying of this disorder and that the blood vessels of the kidneys were more affected than those of any other organ with the possible exception of the spleen. The changes noted were medial hypertrophy, intimal hyalinization, and endothelial hyperplasia. These changes were beautifully illustrated in the study of Moritz and Oldt in 1937 (4). The question of whether these changes preceded the development of an elevated blood pressure was argued back and forth, and since the evidence was based upon the study of autopsy material, the conclusion that the vascular changes of importance antedated the elevation of the blood pressure could not be substantiated. Evidence was lacking concerning the state of the arterioles in living hypertensive patients.

The brilliant experimental work of Goldblatt (5) seemed to support the point of view that vascular disease antedated the development of hypertension. Goldblatt postulated that if renal vascular disease of consequence existed, this would result in a reduction in the renal blood flow, which might in turn be followed by the development of hypertension. If this were true, then it should be possible to simulate the effect of vascular disease and cause a reduction in the renal blood flow by partial constriction of the renal artery with a metal clamp. That constriction of the renal arteries did result in the development of hypertension in animals simulating the so-called essential and malignant forms of the disorder in man is well known to all and has been repeatedly confirmed by many observers, using the Goldblatt technique as well as that of Page (6) and others. These experiments gave strong support to the theory of the renal origin of essential and malignant hypertension in man. However, they did not conclusively prove that pre-existing renal vascular disease of consequence was the invariable precursor of the hypertensive state in man.

The advent of the surgical treatment of hypertensive cardiovascular disease and the development of techniques which permitted the gross inspection of the kidneys and the obtaining of renal biopsies at operation has given an opportunity to further explore the relation between renal vascular disease and the hypertensive state in man. Since 1940 we have had occasion to remove specimens from one or both kidneys of many hypertensive patients for microscopic study. This material has been examined carefully by Castleman, and in 1943 (7) a preliminary report of the findings in the first 100 cases was made. A second report of the findings in the first 500 cases was published in 1948 (8). A very detailed study of this material is now in progress which will correlate the microscopic and clinical findings. This present report will summarize the evidence which has been accumulated to date. It is by way of a forerunner of the much more extensive analysis which will soon be forthcoming.

The Grading of the Vascular Changes in the Renal Biopsies

At first we were somewhat concerned that taking a biopsy from the kidney might result in postoperative complications. So far as we know, there have been none. The biopsies have been taken from the most accessible portion of the kidney, namely, the greater curvature at about the junction of the upper and middle thirds. A wedge-shaped segment is removed, averaging 6 x 5 x 4 mm. in size. The defect is filled with perirenal fat, which is held in place with two or three silk sutures. Each microscopical section contains about 50 cross sections of arterioles and small arteries.

After a careful study of the first 100 biopsies, Castleman decided that there were enough differences in the vascular changes to require 5 grades for classification. The pathological changes varied a great deal from none at all to very severe and were graded from normal to 4 accordingly. The percentage of biopsies in each of the 5 grades in the first 100 and the first 500 cases is given in Table 1. The changes

TABLE 1. The Distribution of Renal Biopsy Grades

Biopsy Grade	Per Cent	
	First 100 Cases	First 500 Cases
Pathological changes none to mild		
N	7	4
1	21	19
2	25	22
Total	53	45
Pathological changes moderate and severe		
3	33	44
4	14	11
Total	47	55

graded 1 or 2 are regarded as minimal and mild and do not appear to be sufficient to cause a marked alteration in the renal blood flow. Those graded 3 and 4 are regarded as moderate and severe and would appear to be sufficient to compromise the renal circulation. Typical examples of Biopsy Grades 1 through 4 are illustrated by Figures 1 through 4. The close correlation between the percentage of cases having each of the biopsy grades in the first 100 and 500 cases is regarded as evidence that about one half of the patients having well-instituted persistent hypertension do not have renal vascular disease of consequence.

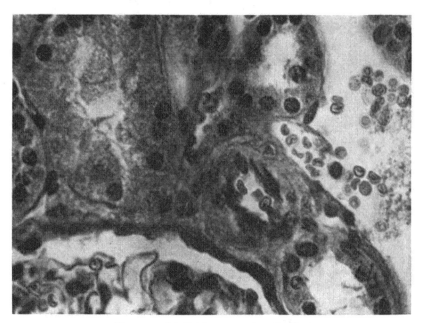

FIGURE 1. Medial hypertrophy, Grade 1.

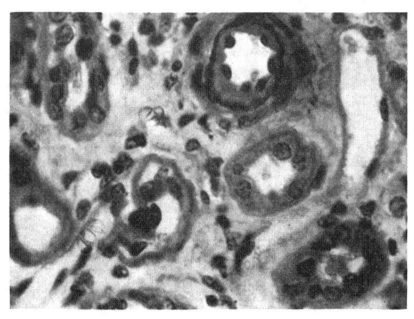

FIGURE 2. Intimal hyalinization, Grade 2.

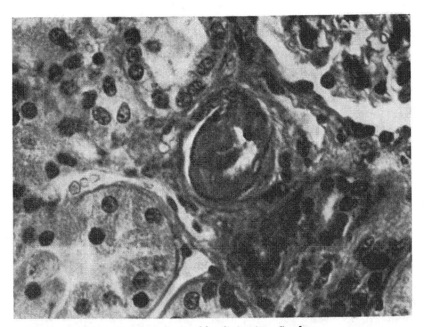

FIGURE 3. Intimal hyalinization, Grade 3.

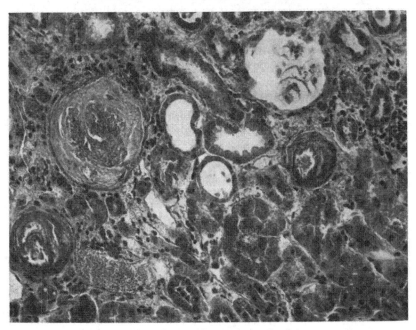

FIGURE 4. Intimal hyperplasia, Grade 4.

In the early years of this study, it was our practice to take a biopsy from one kidney only. More recently, we have obtained a biopsy from both kidneys. A study of the material from the first 100 cases having bilateral biopsies shows a very close correlation between the vascular changes in the two kidneys. This is indicated by Table 2. This finding,

TABLE 2. The Correlation between 100 Bilateral Renal Biopsies

Biopsy Grade	Per Cent
The same	75
One grade different	20
More than one grade different	5

together with the fact that autopsy material indicates that arteriolar disease in a kidney is by and large a generalized process, leads us to believe that a renal biopsy gives an adequate picture of the status of the renal arterioles. This belief gains further support from the split-clearance studies of Chasis and Redish (9), who found that the decrease in the rate of glomerular filtration and effective renal blood flow in hypertensive patients is shared equally by the kidneys.

Renal Function and Renal Vascular Disease

Various ordinary tests of renal function were carried out in all cases. These included urinalysis, a urine concentration test, estimation of phenolsulphonphthalein excretion, non-protein nitrogen determinations, and intravenous pyelography. Of these various tests the excretion of phenolsulphonphthalein administered intravenously appeared to be the most dependable indicator of impaired renal function. If 25 per cent or more of the dye was excreted in 15 minutes and 60 per cent or more in 2 hours, this test of renal function was regarded as normal. It was found that as the evidence of renal vascular disease as judged by the biopsy material increased, the percentage of cases having normal renal function decreased. This is indicated by Table 3.

TABLE 3. The Distribution of Normal Renal Function among
the Renal Biopsies

Biopsy Grade	Per Cent First 100 Cases	Per Cent First 500 Cases
N	100	95
1	81	82
2	64	68
3	58	60
4	7	17

Renal Plasma Flow and Renal Vascular Disease

As a further check upon the accuracy of the biopsy grading it seemed wise to determine the amount of blood flowing through the kidneys for the different biopsy grades. Accordingly a small group of patients were studied by the renal clearance technique of Smith (10). In all, inulin and diodrast clearances were carried out in 20 cases. The biopsy findings were normal in 2 patients, Grade 1 in 4, Grade 2 in 3, Grade 3 in 8, and Grade 4 in 3 patients. The average renal plasma flow for each of the biopsy grades is given in Table 4. As might be

TABLE 4. Renal Plasma Flow for Biopsy Grades

Biopsy Grade	No. of Cases	Average Renal Plasma Flow (cc/minute)
N	2	625
1	4	552
2	3	470
3	8	439
4	3	283

expected, as the evidence of vascular disease increased, the renal blood flow decreased. It was also of interest to note that the filtration fraction was normal in 7 of 9 cases having Biopsy Grades 0, 1, or 2. It was increased in 6 of 11 cases having Biopsy Grades 3 or 4. These findings indicate that constriction of the efferent glomerular arterioles is not necessarily present in the earlier stages of renal vascular disease.

The Effect of Renal Vascular Disease, Cold, and Posture upon the Renal Blood Flow

The estimations of the renal blood flow referred to in the previous section and summarized in Table 4 were made with the patient in the horizontal position and under as nearly basal conditions as could be obtained. Since it is known that in addition to vascular disease vasoconstriction will also cause a reduction in the renal blood flow, an attempt was made in a few cases to study the influence of the upright position and of stimulation by ice water upon the renal circulation.

In studying the blood pressure responses of hypertensive patients in various positions, we have noted that in certain cases the diastolic level rises abnormally when the patient assumes the upright position, as judged by a comparison of the average of five readings of the blood pressure taken at one-minute intervals with the patient first lying and then standing. An average rise of 20 mm. or more in the upright position appears to be abnormal. As has been noted by Hines and Brown (11), most hypertensive patients hyperreact to stimulation by cold as judged by a blood pressure response in excess of 20/15 mm. to a one-minute period of immersion of one hand in ice water. The findings in a patient studied for renal clearance whose blood pressure responses were abnormal to both change of posture and cold are illustrated in Figure 5. The renal blood flow likewise fluctuated a

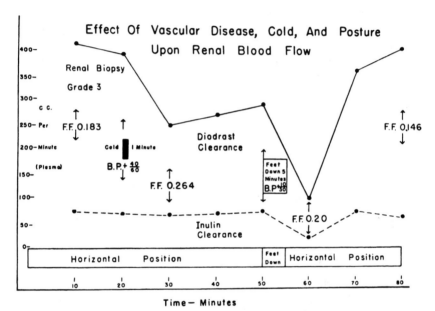

FIGURE 5. The effect of cold and posture upon the renal blood flow in a patient having renal vascular disease Grade 3 is illustrated by this figure. In response to the immersion of one hand in ice water for 1 minute with the patient in the horizontal position, the renal plasma flow decreased from 400 to 250 cc/min. One-half hour later the blood flow was still reduced. At this point the patient was tilted into a foot-down position for 5 minutes. The renal plasma flow decreased to less than 100 cc/min and then returned to the base line in the course of 20 additional minutes. This indicates that physiological factors may cause a striking reduction in the renal blood flow.

great deal under these conditions of study from the highest level noted in the horizontal position. Stimulation by cold caused about a 50 per cent reduction, followed by a slow recovery to the control level, which was already considerably decreased below normal in the horizontal position because of renal vascular disease Grade 3. An assumption of the upright position caused an even more marked reduction in the blood flow, approximating complete ischemia. It was intended to combine the cold and postural stimuli, but this was not done because of the striking effect of posture alone on the urinary output.

These studies were carried out by Dr. John Talbot (12) and were brought to a premature ending when he entered the army in World War II. Facilities for continuing these observations have not been available since. While the evidence is inadequate to permit any conclusions, the findings suggest that physiological factors may profoundly influence the visceral blood flow and may be of fundamental importance. While it has never been shown that splanchnicectomy affects the renal blood flow when measured in the horizontal position, it is conceivable that following operation, downward fluctuations in the blood flow might be minimized. This would increase the blood flow by decreasing the periods of renal ischemia and might influence the renal humoral mechanism. The principal reason for presenting these incomplete data is that some investigator may care to pursue the matter further.

The Relation between the Development of Hypertension and Renal Vascular Disease

One of us has had occasion to study some 3000 patients representing all stages in the development of hypertensive cardiovascular disease. In general this has resulted in the impression that vascular disease of consequence, as judged by careful clinical study of the cerebral, retinal, cardiac, and renal areas, rarely is present until the blood pressure levels have been consistently elevated for a considerable period of time. It also seems quite certain that in the vast majority of cases, persistent hypertension is preceded by years of intermittent or transient hypertension. It also seems highly probable to us that the stage of intermittent hypertension is preceded in many cases by years of unusually variable blood pressure within the normal range. Patients in this latter phase or stage have been classified as normotensive hyperreactors by Hines and Brown.

By far the greater part of our biopsy material is from patients with long-standing persistent hypertension and vascular changes of consequence in one or more areas. We have rarely had occasion to operate upon patients with intermittent or transient hypertension. These are patients who have elevated blood pressure levels when they are up and about and active, but whose blood pressure drops readily to normal on rest. Only rarely does the cardiovascular system of these

patients degenerate. Because this has occurred or because of symptoms difficult to control otherwise or because of the unusual severity
of the upward fluctuations, often simulating paroxysmal hypertension,
splanchnicectomy has been performed in 28 such cases having renal
biopsies. The vascular changes in these cases may be compared with
those noted in patients in a later stage of the disorder. This material
can also be compared with that obtained from hypertensive patients
dying of some complication of the disorder and with autopsy material
obtained from normotensive patients.

TABLE 5. The Relation between the Development of Hypertension and
Renal Vascular Disease

Material Studied	Percentage Having Renal Vascular Disease		
	None to Mild	Moderate	Severe
100 normotensive patients (Moritz and Oldt, 1937)	98	2	0
28 patients with intermittent hyper-tension (Smithwick and Castleman) ...	75	25	0
500 patients with persistent hypertension (Castleman and Smithwick, 1948)	45	44	11
100 patients dying of hypertensive cardio-vascular disease (Moritz and Oldt, 1937) ...		...	47

These findings are given in Table 5. We have used the statistics of
Moritz and Oldt to compare with our two biopsy groups. It is evident
that normotensive patients do not have severe renal vascular disease
at autopsy. Patients who have been operated on in the stage of intermittent hypertension so far have not had severe pathological changes
in the renal arterioles. Moderate vascular changes were noted in 25
per cent of these patients in contrast to 2 per cent of normotensive
patients, indicating that vascular disease of consequence was beginning to develop. It should be emphasized that in 75 per cent of these
patients renal vascular disease was absent, minimal, or mild, and not
sufficient, in our opinion, to be regarded as of importance. When hypertension has been consistently present for years, over half of the
patients show renal vascular disease of consequence, the changes being moderate in 44 per cent and severe in 11 per cent. The surprising
fact is that nearly one half of these patients have no changes or show
the disease graded as minimal or mild.

These findings are interpreted as not being consistent with the
theory that renal vascular disease of consequence usually antedates the

development of hypertension. It seems more likely that in most cases the vascular changes develop along with the hypertension and are partly, at least, the result of it. The fact that at death renal vascular disease of importance is rarely absent in hypertensive patients seems to confirm this view.

Only 3 per cent of patients dying of some complication of the disorder had no evidence of renal vascular disease in the series of Moritz and Oldt, while Bell and Clawson (13) reported that renal arteriolar sclerosis was absent in the small arteries of 10 per cent of their 420 cases. It is of interest that the conclusions drawn by these two sets of authors regarding the relation between renal vascular disease and hypertension are exactly opposite. Moritz and Oldt felt that their data favored the theory that renal vascular disease preceded hypertension. Bell and Clawson stated that "on the whole, the evidence seems to favor the hypothesis that hypertension causes renal arteriosclerosis." We feel that our data offer strong support of the view of Bell and Clawson.

The Relation between the Severity of Hypertension and Renal Vascular Disease

If one divides hypertensive patients according to the severity of the diastolic level, it is found that the higher the level the more frequently is renal vascular disease of importance present in the biopsy material. This finding further tends to confirm the view that the vascular changes are the result of the hypertension, since in the earliest stage and in the milder forms renal vascular changes of importance are absent in the majority of cases, while in the more severe forms of hypertension they are present in most cases. No doubt there is also a relation between the duration of hypertension and the development

TABLE 6. The Relation between the Severity of Hypertension, as Gauged by the Diastolic Blood Pressure, and Renal Vascular Disease

Severity of Hypertension	Percentage Having Renal Vascular Disease	
	None to Mild	Moderate to Severe
Intermittent 75		25
Persistent		
Diastolic blood pressure 90–109 mm. 61		39
Diastolic blood pressure 110–139 mm. ...37		63
Diastolic blood pressure 140+ mm. 29		71

of renal vascular disease, but this cannot be demonstrated because the vast majority of patients with hypertension have no accurate concept of its duration. We have arranged our patients according to the severity of the diastolic level and have calculated the percentage of cases in each blood pressure category having renal vascular changes varying from none to mild as well as from moderate to severe. Patients with intermittent hypertension have diastolic levels commonly above 90 mm. when active, but have levels below this when at rest. Patients with persistent hypertension are divided into three blood pressure zones according to the lowest diastolic level recorded for each patient. The findings are given in Table 6.

The Relation between Renal Vascular Disease and Mortality Rates

The prognosis for patients with renal vascular disease varies according to the severity of the changes noted in the renal biopsies. As might be expected, the mortality rate is lowest for those patients having no vascular changes. The mortality rates for patients having Grade 1 or 2 biopsies is almost identical. For Grade 3 biopsies the mortality rate is much higher than for the lower grades and is highest of all for Grade 4. These findings are given in Table 7. Because the

TABLE 7. The Mortality Rates for the Various Renal Biopsy Grades

Renal Biopsy Grade	No. of Cases	Per Cent Mortality 5–9 Years
N	20	5
1	85	19
2	129	18
3	244	30
4	43	54

mortality rates for Grades 1 and 2 do not differ greatly, the survival rate for these patients is expressed by one curve and that for the other grades in separate curves. These are shown in Figure 6. It is apparent that the prognosis for patients having renal vascular changes ranging from none to mild is significantly better than for those having changes which are moderately advanced or severe.

Summary and Conclusions

1. A study of renal biopsy material taken at operation upon 500 patients having long-standing persistent hypertension reveals that

SURVIVAL RATES FOR RENAL BIOPSY GRADES

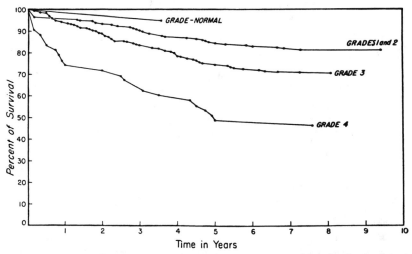

FIGURE 6. The data summarized in Table 7 are presented in the form of survival curves in this figure. Since the mortality rates for Grades 1 and 2 renal biopsies are essentially the same, one survival curve has been constructed for these two grades. It is apparent that there is a relationship between the grade of renal vascular disease and the survival rate. The prognosis for patients having Grade 4 renal vascular disease is much poorer than for patients having changes which are less severe, being best of all for those having no renal vascular disease or Grade 1 and 2 changes, as might be expected.

vascular changes ranging from moderate to severe were present in 55 per cent of the cases. The fact that 45 per cent of the biopsies did not reveal vascular changes of importance indicates that renal arteriolar sclerosis, sufficient to compromise the renal circulation, does not invariably antedate the hypertensive state in man. These data do not seem to support the theory that renal arteriolar sclerosis is the usual cause of essential and malignant hypertension in man. It is possible, indeed highly probable, that much of the vascular change noted in 55 per cent of the cases developed after the onset of persistent hypertension.

2. Renal biopsies were taken from both kidneys of 100 patients. The vascular changes were the same in 75 per cent, one grade different in 20 per cent, and more than one grade different in 5 per cent. Thus the grade of vascular disease in the two kidneys correlated closely in 95 per cent of the cases. This is interpreted as indicating that a kidney biopsy, small as it is, gives accurate information about the status of the renal arterioles and small arteries of a given patient. It also indi-

cates that vascular disease when present in the kidney is by and large a generalized process and that the two kidneys are damaged equally.

3. It was found that as the evidence of renal vascular disease increased, renal function decreased, as judged both by the phenolsulphonphthalein test and by quantitative measurements of the renal blood flow. Severely compromised renal function was particularly apparent in the cases having Grade 4 biopsies.

4. Vasoconstriction resulting from stimulation by cold and by assumption of the upright position may cause a marked reduction in the renal blood flow. It is thus apparent that physiological mechanisms as well as pathological processes may severely compromise the renal circulation.

5. It was found that 75 per cent of the biopsies from patients having intermittent or transient hypertension failed to show vascular changes of importance. If renal vascular disease of consequence antedated the hypertensive state in man, it would be expected that the great majority of the biopsies from patients in this stage of the disorder would show such changes. In the later stages of hypertension and in the more severe forms, as judged by the diastolic level, the percentage of living cases showing important grades of renal vascular disease increases. Renal vascular disease is most marked in hypertensive patients dying of some complication of the disorder and least marked in autopsy material from normotensive persons. Thus renal vascular disease appears to develop in an orderly fashion as one studies material from normotensive patients and from patients in the early, the later, and finally the terminal stages of hypertensive cardiovascular disease. This indicates that most of the vascular disease must develop along with the hypertension, and since it does not appear to antedate it, it presumably is largely the result of the elevated blood pressure. There no doubt are occasional exceptions to this statement, but it is believed that this view holds for the great majority of cases.

6. The prognosis for patients with hypertensive cardiovascular disease is dependent to a large extent upon the amount of cardiovascular damage present at the time of the original observation or at the onset of treatment. With regard to the renal area in particular, the more marked the renal vascular changes, the higher the mortality rate. The prognosis for patients with vascular changes graded 3 and 4 is much poorer than for those having lesser degrees of or no renal vascular disease.

Questions and Discussion

DR. HARRY GOLDBLATT: As a rule, when investigators differ, it is not on the basis of their data. If they differ, it is usually about the interpretation of the data. From the presentations of Dr. Bell and Dr. Smithwick I have obtained considerable comfort.

Dr. Bell, for example, stated very clearly, in the beginning of his talk, that by far the most pronounced vascular disease of real significance affects those vessels that he calls the large and small arteries, and not so much the arterioles, except, of course, in the more advanced stages of the condition.

He talked, however, about arterioles and he did not say much about the large and small arteries. I think that they are of the greatest importance. Dr. Castleman and Dr. Smithwick's observations tell us absolutely nothing about the large and small arteries. Yet, functionally, they are of great significance.

I also derive great comfort from the observations of Dr. Bell to the effect that in the normal group there is a considerable amount of vascular disease. I should have been disturbed had he stated that in the normal group there was no vascular disease and that it occurred only in the hypertensive group. Then the only justifiable conclusion would have been that hypertension comes from some unknown cause and that it, in turn, causes vascular disease. This I do not believe. There is evidently a gradual transition from normal to hypertensive. Vascular disease begins to develop in persons with normal blood pressure, and it affects not only the arterioles, but also the small and large intrarenal arteries.

I derive comfort, for example, from the two slides that Dr. Smithwick showed in which although his interpretation of the causative relationship is different from mine, yet he did show that vascular disease of one degree or another occurred in most of his hypertensive patients. I consider that by the examination of a very small portion

213

of the periphery of the cortex one cannot make a very good estimate of the state of the entire renal vasculature and especially of the hemodynamic state of a kidney.

There are indications, however, from the presentations of Dr. Bell and of Dr. Smithwick that there are changes in other parts of the vascular bed, especially in the large and small intrarenal arteries, and my belief is that there is a causative relationship between the vascular disease, which is primary, and the hypertension.

DR. ELEXIOUS T. BELL: I believe that the biopsies which Dr. Smithwick took are amply sufficient to determine the degree of involvement of the arterioles and prearterioles, but perhaps not that of the small arteries. We should not get any additional information from examining the small arteries, since they show intimal disease in practically all normotensive persons over 50 years of age. If the biopsy shows as many as 10 afferent arterioles, it is adequate.

As regards the interpretations, we have given our data, and you can draw your own conclusions. How can intimal disease of the small arteries be regarded as the cause of hypertension when it is present, often in a severe degree, in practically all normotensive persons over 50 years of age? Over 20 per cent of those who die of primary hypertension without renal insufficiency show no renal arteriolosclerosis. This is a strong argument that hypertension may develop and continue in the absence of renal arteriolosclerosis.

It would be of great interest to see a second biopsy on Dr. Smithwick's patients after a period of years, to determine whether the vascular disease progresses less rapidly in those who are benefited by sympathectomy than in those who do not respond favorably.

I think that Dr. Smithwick can later on give us a good deal more information about the progress of this disease.

DR. SMITHWICK: I naturally am not able to speak with any authority on the subject of pathology, but it is my understanding from what I have read of Dr. Goldblatt's work and from the very excellent discussion of this topic by Moritz and Oldt in 1937 that vascular disease precedes and presumably is an important cause of hypertension. I have gathered the impression, and I hope not erroneously, that all of these people were talking about renal vascular disease of consequence, not these very minimal or minor changes that I have shown.

It is the opinion of Dr. Castleman and Dr. Mallory that these very minor changes, as Dr. Bell has shown, occur in normal people. It is not remarkable, therefore, that a certain percentage of people with hypertension should show these very minor changes graded 1 or 2 in occasional vessels throughout the specimen. The changes are not present in every vessel. You really have to hunt for what we call Grade 1. You can't see it under low power. You have to use high power and you have to search for it. You may find 1 vessel in many sections. When we first published these data, Dr. Moritz, who held the diametrically opposed view, was good enough to go over our material. He changed the grading of some of the biopsies, saying that they had been graded too severely. I think there is really very good evidence from our material and from Dr. Bell's to indicate that in the early stages of hypertensive cardiovascular disease, the degree of vascular damage is inconsequential and the degree to which renal function and the renal blood flow are affected is also inconsequential.

It was my understanding from reading Dr. Goldblatt's work very carefully and many times that when he conceived his experiments, which everybody concedes constitute one of the most brilliant developments in this field, they were based on the concept that not large artery disease but arteriolosclerosis sufficient to produce renal ischemia antedated the hypertensive state.

When he conceived these experiments, which simulated renal vascular disease through the clamping of the renal arteries in such a way as significantly to reduce the renal blood flow, that was his concept. I may be entirely wrong, but I believe that is what he wrote. I feel that his view is not in keeping with the facts which Dr. Bell and I have presented this morning.

· · · · · · · · · · · · · · · · · · *by* GEORGE E. FAHR

The Mechanism of Hypertension in Chronic Genuine Nephrosis

HYPERTENSION develops when the circulation through the kidneys is experimentally obstructed by means of clamps on the renal veins or arteries (1, 2). There are a number of pathological mechanisms that obstruct the circulation going through the kidneys, with a resulting production of renal hypertension. The best-known mechanism is the obstruction of the renal circulation brought about by endothelial cell proliferation within the capillaries of the glomeruli in acute and chronic glomerulonephritis. I shall discuss today the mechanism of the production of hypertension in cases of subacute and chronic genuine or lipemic nephrosis, because this mechanism is not widely understood as yet.

The literature shows knowledge of the fact that some cases of chronic genuine nephrosis eventually develop hypertension, but the mechanism was never elucidated, probably because the Mallory-Heidenhain azo-carmine stain was not used in studying the glomeruli and Bell and Goldblatt's work on experimentally produced renal hypertension was still unpublished.* Making use of the Mallory-Heidenhain azo-carmine stain, Dr. E. T. Bell (3) showed that in chronic genuine or lipemic nephrosis in adults, one sometimes finds focal or, in most cases, a very moderate degree of diffuse thickening of the basement membrane of the glomerular capillaries. It was not until 1932 that we became aware of the mechanism of hypertension in chronic lipoid nephrosis through the staining of the kidney sections with azo-carmine stain and from the results obtained in producing hypertension in animals experimentally by throttling the circulation through the kidneys.

* Some of Th. Fahr's illustrations (in Henke-Lubarsch: Handbuch d. Path. Anatomie, Vol. VI-1) of the glomeruli in chronic lipemic nephrosis stained with hematoxylin and eosin undoubtedly show the thickening of the membrane, but were not accurately interpreted by him in 1925.

Our first case was a 37-year-old physician who had developed a severe albuminuria with hydrops five years before his death in uremia accompanied by hypertension. In 1927 he came to see me. He had a moderately severe edema, ascites, and mild hydrothorax. The urine was examined on numerous occasions very carefully and never showed more than from 1 to 3 red blood cells in an occasional high-power field. Most of the high-power fields showed no red blood cells. A few (5–20 per h.p. field) pus cells were always found in the urine. There were numerous hyaline and granular casts; the specific gravity ranged from around 1.030 to 1.036. There were numerous highly refractive small globules in the urine, and the plasma was lipemic. The daily output of albumin, as measured with the Esbach, ranged around 10–16 gm. per 24 hours. The serum albumin was 2.2–2.6 gm. per cent. The serum globulin was 1.8–2.5 gm. per cent. The colloid osmotic pressure, calculated for this plasma, is 9–12 mm. Hg. The P.S.P. test showed an output of 45 per cent in one hour and 65 per cent in two hours, when the bladder was washed out with saline in order to collect all of the dye that came down from the kidneys during the test periods. There was no sign of any renal insufficiency as measured by the concentration test after correcting for the albumin effect on the urinary specific gravity. The blood urea nitrogen was 18 mg. per cent. The blood cholesterol was 340 mg. per cent. Blood pressures as taken by me ranged between 114 and 126 mm. Hg systolic and between 76 and 82 diastolic. After careful study, the diagnosis of chronic genuine nephrosis was made.

This diagnosis was confirmed after a six months' observation in the Rockefeller Hospital, where the patient was very thoroughly studied in 1929. The late Dr. John Phillipps, of the Cleveland Clinic, also studied this patient in 1929 and confirmed the diagnosis of chronic genuine or lipemic nephrosis. I examined this patient's urine with my technician on numerous occasions; a microscopic hematuria was never observed. On a low salt intake, the patient's edema was very moderate. In 1929 the patient went off total and permanent disability and returned to his practice. I did not take his blood pressure in 1930, but it was found to be 120/76 in May 1930, when he entered the Rockefeller Hospital for the second time. His standard urea clearance was 23 per cent of the average normal on this occasion, and the P.S.P. was 26 per cent in one hour and 37 per cent in two hours. In July 1931, at the time of the kidney symposium at the University of Minnesota, the patient was shown to Professor Volhard, of Germany, and, much to my surprise and chagrin, the blood pressure ranged around 180

systolic and 110 diastolic. There were at this time no red blood cells
in the urine. There was very little edema present. The patient did not
concentrate his urine beyond 1.018 after correcting for the effect of
the urinary albumin on the urinary specific gravity. Despite the fact
that there was no hematuria, Professor Volhard would not accept the
diagnosis of chronic genuine nephrosis, preferring to call the case a
subchronic glomerulonephritis. During the next year the blood pressure rose steadily, and at the time of the patient's death in July 1932
it ranged as high as 250 systolic. Shortly before his death a creatinine
clearance test showed only 10 per cent of normal clearance. The patient
died of heart failure and uremia. There was marked enlargement of
the heart, and the liver was slightly enlarged from passive congestion.

The autopsy revealed no edema, no cyanosis, no jaundice. The peritoneal cavity was free from fluid. There was 300 cc. of straw-colored
fluid in each pleural cavity. There was a normal amount of pericardial
fluid. The transverse diameter of the heart was 15 cm., whereas the
normal diastolic transverse diameter for a man of his size is 12.8 cm.
The heart weighed 500 gm. The valves were normal. The aorta showed
a small amount of atheroma. The descending branch of the left coronary artery was markedly sclerotic. The myocardium showed no
fibrosis or softening. The lungs showed marked edema on section. The
right lung weighed 800 gm. and the left 750. There was some congestion of the spleen. The liver weighed 2000 gm. and showed slight passive congestion. The right kidney weighed 100 gm. and the left 125.
There was a granular appearance after the capsules were stripped off
and they were moderately contracted, otherwise normal, on macro-
scopic examination. There was moderate atherosclerosis of the abdominal aorta. Dr. Bell's diagnosis was "lipoid nephrosis with uremia,
coronary sclerosis, edema of the lungs, pleural effusion, hypertrophy
of the heart, and slight passive congestion of the liver. On microscopic examination it was noted that a very large proportion of the
glomeruli were hyaline and their associated tubules markedly atrophic.
The persistent glomeruli showed a marked thickening of the capillary
basement membrane. The process of obliteration of the glomeruli was
a thickening of the basement membrane. There was no increase in the
endothelial nuclei."

In Figure 1 we see a photomicrograph of three of the glomeruli in
this case stained with azo-carmine stain. There is a remarkable thickening of the basement membrane, of such a nature that most of the
capillaries are nearly completely obliterated and the glomeruli hyalinized by the thickening of the basement membrane. In this case the

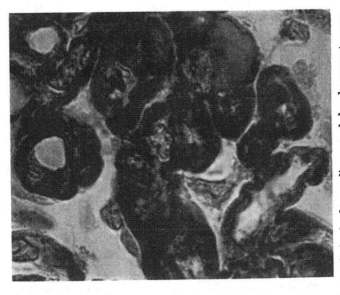

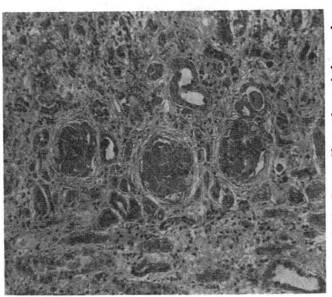

Figure 1 (left). Case 1. Shows three of the nearly completely hyalinized glomeruli, caused by basement membrane thickening. Atrophic tubules. Kidneys macroscopically small and granular. Figure 2 (right). Case 2. High magnification of a small part of a glomerulus. Lumen of the capillaries very much narrowed by basement membrane thickening of very high degree. Kidneys granular and of normal size. The patent loops of both Cases 1 and 2 are all very much like this. (Figures 1 through 4 are reproduced, by permission of the copyright owner, from E. T. Bell: Renal Diseases, ed. 2, Philadelphia, Lea & Febiger, 1950.)

majority of the glomeruli are very much like these three, but there are other glomeruli in which there is more passageway for the blood, as shown in the capillaries of Figure 2. The lumen in some of these capillaries is cut down to less than one half the normal diameter, which increases the resistance to the blood flow 16 times, according to Poiseuille's law. The lumen of each capillary in Figure 2 has its own Bell-Goldblatt clamp put on by the thickening membrane. Figure 2 is a photomicrograph of a section of kidney of my second case, but shows well the membrane thickening as found in about 20 per cent of the glomeruli in Case 1. In fact, the patent glomeruli in Case 1 look exactly like the patent glomeruli in Case 2. It is to be noted that the total filtering surface in these kidneys is remarkably reduced, because most of the glomerular capillaries are closed or nearly closed.

It is easy to see from these slides that there was a remarkable obstruction to the flow of blood through the glomeruli and a very great reduction in the filtering surface. We believe that the hypertension was determined by the throttling of the blood flow through the kidneys. The renal insufficiency was produced by the marked reduction in the filtering surface as well as by the slowing up of the circulation volume through these kidneys.

The next patient was a 45-year-old man who had six months previously developed a decreased appetite and edema. Four months before entering the Minneapolis General Hospital he had noticed oliguria, puffiness of the face and eyes, and severe edema of the legs. Albuminuria was present, but no increase in the blood pressure over 110–120 mm. Hg systolic was found by his private physician. Three months before entrance to the hospital he developed swelling of the abdomen and dyspnea, both of which increased gradually. The systolic pressure rose to 150 mm. Hg toward the end of this period, and he was sent into the Minneapolis General Hospital in September 1930. The symptoms had all developed gradually. The patient had been in bed at home for 4 months. Throughout the next 18 months he entered the hospital five times for periods of from 2 to 4 months, excepting the last admission of 2 days, when he was definitely in uremia.

Physical examination on his first hospital admission revealed a somewhat pale man with swollen eyes and face. The abdomen was much distended with fluid. There was marked edema of the legs and scrotum.

The urine showed 4+ albumin, specific gravity 1.031–1.034. Other findings were as follows: Daily output of albumin in urine 5–20 gm. Serum albumin 2.1–2.4 per cent. Serum globulin 2.4–2.8 per cent. Hemoglobin 98 per cent on entrance; 7 months later 60 per cent.

Erythrocytes 4,700,000 on entrance; 7 months later 3,000,000. After this period there was very little reduction in the hemoglobin and red count despite the development and increase of uremic poisons in the blood. The blood pressure on entrance was 150/100; 1 year later it was 180/130. The B.U.N. on entrance was 20 mg. per cent. At the time of death 18 months later it was 139 mg. per cent, with creatinine 7.5 mg. per cent. Twenty-seven out of 112 microscopic* examinations of the urinary sediment showed no red cells present. Nineteen examinations out of 112 showed 0–1 red cell in high-power fields. Fifteen examinations out of 112 showed 1–3 red cells per high-power field. Twelve microscopic examinations of the urinary sediment showed 2–3 red cells per high-power field. Two examinations showed 4–5, three examinations showed 5–8, one examination showed 6–10, and one examination showed 15–20. The average number of red cells per high-power field was 1–2 for 112 examinations. If we remember that the urinary output during these examinations was only 250–500 cc. in 24 hours, we can see that this urinary sediment was three times as concentrated as in a normal urine volume. Therefore, we should divide the number of cells in the urinary sediment by three to get an estimation of the number of red cells in his urine. In other words, there was very little, if any, hematuria present.

The P.S.P. test on entrance was practically normal (45 per cent for two hours).† At the time of death the test was too light to read. The concentration test on entrance was normal, taking into consideration the effect of the albumin in the urine. At the time of death the specific gravity of the urine was 1.014, with a protein content of 1 per cent, which would make the urine practically isosthenuric. The original clinical diagnosis was subchronic glomerulonephritis with a very strong nephrotic component. At the time of this patient's death, we supposed that he had had a very mild degree of hematuria, which caused us to hesitate in making this a case of pure genuine nephrosis. If we assume that this patient lost ⅓ cu. mm. of his blood per 24 hours in 300 cc. of urine, then the sediment in a 15 cc. centrifuge tube would contain 80,000 red blood cells, and search with a high dry lens giving a magnification of 250 would give a scattering of red blood cells very much like what our laboratory found in the 112 examinations of the urinary sediment. An output of 1,600,000 red cells in a 24-hour specimen of

---

*Each examination consisted in the scanning of 10 high-power fields. The 112 examinations were made on the urine specimens of 112 days.

†The bladder was not washed out in this determination, and the output of urine was only 40 cc. Therefore, the residual urine in the bladder was a goodly percentage. The P.S.P. output from the kidney must have been normal.

urine is far below what Addis has found in the latent stage of many cases of chronic glomerular nephritis. This is also my very much less extensive experience. At the present time I should hold out for a diagnosis of chronic genuine nephrosis with perhaps some slight tendency to endothelial cell proliferation in the glomeruli.

The autopsy revealed normal-sized, pale kidneys, with difficult stripping of the capsules. There was no increase in endothelial cells in the glomerular capillaries.* There was a high degree of thickening of the basement membranes of the glomerular capillaries, causing a marked throttling of the kidney circulation. There was a high degree of tubular atrophy, and approximately 50 per cent of the glomeruli were hyalinized. This is a typical picture of pure genuine nephrosis: marked thickening of the capillary basement membrane, consequent decreased circulation through the kidneys and a decreased glomerular filtration surface, marked atrophy of the tubules and hyalinization of many glomeruli, and no increase in endothelial cell proliferation. Figure 2 shows a photomicrograph of the kidney.

My third case was a 47-year-old man whose symptoms began in December 1930 with fatigability and lack of appetite. Then mild edema was noted, with moderately severe albuminuria, in February 1931. His private physician assured me that his blood pressure had been around 120–130 systolic until the end of April 1931, when his edema became more pronounced and his abdomen began to show a marked swelling. The diagnosis of his physician was ascites. The diaphragm was pushed up by the ascites, and the patient complained of shortness of breath. His blood pressure was now in the neighborhood of 140 systolic. The family physician said that all this time there was heavy albuminuria but no hematuria microscopically. He entered the hospital on May 5, 1931, with an enormous ascites and dyspnea. In addition there was pitting edema of the legs. His phenolsulphonphthalein output in two hours was 55 per cent. Urine examinations showed a specific gravity of 1.030–1.040. There was 3–4 per cent of albumin in the urine. Some urine specimens showed no red cells on microscopic examination. Some showed a "few red blood cells." Red blood cells were more frequently absent than present in quantities designated as "few." There were an increased number of white blood cells in the urine at all times. There were many hyaline and granular casts at all times. The blood non-protein nitrogen was normal until

*Endothelial and epithelial cell proliferation are the accepted histological criteria of glomerular nephritis!

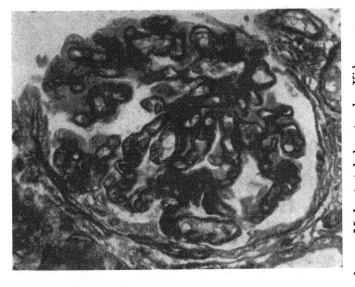

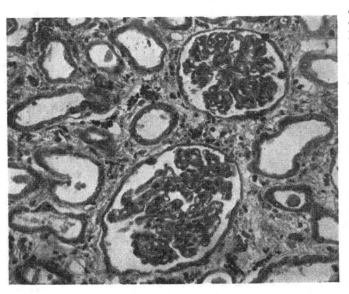

FIGURE 3 (left). Case 3. Two glomeruli with thick basement membranes. Moderate tubular atrophy. Kidneys were macroscopically large and smooth. FIGURE 4 (right). Case 3. Another glomerulus, under higher magnification. Capillary narrowing from basement membrane thickening, but many capillaries not completely closed.

five days before the patient's death on August 18, 1931. It rose to 75 mg. per cent on August 13 and was 95 mg. per cent on August 18, the day of his death. In my opinion, he died of inanition. His average daily caloric intake was 400 for three months, as determined daily by the head dietitian of the hospital. His blood pressure on May 5, 1931, was 148/102, and was 162/100 on May 8. It remained in this range until shortly before his death, when it dropped to 130/80.

Figures 3 and 4 are photomicrographs of his glomeruli. They show a moderately severe degree of diffuse basement membrane thickening but no endothelial cell proliferation. There was a very moderate degree of tubular atrophy. The heart weight was normal. This is a case of pure subacute genuine nephrosis without any doubt, in which a moderate degree of hypertension developed during a period beginning about 3 months after the onset, death occurring from inanition 7 months after the onset. The rise in blood non-protein nitrogen a week before his death was probably due to the premortal body protein destruction of severe starvation as well as a moderate degree of renal insufficiency in the last few weeks of his life.

These 3 cases of "pure" chronic genuine nephrosis are as good evidence for the thesis that a "throttling of the circulation through the kidneys results in hypertension" as the experiments on animals making use of clamps on the renal arteries or veins. In the first case high blood pressure developed 4 years after the onset of nephrosis and increased throughout a period of 1 year. There was no evidence from small artery and arteriolar sclerosis of the kidney to support a diagnosis of essential hypertension. In the second case the nephrosis started at a time when the blood pressure was normal. Within 6 months hypertension developed, and it increased in the next 18 months. There was no evidence in the renal vessels to support a diagnosis of essential hypertension. In the third case, hypertension showed up 3 months after the onset of the nephrosis and increased in intensity in the next 4 months. The kidneys showed no evidence to support a diagnosis of essential hypertension.

I have, up to now, personally seen 31 cases of chronic nephrosis that will pass my very rigorous clinical definition of chronic genuine nephrosis. Therefore, 10 per cent of all my cases have developed hypertension. There are 4 other cases of mine which I have not included in the calculation of the incidence of hypertension because they have not fulfilled all the criteria necessary for rigorous proof. One case that I saw in 1923 was clinically a pure case, but he died in a small town in the western part of the state, without an autopsy, so that this evidence is lacking. His physicians said on inquiry that he developed high blood pressure and uremia before he died. One case seen in consultation would satisfy the clinical definition, but high blood pressure was present at the time I first saw him. There is, therefore, no evidence that the blood pressure was normal before the onset of nephrosis. His blood pressure was then only mildly elevated; in 2 years it became very high. Death was in uremia. Microscopic examination showed glomerular basement membrane thickening but no endothelial cell proliferation. One General Hospital case of mine showed mild hypertension on entrance. Again, proof of normal blood pressure before the onset of nephrosis is lacking. She died 2 years later in uremia. Examination of the kidneys showed basement membrane thickening and no endothelial cell proliferation. One General Hospital case showed hypertension on entrance, and the microscopic examination of the kidneys showed typical basement membrane thickening but no endothelial cell proliferation. Dr. Bell classes these 4 anatomically as lipemic nephrosis.

If these 4 cases are accepted, my material shows that at least 22 per cent of my cases of chronic genuine or lipemic nephrosis developed hypertension. On the other hand, I have no follow-up information on 16 of my patients, and there is no prospect of getting it. If we accept the 7 cases as chronic genuine nephrosis and base the calculation of the incidence of hypertension on the 15 cases which I have been able to follow, there is a 47 per cent incidence of hypertension in chronic genuine nephrosis. As the average age of the patients was about 37 years, this is more than three times higher than the incidence of hypertension in the population of this age in the country. This is, in my opinion, one more proof of the thesis that thickening of the basement membrane in chronic genuine nephrosis, causing obstruction in the kidney circulation, is a cause of the hypertension seen in chronic genuine nephrosis. If we remember that obstruction in the kidney circulation as here demonstrated would undoubtedly cause hypertension, and if we remember that there was no anatomical evidence in these kidneys to support a diagnosis of hypertension, our thesis seems very well supported.

Questions and Discussion

DR. EDGAR V. ALLEN: Do you think there is any prospect that these were patients who had genuine nephrosis and who coincidentally developed hypertension? Would you discuss this question?

DR. FAHR: I should have read my paper in entirety because I take this question up in the paper.

There is no evidence of small artery sclerosis or arteriolosclerosis in these kidneys. This is evidence that the hypertension was not present for a long period. The thickening of the basement membrane of the glomerular capillaries would without much doubt produce hypertension through the experimentally proved Bell, Goldblatt mechanism of obstructing the flow through the blood vessels of the kidney. When primary hypertension brings on renal insufficiency and uremia rapidly, we get the picture that Dr. Bell showed this morning of the necrosis and the endarteritis of the small arteries and the arterioles. There was none of that in these cases.

Moreover, the incidence of hypertension in genuine nephrosis is greater than in the same age group of the population.

· · · · · · · · · · · · · · · · · · · *by* HERBERT CHASIS

Renal Hemodynamics in Essential Hypertension

THE pattern of alteration in the renal circulation is fairly typical in the majority of patients with hypertensive disease and consists in a decrease in the renal blood flow, a diminished capacity of the tubules to remove diodrast and p-aminohippurate from the postglomerular blood, an eventual decrease in the rate of glomerular filtration, an increase in the fraction of plasma filtered at the glomerulus, an increase in renal resistance, a decrease in the renal fraction of the cardiac output, and a normal renal oxygen arterial-venous difference. In some hypertensive patients the renal circulation and function are in the normal statistical range as measured by our present methods, and the temporal relationship between the onset of essential hypertension and the first change in renal hemodynamics is unknown.

Data obtained from normal subjects and hypertensive patients by clearance, saturation, and titration techniques have for the most part supplied the basis for this description of the pattern of disturbance in the renal circulation and function in essential hypertension (20, 13, 21). More recently, the validity of the clearance technique as a measure of the renal blood flow in essential hypertension has been established by Bradley *et al.* (5), Reubi and Schroeder (17), and Cargill (6), who found that the PAH renal extraction ratio is well maintained except in patients with advanced renal injury. It is safe to assume, therefore, that if the diodrast or PAH clearance is about 300 cc. per minute or more, it represents a dependable measurement of the renal plasma flow.

The renal blood flow, as measured by diodrast (C_D) and p-aminohippurate (C_{PAH}) clearances, and the maximal tubular excretory capacity (Tm_D or Tm_{PAH}) are occasionally in the normal range in some hypertensive patients, but in the large majority there is moderate to marked reduction. The glomerular filtration rate as measured by the inulin clearance (C_{IN}), however, is frequently in the normal range and tends

227

to stay in the lower range of normal until there is marked reduction in Tm_D.

Since there are variations in the amount of functional renal tissue in different hypertensive patients as well as variations in the same patient in different phases of the disease, it is important to relate changes in the renal circulation and function to a standard quantitative measurement of the amount of functioning renal tissue such as Tm. In presenting observations on the renal hemodynamic pattern in hypertensive patients, we (13) therefore related changes in the renal blood flow and filtration rate to tubular excretory capacity. The distribution of the C_D/Tm_D ratio in 60 hypertensive patients when plotted against a background of our data obtained in normal subjects revealed a preponderant distribution below the mean normal value, a result indicating that some factor in these hypertensive patients was causing relative ischemia of the residual functional tissue. When the filtration rate was related to Tm_D we observed that this ratio exceeded the mean normal value in about 75 per cent of the 60 patients. We are unable to determine whether an increased mean arterial pressure or the formation of impotent nephrons—that is, nephrons that have lost their excretory power but continue to serve as conduits conveying glomerular filtrate to the urine—accounts for the maintenance of the relatively high filtration rate. Whichever is the cause, the result upon the blood flow to the residual functional tissue will be the same, since both will produce apparent hyperemia in this tissue. A patient with an abnormally high value for C_{IN}/Tm_D may therefore be expected to have a high blood flow per Tm_D ratio, and when we deleted such patients from the analysis, over 90 per cent of the remaining 39 subjects had a C_D/Tm_D ratio below and some far below the mean normal value. This finding again indicated that there is a mechanism operating in patients with hypertensive disease which produces relative ischemia in the kidneys.

Examination of the filtration fraction (C_{IN}/C_D) in patients with hypertension revealed an abnormal elevation in the majority of patients. The elevation in some patients was excessively high relative to the behavior of the normal kidney during the action of adrenalin, a result to be expected if there exist in these patients impotent nephrons or if the filtration rate in some nephrons is increased by an elevated glomerular pressure. The deletion of those patients with excessively high C_{IN}/Tm_D ratios indicated that in the remaining hypertensive patients there was an abnormal elevation of the filtration fraction, quantitatively similar to the normal kidney's response to adrenalin, a drug that acts predominantly by changing the caliber of the vascular channels of the kidney. This abnormal elevation of the filtration fraction led us to conclude that in hypertensive disease there is from moderate to severe arteriolar constriction. We suggested that this change in the renal circulation might represent the renal component of the generalized vasoconstriction believed to be responsible for the increased total effective peripheral resistance observed in patients with essential hypertension. Since all these patients had an abnormally elevated mean systemic blood pressure, it is suggested that the cause of the relative ischemia to the residual functional tissue is an increase in the resistance to perfusion offered locally in the kidney.

The total renal resistance in normal subjects and in patients with essential hypertension has been calculated by Gomez (14) as the effective perfusion pressure divided by the blood flow:

$$R = \frac{Pm - Pv}{Q} \times 1328$$

where R = total renal resistance (dynes sec. cm.$^{-5}$); Pm = mean arterial pressure (mm. Hg); Pv = renal venous pressure (mm. Hg); and Q = renal blood flow (cc/sec). The factor 1328 serves to convert blood pressure units into absolute units of resistance. This equation yields the total renal resistance, R, through the clinically determinable values Pm, Pv, and Q. The average value of 22 normal subjects was calculated to be 6281 dynes sec. cm.$^{-5}$ as compared with an average value in 16 hypertensive patients of 16,720 dynes sec. cm.$^{-5}$. This increase in the total renal resistance by 166 per cent confirms and quantitates the conclusion drawn from data obtained by indirect methods that the kidney participates in the generalized increase in systemic vascular resistance in hypertensive disease.

In the original mathematical treatment of renal resistance, we (19) made certain assumptions that are now questioned: namely, that filtration equilibrium is necessarily reached in the glomerulus and that filtration pressure in the glomerular capillaries is opposed only by interstitial and oncotic pressures, the opposition of the renal venous pressure having been neglected. Lamport also assumed that filtration equilibrium is reached in the glomerulus when he calculated that the afferent constriction outweighed the efferent arteriolar constriction in 17 patients with essential hypertension (15). Smith (18) cites Gomez (14), who has reworked the original data and added observations by Bolomey et al. (3). The total renal resistance is here calculated as being equal to the sum of the afferent arteriolar, efferent arteriolar, and venular resistances, which Gomez defines and for the calculation of which he gives formulas. Hemodynamic theory does not permit calculation of the local resistance of the glomerular and peritubular capillaries as individual segments, but their absolute contribution to resistance is believed to be small compared to that of the afferent and efferent arterioles and venules because of the relatively large number of these capillaries. Gomez calculated the afferent and efferent arteriolar and venular resistances in a group of 16 patients with essential hypertension, who were not in congestive heart failure and in all of whom the glomerular filtration rate was above 60 cc. per minute and the renal plasma flow above 250 cc. per minute. He found that the average value for all 16 patients was greater for each of these three resistances than the values for the normal control group. The afferent arteriolar resistance was consistently increased and represented the largest portion of the increase in the total renal resistance. Although some of these 16 patients had elevated filtration fractions, the average for the group was 22.8 per cent, only slightly higher than the value for the average of his normal subjects of 20.3 per cent. This selected group, then, differs from the mixed group of hypertensive patients reported by Goldring et al. (13), in which the filtration fraction was increased more frequently and to a greater degree.

It seems safe to assume that the total renal resistance is abnormally increased in essential hypertension, but the secondary problem of the individual contribution of each intrarenal segment to the total apparently requires an extension of methods to supply direct quantitative data on such important gaps in our knowledge as glomerular pressure and permeability. At the present time it appears that the increase in the renal resistance is due to increases in the resistance offered by all segments and that the major contribution is made by the afferent arteriole. The combination of afferent arteriolar vasoconstriction and increased mean arterial pressure results in a sort of physical resetting of the glomerular circulation. The increased tone of the efferent arteriole then acts to increase the glomerular pressure and accounts for the increased filtration fraction observed in patients with hypertensive disease, assuming that glomerular permeability remains unchanged.

The cause of the increased renal resistance in essential hypertension is unknown. It seems unlikely that the resistance is increased by structural obstructive lesions. Bell (2) found that over 20 per cent of hypertensive patients who died showed no structural change in the arterioles and no greater involvement of the large and small renal arteries than did non-hypertensive controls of corresponding age. That the increase in resistance is due at least in some part to a reversible process such as an increased renal arteriolar tonus is indicated by the fact that we were able to increase the renal blood flow and lower the filtration fraction by agents which produced these effects in the normal kidney (13). That this hypertonus is not of neurogenic origin is suggested by the fact that surgical renal denervation fails in general to increase the renal blood flow or lower the filtration fraction in hypertensive patients (1, 9, 10, 23, 11).

However, a neurogenic component cannot be excluded on the evidence at present since we cannot be certain of complete renal denervation. The anticipated hypersensitivity to adrenalin which follows when the smooth muscle of an arteriolar wall is deprived of its nerve supply was not demonstrated shortly after unilateral sympathectomy in hypertensive patients (12). The reduction in the renal blood flow following the administration of adrenalin was no greater in the sympathectomized kidney than in the control unoperated kidney, a fact that suggests the possibility that unilateral lumbodorsal sympathectomy does not completely denervate the kidney. But even if we could denervate successfully, resultant changes in the renal circulation might be obscured by assumption of autonomous control, since the kidneys in hypertensive patients may retain the same autonomy of their circulation which characterizes the normal kidney (22).

At this time it seems likely that one or more humoral vasoconstrictor agents are present in patients with essential hypertension that are primarily responsible for the increase in the renal resistance, although their identity, nature, and mode of activity remains to be described. It is realized that the possibility of a local vascular defect has not been excluded as the cause of the increased resistance.

In normal subjects the kidneys receive somewhere between 15 and 20 per cent of the cardiac output. The data of Bolomey et al. (3) show that the renal fraction of the cardiac output is reduced to 2 per cent or less in patients with advanced hypertensive disease, a fact indicating that the cardiac output does not decrease as the renal circulation is progressively impaired.

Cargill and Hickam (7) found the renal oxygen arterial-venous difference to be within the normal range in hypertensive patients whose renal blood flow ranged from 1237 to 212 cc. per minute, oxygen consumption decreasing at the same rate as the renal blood flow was reduced. Smith (18) interprets this finding as indicating that residual functional renal tissue presumably metabolizes at the normal rate and that the defunct tissue is in effect metabolically nonexistent. In 4 patients with established hypertension Cargill and Hickam found the renal blood flow and oxygen consumption normal, a finding suggesting that in these patients total renal metabolic activities were being carried on at the normal level.

The changes in the renal circulation and function which have been discussed so far were based on observations of the combined activity of both kidneys. Observations which were made to determine the extent of these changes in each kidney by means of ureteral catheterization revealed that the decrease in the renal blood flow and maximal tubular excretory capacity was shared equally by the two kidneys and that the C_D/Tm_D ratios were similar in the two kidneys (8). These results indicate that the impairment of the renal circulation and function progresses equally in the two kidneys in hypertensive disease. The fact that these changes proceed to an equal degree and at a parallel rate in both kidneys is evidence for the thesis that renal injury is a sequela of hypertensive disease and evidence against the thesis that renal vascular disease is primary in the genesis of hypertension.

Changes in the renal circulation and function can be explained in part on the basis of physiological and anatomical alterations that occur in the course of essential hypertension. An increase in the mean systemic blood pressure and arteriolar constriction tend to maintain the rate of glomerular filtration in the normal range; variations in the filtration rate in this stage may be expected, since blood pressure levels and arteriolar tone are labile. A decrease in the filtration rate occurs as the disease progresses because the glomerular filtering bed is progressively obliterated as a result of irreversible organic vascular changes. If there are changes in glomerular permeability, we cannot at this time evaluate quantitatively their result on effective filtration pressures. Our data indicate that the decrease in the renal blood flow observed early in the disease is due to an increased arteriolar tone and later on to the obliteration of vascular channels.

The maintenance of maximal tubular reabsorptive capacity for glucose (Tm_G) indicates no specific impairment of tubular reabsorption of glucose. When Tm_G is reduced late in the course of the disease, the C_{IN}/Tm_G ratio remains in the normal range, a fact indicating that Tm_G is reduced only when the glomerulus of a nephron is obliterated by vascular changes and its appertaining tubule is cut off from reabsorptive activity. The decrease in tubular excretory capacity for diodrast and PAH under conditions of saturation observed early in the course of the disease appears to be due to the impairment of a specific tubular function and may represent a change in the metabolic activity of the tubular cells. We think it improbable that the reduction in Tm_D observed early in the course of the disease is a manifestation of ischemic injury due to obliterative arteriolar lesions, because of the high C_{IN}/Tm_D and normal C_D/Tm_D ratios observed in some subjects with only moderate renal injury. We believe that early decreases in Tm_D are due to loss of specific function rather than to tubular obstruction or obliteration because of the tendency of the C_{IN}/Tm_D ratio to rise to supernormal levels, and this interpretation is supported by the fact that Tm_G does not decrease in proportion to Tm_D. The cause of the impairment of tubular excretion of diodrast and PAH is unknown. The moderate and marked decreases in tubular excretory capacity observed later in the course are a manifestation of severe tubular injury as well as of a progressive decrease in the number of functioning nephrons.

The degree of renal hyperemia induced by the administration of pyrogen in hypertensive patients is comparable to that observed in normal subjects (13). The level of Tm_D during hyperemia so induced has special significance, since tubules which are ischemic under basal conditions might become active. A particular tubule will contribute to Tm_D at a maximal rate only so long as the plasma flow to the tubule is adequate to effect saturation at the existing diodrast plasma concentration. Detecting ischemic tubules by Tm_D, then, is dependent on the plasma concentration of diodrast in the sense that the higher the concentration the lower the blood flow must be to ischemic tissue before the latter will cease to contribute to Tm_D. Smith (18) defines the load of diodrast carried to the tubules as the product of plasma flow times plasma concentration minus the quantity of diodrast excreted through the glomeruli. In our observations on hypertensive patients (13) the load/Tm_D ratio was with few exceptions greater during hyperemia than during basal conditions, a circumstance that would operate to effect the saturation of tubules which might have been unsaturated as a result of ischemia during the basal state. A comparison between Tm_D measured under basal conditions and during hyperemia revealed no significant increase in the majority of hypertensive patients. In some patients, however, there was an increase in Tm_D by more than 10 per cent, indicating that portions of the renal parenchyma capable of excreting diodrast were not available to perfusion under basal conditions. The presence of focal ischemic areas in an occasional hypertensive patient has also been indicated in an analysis of our data obtained by glucose and diodrast titration methods (21). We suggested that although arterial lesions may affect large numbers of glomeruli adversely, tubular perfusion is usually maintained uniformly and focal tubular ischemia is the exception rather than the rule. Bradley (4) believes that since PAH extraction is high, true arteriovenous shunting must be excluded as a possible cause of localized ischemia and that focal ischemia results from the development of structural lesions.

Observations in the experimental animal indicating an ability to divert blood from the cortex to the juxtamedullary region of the kidney have led to the suggestion that such a mechanism might operate in man to produce cortical ischemia and be concerned in the genesis of essential hypertension (24). But Maxwell et al. (16) reviewed the significance of the renal juxtamedullary circulation and concluded that there is no positive evidence at hand of the diversion of any appreciable quantity of blood through uncleared channels in man or dog. A large shunt from cortex to medulla would tend to arterialize the renal venous blood, but that this does not occur is demonstrated by the fact that the PAH extraction ratio is normal until hypertensive disease is far advanced and by the fact that the renal oxygen arterial-venous difference does not vary significantly from the normal. This failure to obtain evidence of arterialization of the renal venous blood, the presence of a normal renal circulation in some hypertensive patients, and the demonstration that no large amount of functioning renal parenchyma capable of excreting diodrast is deprived of blood lead us to conclude that a juxtamedullary shunt is not involved in the genesis of hypertensive disease.

It has been suggested that the alteration in renal hemodynamics is causally related to the genesis of hypertensive disease. Even if it were admitted that this is so, it would have to be recognized that the functional or structural renal vascular disease which would neces-sarily precede the changes in the renal circulation would itself remain unexplained. Our data supply three pieces of evidence against this view. The failure to demonstrate changes in the renal circulation early in hypertensive disease, the fact that with the progress of the disease there is an accompanying deterioration in the renal circulation explained satisfactorily by the decrease in the number of vascular channels and functioning nephrons, and the fact that the changes in the renal circulation proceed to an equal degree and at a parallel rate in the two kidneys have led us to conclude that the change in renal hemodynamics is a sequela rather than the cause of essential hyper-tension.

Questions and Discussion

DR. MAURICE B. VISSCHER: Dr. Chasis has presented a beautiful account of the type of study that every physiologist is pleased to see. He has pointed out that there is, with the progress of the disease, a proportionately greater increase in resistance in the vascular bed in the kidney than in other organs of the body in hypertension. He suggests that this progressively increasing resistance in the vascular bed may be accounted for on the basis of the structural changes that take place in the renal blood vessels with the progression of the disease. I should like to ask him to elaborate a little more on the question of positive proof that the differential increase in resistance in the renal bed versus other beds is on a morphological basis rather than on the basis of some physiological susceptibility of the renal blood vessels to a circulating vasoconstricting agent, as compared with other blood vessel beds.

Now if you will recall what Dr. Kubicek said yesterday concerning the renal blood flow in dogs with elevated blood pressures produced by chronic electrical stimulation of the renal pedicle nerves or the sympathetic trunk nerves, you will recall that the early effect of such stimulation was a decrease in the renal plasma flow, but that after hypertension became established the renal plasma flow rose to normal. I make the suggestion that there may be homeostatic mechanisms so arranged that the blood pressure will be raised to a point where the renal blood flow is restored to a value providing adequate pressure for glomerular filtration to maintain the animal in a constant state.

I am inclined to the view that we cannot exclude the possibility that small changes in the renal blood flow due to a circulating vasoconstricting agent could bring about the elaboration within the kidney of the same sort of substances that are liberated early after the application of the Goldblatt clamp.

I do not believe we are justified in assuming that there must be a very large decrease in the renal blood flow maintained over 24 hours if these vasoactive substances are to be liberated from the kidney. A relatively small decrease in the blood flow, which might be difficult to pick up in a chronic situation, could accomplish such effects, it seems to me.

But I should like to have Dr. Chasis, if he will, elaborate a little further on the question I have raised.

DR. ELEXIOUS T. BELL: I am quite sure that Dr. Visscher misunderstood Dr. Chasis. In fact, Dr. Chasis said quite the opposite of what he was quoted to have said. He is on my side of this argument, and I should not like to have him as an opponent.

I want to call attention to some of the things Dr. Chasis said. I think he has made one of the most important contributions that we have ever had to the pathological physiology of hypertension.

He has shown that there is decreased blood flow and increased renal resistance in certain stages of hypertension. But under the influence of pyrogens the blood flow will return temporarily to normal. That is, these vessels will dilate. They dilate under the influence of pyrogens. Now it is much easier to think of a normal arteriole dilating than one that is rigid with hyalin. It is quite hard to think of a rigid hyalin arteriole responding in that way. I think this is an excellent argument that hypertension is initiated by spastic and not by organic changes in the vessels.

DR. ROBERT W. WILKINS: One always hesitates to draw any conclusions from one case. However, we have had an opportunity to study thoroughly a case of pheochromocytoma in a young man of 24 with symptoms of approximately 4 years' duration. He had what we termed an "intermittent normotension" rather than an intermittent hypertension. By that we meant that his blood pressure was only rarely normal and usually was elevated at quite high levels. Because we were positive of the diagnosis, or as positive as we could be before operation, we subjected him to rather elaborate physiologic studies, including the techniques of Drs. Chasis, Goldring, and Smith.

We were interested to find that this young man, whose hypertension was due to pheochromocytoma (since it was completely relieved by operation), had the typical renal hemodynamic changes of essential hypertension, with a moderately reduced renal blood flow and an increased filtration fraction. By taking renal venous samples, we also showed that there was no shunting of blood past functioning tissue in the kidney, since the extraction of PAH was virtually complete, both before and after the removal of the tumor.

Therefore, we were quite hopeful that this patient would show us how the kidney responds to the relief of intermittent hypertension of some standing. Dr. Reginald H. Smithwick removed a pheochromocytoma and also took a renal biopsy. The kidney showed definite, though mild, morphologic changes in the prearterioles, the arterioles, and the glomeruli themselves, on which the pathologist was unwilling to commit himself finally.

When we retested his renal clearances 6 months and again 18 months after the removal of this tumor, during which time the patient's pressure had remained normal, we found to our disappointment, but great interest, that the blood flow and filtration rate were just about what they had been before the removal of the tumor. However, the calculated resistance through the kidney, of course, was greatly decreased since his arterial pressure was normal.

We thought these findings might be explained by the side of the argument that you have heard upheld this morning, namely, that while this man had certain functional disturbances in his kidney due to the circulating epinephrine, norepinephrine, or whatever pressor substances were present before operation, he had in addition, certain morphologic abnormalities visible under the microscope. These structural abnormalities we believed were due to the long-lasting hypertension and, in turn, caused further functional defects that were not reversible; at least, 18 months after operation they were still manifested by a moderately increased resistance to blood flow in the kidney and an increased filtration fraction. It will be of interest to test him again in 2 years.

What this all means with respect to essential hypertension is not completely clear, but it does suggest that long continued periods of even intermittent hypertension may cause structural and functional changes which are only slowly reversible, if reversible at all.

DR. MARK NICKERSON: In the preface to his remarks Dr. Chasis mentioned that the line between the conceptions of kidney changes as primary or secondary in essential hypertension was clearly drawn and that he was on the secondary side. I feel that this line should not exclude a synthesis of these two points of view. Perhaps there is a close relationship between the evidence which indicates that the kidney is the culprit in the development of essential hypertension and that which depicts it as the victim. Data are gradually accumulating, although obviously they are far from complete, indicating that the kidney may be first the victim and later the culprit in the same case. Dr. Wilkins' case of pheochromocytoma is an interesting and valuable addition to this evidence. In such cases it appears to be quite possible that intermittent periods of an increased blood pressure and renal vasoconstriction may induce lasting changes in renal structure or function so that the kidney may then be an etiological factor in the maintenance of the elevated blood pressure.

Those of you who were here last night will recall Dr. Braun-Menendez's statement which very nicely summarizes this idea. He pointed out that the kidney is undeniably involved in a great many cases of hypertension, both human and experimental. Some people feel that it is the culprit, others that it is the victim, but whatever its initial role may be, it has a great propensity to join the gang.

DR. CHASIS: Dr. Allen is bigger than I am and wields a big stick, so in attempting to keep within the time allotted me, I read my paper much too fast. That probably explains why Dr. Visscher misunderstood what I said. We believe that the increase in renal resistance in hypertensive disease is functional and not anatomical. When we administered pyrogenic inulin or triple typhoid vaccine, the renal blood flow increased and the filtration fraction decreased in hypertensive patients as it did in normal subjects.

It is probable that as the disease progresses and the vascular lesions result in obliteration of the filtering bed, both functional and anatomical factors contribute, but the early and significant increase in renal resistance is a functional and reversible manifestation of hypertensive disease.

· · · · · · · · · · · · · · *by* BENJAMIN J. CLAWSON

The Heart in Essential Hypertension

THE cardiac deaths due to hypertension and coronary disease as determined by 50,730 autopsies from the records in the Department of Pathology of the University of Minnesota (1910–1947) are here being reported on. This large group (6512 cases) of diseases of the heart is commonly referred to as arteriosclerotic heart disease. There is some objection to this terminology in the hypertensive cases, where death is not due primarily to coronary disease since in this group the coronary arteries are relatively good in a high percentage of the cases. We agree with Levine (1) that this term should be given up. These cardiac cases are analyzed with respect to general incidence, incidence by types, incidence by age and sex, and gross and microscopic pathological findings.

General incidence. The total group of 6512 cases comprises 12.83 per cent of the deaths in the autopsy series during 1910–1947. The group is 66.89 per cent of the 9585 deaths from noncongenital cardiac disease.

Incidence by types. In this analysis the total number of cases are divided into two groups: (1) hypertensive heart disease in which death was primarily due to or associated with congestive heart failure, cerebral hemorrhage, or uremia and (2) coronary disease where death resulted chiefly from coronary insufficiency (Tables 1 and 2). As will be observed, the two groups overlap considerably. In about a fourth of the coronary cases no evidences of hypertension were noted. These cases, however, were included in the analysis because of the close relationship between coronary disease and hypertension.

The incidence of the types in the hypertensive group is noted in Table 1. This is the largest group among all cardiac deaths. There were 5935 cases among 9585 cardiac deaths (61.91 per cent) and among the 50,730 autopsies (11.69 per cent).

Depending upon the primary cause of death, this hypertensive

TABLE 1. Types of Hypertensive Heart Disease (5935 Cases) among 9585 Cardiac Deaths and among 50,730 Autopsies during the Years 1910–1947

Types	No. of Cases	Per Cent of Group	Per Cent of Cardiac Deaths	Per Cent of Autopsies
Myocardial insufficiency 2221		37.42	23.17	4.37
Coronary sclerosis 2507		42.24	26.15	4.93
Cerebral hemorrhage 847		14.27	8.83	1.66
Uremia 360		6.06	3.75	0.71
All types 5935		99.99	61.91	11.69

TABLE 2. Types of Coronary Sclerosis (3084 Cases) among 9585 Cardiac Deaths and among 50,730 Autopsies during the Years 1910–1947

Types	No. of Cases	Per Cent of Group	Per Cent of Cardiac Deaths	Per Cent of Autopsies
With hypertension 2507*		81.29	26.15	4.93
Systolic blood pressure 150 or over	877			
Systolic blood pressure unknown or below 150; male heart weight above 400 gm., female above 350 gm.	1630			
Without hypertension 577		18.7	6.01	1.13
Both types 3084		100.00	32.17	6.07

*Included in the hypertensive group.

group is divided into four types: myocardial insufficiency, coronary sclerosis, cerebral hemorrhage, and uremia (Table 1).

There were 2221 cases of myocardial insufficiency (37.42 per cent) among the hypertensive group, 23.17 per cent of all cardiac deaths, and 4.37 per cent of all autopsies (not including stillbirths). These 2221 cases, with a few exceptions, were classified as hypertensive hearts either because a systolic blood pressure of 150 mm. Hg or more was recorded or because even though there was a recorded normal blood pressure, the male hearts weighed 500 gm. or more and the female hearts 450 gm. or more. It is this latter group, in which the blood pressure is recorded as normal or below, that is often referred to as showing adult idiopathic cardiac hypertrophy. Of these 2221 cases, where death was practically always associated with left and right heart failure, there were 219 (8.86 per cent) in which the systolic blood pressure recorded was always below 150 mm. Hg. In all of these 219 cases the hearts were large, 500 gm. or more in the males and 450 gm. or more in the females.

There has been a great deal of discussion among internists and pathologists whether the hypertrophy and final failure are caused by high blood pressure at some time or by some other cause as yet unknown. In 1944 Levy and Von Glahn (2) reported 10 cases and stated that previously there had been only 14 such cases reported in the literature. In 4 of Levy and Von Glahn's 10 cases there was a systolic blood pressure of 150 mm. Hg or more, with a diastolic pressure of from 90 to 110. In 3 other cases with a systolic blood pressure below 150 there were diastolic pressures of 90, 90, and 105 respectively. Hearts of this type have been intensively studied. Apparently all of them begin with left ventricular hypertrophy and end with dilatation. The stigma of a high blood pressure (high diastolic pressure of from 90 to 115 mm. Hg) was present in 98 of the 219 cases (44.74 per cent). The remaining 121 cases are 5.44 per cent of the 2221 in which death resulted from myocardial insufficiency. It seems fairly reasonable to regard most of this so-called idiopathic group as hypertensive cases in which the systolic blood pressure has temporarily dropped or as cases which are in some way tied up with hypertension. White (3) in discussing cardiac enlargement emphasizes the importance of strain as the cause of hypertrophy. There are relatively few hearts in which the cause of the enlargement and failure is not apparent. The small percentage in which the cause is not known need further study to determine whether the cardiac enlargement is due to muscular hypertrophy, to diffuse fibrosis, or to some other condition.

The second type of hypertensive cardiac disease is that in which death resulted primarily from coronary sclerosis with or without coronary thrombosis. About 75 per cent of all coronary arterial deaths gave evidence of hypertension. There were 2507 cases of coronary sclerosis with hypertension (42.24 per cent of the entire hypertensive cardiac group, 26.15 per cent of all cardiac deaths, and 4.93 per cent of all autopsies).

The third type of hypertensive cardiac disease is made up of the cases in which death was finally caused by cerebral hemorrhage. In most of these there were evidences of cardiac failure both clinically and at autopsy. Death would evidently have resulted from cardiac failure in most of these had life not been terminated by the cerebral hemorrhage. Of this type there were 847 cases (14.27 per cent of the hypertensive cardiac group, 8.83 per cent of all cardiac deaths, and 1.66 per cent of all autopsies). These cases either had a history of a systolic blood pressure of 150 mm. Hg or more or, among the males, had hearts weighing 500 gm. or more and, among the females, 450 gm. or more. It is possible, if not probable, that some other cases in the autopsy series where death was from cerebral hemorrhage should have been included in this type.

Death from renal insufficiency associated with and resulting from hypertension is the fourth type. Clinically symptoms of myocardial failure were commonly present, but all of these finally died from uremia. As with the apoplectic type, there was either a recorded history of a systolic blood pressure of 150 mm. Hg or more or, among the males, hearts of 500 gm. or more and, among the females, of 450 gm. or more. Of this renal type there were 360 cases (6.06 per cent of the hypertensive group, 3.75 per cent of the cardiac deaths, and 0.71 per cent of the autopsies).

In the total group of 6512 cases there were 3084 in which death was due in the end to coronary sclerosis with or without coronary thrombosis (Table 2). Of these 2507 were included in the hypertensive group because of the recorded high blood pressure or weight of the heart (males 400 gm. or more and females 350 gm. or more). In 577 cases (18.7 per cent) of the 3084 it appeared that there probably had not been hypertension (Table 2). It is likely that this percentage should be somewhat higher since a few in the lower brackets with hearts, among the males, of 400–450 gm. and, among the females, of 350–400 gm. probably were not hypertensive cases. It appears reasonable to conclude that about 75 per cent of the people who died from coronary disease had high blood pressure. The total group of coronary cases comprised 32.17 per cent of the 9585 noncongenital cardiac deaths and 6.07 per cent of the 50,730 autopsies.

Incidence by age and sex. In the entire number of 6512 cases most of the deaths in both sexes occurred in the fourth through the ninth decades (Table 3). The sex differences are seen in Table 4. There was no significant sex difference in the type in which death was due to cardiac failure in any of the decades except the eighth, in which the females predominated. There was a total of 44.87 males and 41.82 females per thousand autopsies on the respective sexes, a ratio of 1.07 males to 1 female. This difference was on the borderline of significance.

In the type in which death was primarily caused by coronary disease the males predominated significantly in the fourth, fifth, sixth, and seventh decades (Table 5). The number of females was greater in the eighth, ninth, and tenth decades, but this difference was not a significant one. The total number of males was significantly greater than that of the females per thousand autopsies on the respective

TABLE 8. The Incidence of Death by Age Decade among Hypertensive Cases of 4 Types (Divided according to the Cause of Death) and Non-Hypertensive Cases of Coronary Sclerosis

Age Decade	Myocardial Failure (2221)		Coronary Sclerosis (2507)		Cerebral Hemorrhage (847)		Uremia (360)		Non-Hypertensive Coronary Sclerosis (577)	
	M (1459)	F (762)	M (1900)	F (607)	M (509)	F (338)	M (217)	F (143)	M (493)	F (84)
1	0.0%	0.0%	0.0%	0.0%	0.0%	0.0%	0.0%	0.0%	0.0%	0.0%
2	0.0	0.0	0.0	0.0	0.0	0.9	1.4	2.1	0.0	0.0
3	0.4	0.1	0.1	0.0	1.4	1.5	1.8	4.9	1.2	0.0
4	2.6	3.8	1.5	0.7	3.9	4.1	7.8	20.3	7.1	1.2
5	10.4	10.5	12.7	2.0	13.4	20.4	23.0	25.9	20.5	13.1
6	25.2	19.5	26.1	14.7	32.0	23.4	31.3	16.8	24.5	17.9
7	28.1	27.2	31.4	31.5	27.1	27.8	23.0	18.2	21.1	20.2
8	23.5	27.8	21.4	37.7	19.4	16.0	10.1	7.7	17.7	30.9
9	9.1	10.7	6.5	12.1	2.7	5.3	1.4	3.5	7.1	15.5
10	0.6	0.4	0.2	1.1	0.0	0.6	0.0	0.6	0.8	1.2

243

TABLE 4. The Incidence of Death by Sex and by Age Decade among 2221 Hypertensive Cases of Myocardial Failure, as Determined per Thousand Autopsies

Age Decade	Males (1459)			Females (762)		
	Total No. of Autopsies	No. of Cases	Cases per Thousand	Total No. of Autopsies	No. of Cases	Cases per Thousand
1	4293	0	0.00	3123	0	0.00
2	941	0	0.00	811	0	0.00
3	1819	6	3.29	1609	2	1.24
4	2831	39	13.77	1877	29	15.45
5	4498	152	33.79	2207	80	36.24
6	5934	368	62.01	2597	149	57.37
7	6064	409	67.44	2718	206	75.78
8	4518	343	75.91 *	2330	212	90.98 *
9	1521	133	87.44	867	81	93.42
10	94	9	95.74	77	3	38.96
11	0	0	0.00	1	0	0.00
All decades ...32,513		1459	44.87	18,217	762	41.82

* A significant difference.

TABLE 5. The Incidence of Death by Sex and by Age Decade among 2507 Hypertensive Cases of Coronary Sclerosis, as Determined per Thousand Autopsies

Age Decade	Males (1900)			Females (607)		
	Total No. of Autopsies	No. of Cases	Cases per Thousand	Total No. of Autopsies	No. of Cases	Cases per Thousand
1	4293	0	0.00	3123	0	0.00
2	941	0	0.00	811	2	2.46
3	1819	2	1.09	1609	0	0.00
4	2831	28	9.89 *	1877	4	2.13 *
5	4498	242	53.80 *	2207	12	5.43 *
6	5934	496	83.58 *	2597	89	34.27 *
7	6064	596	98.28 *	2718	191	70.27 *
8	4518	408	90.30	2330	229	98.28
9	1521	124	81.52	867	73	84.19
10	94	4	42.55	77	7	90.90
11	0	0	0.00	1	0	0.00
All decades ...32,513		1900	58.43 *	18,217	607	33.32 *

* A significant difference.

sexes (58.43 males and 33.32 females). This is a ratio of 1.7 males to 1 female among the 2507 deaths from coronary sclerosis with hypertension.

In the type of hypertension where death was due to cerebral hemorrhage the females predominated significantly in the fifth, seventh, and ninth decades (Table 6). The total number of males and females per thousand autopsies on the respective sexes was also significantly different (15.65 males and 18.55 females). Evidently

TABLE 6. The Incidence of Death by Sex and by Age Decade among 847 Hypertensive Cases of Cerebral Hemorrhage, as Determined per Thousand Autopsies

Age Decade	Males (509)			Females (338)		
	Total No. of Autopsies	No. of Cases	Cases per Thousand	Total No. of Autopsies	No. of Cases	Cases per Thousand
1	4293	0	0.00	3123	0	0.00
2	941	0	0.00	811	3	3.69
3	1819	7	3.84	1609	5	3.10
4	2831	20	7.06	1877	14	7.45
5	4498	68	15.11 *	2207	69	31.26 *
6	5934	163	27.46	2597	79	30.41
7	6064	138	22.75 *	2718	94	34.58 *
8	4518	99	21.91	2330	54	23.17
9	1521	14	9.20 *	867	18	20.76 *
10	94	0	0.00	77	2	25.97
11	0	0	0.00	1	0	0.00
All decades 32,513		509	15.65 *	18,217	338	18.55 *

* A significant difference.

TABLE 7. The Incidence of Death by Sex and by Age Decade among 360 Hypertensive Cases of Uremia, as Determined per Thousand Autopsies

Age Decade	Males (217)			Females (143)		
	Total No. of Autopsies	No. of Cases	Cases per Thousand	Total No. of Autopsies	No. of Cases	Cases per Thousand
1	4293	0	0.00	3123	0	0.00
2	941	3	3.18	811	3	3.69
3	1819	4	2.19	1609	7	4.35
4	2831	17	6.00 *	1877	29	15.45 *
5	4498	50	11.11 *	2207	37	16.76 *
6	5934	68	11.45	2597	24	9.24
7	6064	50	8.24	2718	26	9.56
8	4518	22	4.86	2330	11	4.72
9	1521	3	1.97	867	5	5.76
10	94	0	0.00	77	1	12.98
11	0	0	0.00	1	0	0.00
All decades 32,513		217	6.67	18,217	143	7.84

* A significant difference.

cerebral hemorrhage occurs more commonly in women than in men with hypertension.

In the hypertensive type in which death was finally due to uremia the females predominated significantly in the fourth and fifth decades only (Table 7). The total number of each sex per thousand autopsies (6.67 males and 7.84 females) showed no significant sex difference.

In the type of coronary sclerosis in which no evidences of hypertension were present there was a significant male preponderance in

TABLE 8. The Incidence of Death by Sex and by Age Decade among 577 Non-Hypertensive Cases of Coronary Sclerosis, as Determined per Thousand Autopsies

Age Decade	Males (493)			Females (84)		
	Total No. of Autopsies	No. of Cases	Cases per Thousand	Total No. of Autopsies	No. of Cases	Cases per Thousand
1	4293	0	0.00	3123	0	0.00
2	941	0	0.00	811	0	0.00
3	1819	6	3.29	1609	0	0.00
4	2831	35	12.36 *	1877	1	0.53 *
5	4498	101	22.45 *	2207	11	4.98 *
6	5934	121	20.39 *	2597	15	5.77 *
7	6064	104	17.15 *	2718	17	6.25 *
8	4518	87	19.25	2330	26	11.15
9	1521	35	23.01	867	13	14.99
10	94	4	42.55	77	1	12.98
11	0	0	0.00	1	0	0.00
All decades	32,513	493	15.16 *	18,217	84	4.61 *

* A significant difference.

the fourth through the seventh decades (Table 8). The total number of males greatly outnumbered that of the females per thousand autopsies on the respective sexes (15.16 males to 4.61 females). This ratio of 3.3 males to 1 female is higher than in the cases of coronary deaths where hypertension was present, and is a marked significant sex difference. One thing to be noticed in coronary cases with and without hypertension is that there does not appear to be a decade beyond which one is safe from coronary death.

Pathology. Excluding the cases in which death was due to coronary disease, the chief gross pathological changes noted in the heart in the hypertensive group were hypertrophy with dilatation, variable degrees of coronary atherosclerosis, and pericarditis in the uremic and coronary types. Coronary thrombosis and myocardial infarction in the types with death from myocardial failure, cerebral hemorrhage, or uremia were rarely found (3 per cent).

In Table 9 the degree of cardiac hypertrophy indicated by the weights of the hearts is noted in 1588 cases in which death was due to myocardial failure. It is to be observed that in a few (4.84 per cent) even with a recorded hypertension, hypertrophy did not take place. In a large majority the weights of the hearts were 500 gm. or more in the males and 450 gm. or more in the females. These large male hearts ranged from 500 gm. to an occasional one of over 1000 gm. The female hearts weighed less than the male by 50 gm. or more.

All the hearts listed in the types where death was from cerebral hemorrhage or uremia with no high blood pressure recorded weighed 500 gm. or more in the males and 450 gm. or more in the females. The weights of the hearts, indicating the degree of hypertrophy, in 3071 of the total group of 3084 coronary cases with and without hypertension are seen in Table 10. It is to be noted that 718 (23.3 per cent) have hearts weighing below 400 gm. among the males, and below 350 among the females. A few of the male hearts of 400 gm. and the

TABLE 9. The Weights of the Hearts in 1588 Cases of Hypertension (Systolic Blood Pressure 150 mm. Hg or more) in Which Death Was Due to Myocardial Failure

Heart Weight in Grams	Number	Per Cent
M 500 or more F 450 or more	1174	73.92
M 400–499 F 350–449	 337	21.22
M below 400 F below 350	 77	4.84

TABLE 10. The Weights of the Hearts in 3071 Cases of Coronary Sclerosis, with and without Hypertension

Heart Weight in Grams	Number	Per Cent
M 500 or more F 450 or more	1172	38.1
M 400–499 F 350–449	1181	38.4
M below 400 F below 350	 718	23.3

female hearts of 350 gm. or slightly over may not have been hypertrophied. It appears that in about 25 per cent of the coronary deaths cardiac hypertrophy was not present. This is an important observation to be taken into account in considering whether coronary disease is a factor in the pathogenesis of cardiac hypertrophy. Kahn and Ingraham (4) analyzed 1000 cases with prolonged hypertension and found that the weights of the hearts with moderate to marked coronary sclerosis were significantly greater than those of the hearts with little or no coronary sclerosis. In our material the hypertrophy in the hypertensive hearts with coronary sclerosis was as a rule not so great as in the hypertensive hearts where death resulted from myocardial insufficiency following hypertension.

TABLE 11. Coronary Sclerosis and Myocardial Fibrosis among 139 Cases of
Hypertensive Heart Disease of 4 Types

	Myocardial Failure (78)		Coronary Sclerosis (37)		Cerebral Hemorrhage (16)		Uremia (8)	
	No.	Per Cent	No.	Per Cent	No.	Per Cent	No.	Per Cent
Coronary sclerosis								
Severe 12		15.5	37	100.0	6	37.5	1	12.5
Slight 54		69.0	0	0.0	8	50.0	5	62.5
None 12		15.5	0	0.0	2	12.5	2	25.0
Myocardial fibrosis								
Severe 2		2.5	18	48.5	0	0.0	0	0.0
Slight 35		45.0	17	46.0	6	37.5	1	12.5
None 41		52.5	2	5.5	10	62.5	7	87.5

Gross and microscopic myocardial fibrosis in its relation to the
degree of sclerosis in the coronary arteries is recorded in Table 11.
This table shows a segment of 139 cases in which a gross examination
of each heart and microscopic examinations of 5 blocks from each heart
were studied for evidences of fibrosis. The degree of coronary sclerosis
was also noted and was found to be greatest in Group 2, or the cases
in which death followed coronary insufficiency. In the other three
types—myocardial insufficiency, cerebral hemorrhage, and uremia—
there was a relatively low percentage of severe coronary sclerosis.
Severe myocardial fibrosis was seen most commonly in the coronary
sclerotic type (48.5 per cent). In the myocardial insufficiency type,
fibrosis to a severe degree was present in only 2.5 per cent. Severe
fibrosis did not occur in the apoplectic and uremic types. The degree
of myocardial fibrosis corresponded, in general, with the degree of
coronary sclerosis. The myocardial fibrosis in all cases of hypertension
appears to be due to an anatomic narrowing of the lumen of the
coronary arteries. It is of interest to note that even in the cases in
which death resulted from coronary disease, severe myocardial fibrosis
was seen in less than half the cases.

Infarction of the myocardium is relatively rare (3 per cent) in
deaths due to hypertension except in the cases in which the final cause
of death is coronary disease. Infarction occasionally occurs in large
hearts with fairly good coronary arteries. In the cases of death from
coronary disease, infarction (43.75 per cent) occurred less frequently
than coronary thrombosis (53.84). The patients with coronary thrombosis not infrequently die before an infarction can take place. Frequently microscopic evidences of an infarct can be detected before
gross evidences are manifested. In case the patient with coronary

thrombosis does not die soon, infarction of the muscle of the heart is generally found. The infarct may heal and leave well-defined fibrous areas. The rather indefinite fibrous areas in the heart appear to be due to a slow fraying out of the muscle, with replacement by connective tissue, resulting from ischemia from coronary narrowing.

The frequency of myocardial infarction, with or without thrombosis, among 3065 cases of coronary deaths is recorded in Table 12. There

TABLE 12. The Incidence of Myocardial Infarction among 3065
Cases of Coronary Sclerosis

	Number	Per Cent
Infarction without thrombosis 367		11.97
Infarction with thrombosis 974		31.77
All cases of infarction 1341		43.75

were 974 (31.77 per cent) in which infarction occurred with coronary thrombosis and 367 (11.97 per cent) without a demonstrable thrombus. It is quite possible that in some of these the thrombus might not have been found. However, it appears evident that in some cases, at least, infarction may take place without the presence of a thrombus. Infarction was demonstrated in 1341 of the 3065 cases (43.75 per cent).

The microscopic picture of cardiac infarction depends upon the age of the infarct. In an early infarct the muscle fibers lose their striations and become hyalinized in appearance. There is a rapid infiltration with polymorphonuclear leucocytes. The appearance may approach that of the wall of an abscess. Later the polymorphonuclear leucocytes disappear and an increasing number of fibroblasts are noted. Blood pigment is commonly found. The end stage shows a scar fairly well circumscribed, differing in this respect from scattered areas of fibrosis due to atrophy of muscle fibers with connective tissue replacement. The fibrous tissue may stretch and produce a bulging cardiac aneurysm. Whether infarction or scattered areas of fibrosis occur depends upon whether the coronary arteries close slowly with muscular atrophy and connective tissue replacement or rapidly when infarction results. Myocardial fibrosis due to coronary insufficiency is, as a rule, not located immediately around the blood vessels. In this respect the fibrosis differs from that seen in rheumatic hearts, in which the fibrosis is periarterial in location.

The changes noted in the coronary arteries in cases of coronary deaths are atherosclerosis and thrombosis. The degrees of atherosclerosis in the left and right coronary arteries in 2952 cases in which

TABLE 13. The Degree of Sclerosis in the Coronary Arteries among 2952 Cases in Which Death Was Due to Coronary Disease

Degree	Number	Per Cent
Both +++ to ++++ 2114		71.61
L ++++ R ++ 396		13.41
L ++++ R + ... 163		5.52
L ++++ R 0 6		0.20
L +++ R ++ 169		5.72
L +++ R + ... 53		1.89
L +++ R 0 1		0.03
L ++ R ++ 27		0.90
L ++ R + ... 5		0.16
R ++++ L ++ 7		0.23
R ++++ L + ... 4		0.13
R +++ L ++ 5		0.16
R +++ L + ... 1		0.03
R +++ L 0 1		0.03
R ++ L + ... 0		0.00

death was due to coronary disease are shown in Table 13. The left coronary artery, generally its descending branch, is the one most commonly affected. A severe involvement of the right artery occurred in 181 of the 2952 cases (6.13 per cent). It is to be seen that death in cases with coronary atherosclerosis of less than 3 plus in one or both of the arteries is rare.

Microscopic examination of the arteries reveals atherosclerosis, diffuse or localized. This sclerosis may occur in short plaques and can be missed easily unless the arteries are cut transversely at short intervals apart. Paterson (5) found intimal hemorrhage to be a commonly observed condition. Lymphocytic infiltration in the adventitia is also common. No relation can be demonstrated between this adventitial lymphocytic infiltration and syphilis.

Thrombosis of one or both coronary arteries is a common complication of coronary sclerosis. Thrombosis without sclerosis is rare, but occasionally it may occur with infection. Coronary emboli, except small emboli as in subacute bacterial endocarditis, are seldom found.

TABLE 14. The Incidence of Thrombosis among 2851 Cases of Coronary Sclerosis

	Number	Per Cent
Left coronary artery 1073		37.63
Right coronary artery 330		11.57
Both coronary arteries 132		4.63
All cases of thrombosis 1535		53.84

Gross infarcts are not produced by these small emboli. The incidence of gross thrombosis of sufficient degree to be seen easily at autopsy or to cause clinical symptoms or sudden death is seen in Table 14. Among 2851 cases thrombosis of the left coronary alone was present in 1073 (37.63 per cent), of the right artery in 330 (11.57 per cent), and of both in 132 (4.63 per cent). In the entire group of 2851 cases thrombosis of one or both of the arteries was observed in 1535 cases (53.84 per cent). A thrombosis of the coronary artery if the patient survives becomes organized and canalized. Grossly it may have the appearance of a fresh thrombus at autopsy for as much as a year or more after its formation because of the blood in the canals. The thrombus may cause sudden death or it may result in an infarct which may heal or, not infrequently, may soften and rupture with massive hemorrhage in the pericardial cavity (tamponade). Edmondson and Hoxie (6) among 25,000 autopsies observed 865 cases of acute myocardial infarction, 72 (8 per cent) of which had myocardial rupture with hemopericardium. Friedman and White (7) reported 105 cases of infarction, 10 of which (9.5 per cent) had myocardial rupture. In a series of 22 cases of recent infarction in patients in a mental institution, Jetter and White (8) noted myocardial rupture in 16 (73 per cent). The incidence of rupture of the heart with hemopericardium among all coronary deaths and among the cases with infarction of the myocardium in our series is listed in Table 15. Of the total num-

TABLE 15. The Incidence of Rupture of the Heart with Hemopericardium among All Coronary Deaths and among Coronary Deaths with Myocardial Infarction

	Number	Per Cent
Among all coronary deaths (3065) 122		3.98
Among coronary deaths with myocardial infarction (1341) 122		9.1

ber of coronary deaths (3065) studied there were 122 (3.98 per cent) in which the heart ruptured. This number (122) was 9.1 per cent of the cases which had infarction of the myocardium.

Pericarditis, except in the uremic type and with myocardial infarction, is rarely seen in death from hypertension and coronary disease. In hypertensive cases dying from uremia, fibrinous pericarditis was present in 31 per cent of the cases. This pericarditis is believed by many people to be the result of uremia and is commonly called chemical pericarditis. Why this inflammation occurs on the pericardium and not on other serous surfaces is not known. Localized and sometimes generalized pericarditis was generally present in cases of myocardial infarction.

Summary and Conclusions

The group of hypertensive and coronary arterial heart disease includes about two thirds of all cardiac deaths and a high percentage (12.83) of the deaths in the autopsy material.

The term arteriosclerotic heart disease that is now used to include the above two groups is not a good one since the coronary arteries in many of the cases where death is due to myocardial failure, cerebral hemorrhage, or uremia are only slightly affected and often not at all.

Death in the total group of hypertensive and coronary arterial diseases, in order of frequency, finally results from coronary disease (47.35 per cent), myocardial failure (34.10 per cent), cerebral hemorrhage (13 per cent), and uremia (5.52 per cent).

Most deaths in both sexes occurred in the fifth through the ninth decades. The sexes showed the greatest difference of involvement in the coronary deaths, where the males far outnumbered the females. The females predominated significantly in the apoplectic type and in the fourth and fifth decades in the uremic type. There is no age beyond which one can be considered exempt from hypertensive or coronary death.

The so-called adult idiopathic hypertrophic heart is a rare condition if it occurs at all. The large heart with myocardial failure without a recorded high blood pressure (about 5 per cent in the series) needs further study to determine the actual cause of the cardiac enlargement.

The chief gross pathological changes noted were atherosclerosis and thrombosis in the arteries, and hypertrophy, fibrosis, and infarction in the myocardium. About 25 per cent of the coronary cases did not have myocardial hypertrophy.

Coronary sclerosis, with few exceptions, was not extreme except among coronary deaths. Coronary thrombosis was rarely seen except in the coronary cases, where it was present in over half. It was always associated with severe coronary sclerosis.

The left coronary artery was much more commonly and extensively involved than the right.

Myocardial fibrosis corresponded in frequency and degree with the degree of coronary sclerosis. Infarction of the myocardium rarely occurred except among coronary deaths, where it was noted in 43 per cent. Occasionally infarction was present without a demonstrable thrombus. Rupture of the myocardium was present in 9 per cent of the cases with myocardial infarction. This percentage has decreased since 1939, when the incidence of rupture in 281 cases of infarction was 16 per cent. Whether this reduction is due to the use of dicumoral or other anticoagulants in recent years or to other causes needs further analysis.

Pericarditis with fibrinous exudation was seen only in the cases dying from uremia (31 per cent) or in the coronary cases having myocardial infarction.

With the exception of rupture of the myocardium with hemopericardium following infarction, there is not a sufficient amount of anatomic change noted in the above groups of hearts, as a rule, to account for the cardiac deaths.

· · · · · · · · · · · · · · · · *by* GEORGE A. PERERA

The Adrenal Cortex and Hypertensive Vascular Disease

IT HAS been said by some that the adrenal cortex governs the cell, the psyche, sex, and the soul, not to mention most of the diseases of man that hitherto have been of unknown etiology. As the subject of the adrenal and hypertension has been reviewed elsewhere in more detail* and as Dr. Selye and Dr. Braun-Menendez have already discussed certain aspects of the problem, I shall deal principally with our own studies in patients with hypertensive vascular disease.

As background, however, I should like to remind you that the adrenal—and practically every other organ and structure—has been related to hypertension for half a century. It has been involved in almost every experimental approach. For example, Dr. Goldblatt made the initial observation that bilateral adrenalectomy interfered with the development or maintenance of experimental renal hypertension. Dr. Shorr finds it necessary to consider the adrenals in his studies of vasotropic principles. Epinephrine injection alters the output of cortical hormones. The adrenal cortex, moreover, is closely related to sodium metabolism, and there are many suggestions of a disturbance in the salt and water metabolism in hypertensive animals. In addition, elevation of the blood pressure has been reported following the administration of various sterols. And finally, in 1939, Loeb and his associates first noted a rise in the blood pressure in association with the injection of desoxycorticosterone esters, followed by Dr. Selye's descriptions of the many profound morphological changes which can be produced by large doses of this steroid.

You are all familiar, I am sure, with the association in man of hypertension and adrenal cortical tumors and of the reduced blood pressure in Addison's disease. However, it is no longer held that

---

* George A. Perera: The adrenal cortex and hypertension, Bull. New York Acad. Med. 26: 75, 1950.

adenomatous or nodular hyperplasia of the adrenal cortex is the rule
in essential hypertension, although the literature contains numerous
references to this effect. You are all familiar and will hear more of the
story of salt and low sodium diets, and the adrenal implications of
such therapy are obvious.

Our own studies stem from the repeatedly confirmed observation
that desoxycorticosterone may give rise to hypertension in the course
of the treatment of Addison's disease. Today, for example, the majority
of patients with adrenal cortical insufficiency who have been maintained on this steroid are, or have been, hypertensive at some time.
One has developed transitory retinal hemorrhages; others, although
the role of coincidence cannot be overlooked, have sustained myocardial infarctions. All observations were made in patients with established but uncomplicated hypertensive vascular disease on a balanced
regimen employing identical menus and regulated sodium and fluid
intakes. "Resting" blood pressures were determined—multiple morning readings by the same observer on a resting patient after at least
a 3-week base line period—further to substantiate the significance of
smaller changes, and the effects of psychotherapeutic influences were
eliminated by various techniques. It should be emphasized that all the
blood pressure modifications reported today reflect alterations in the
peripheral resistance rather than in the cardiac output or plasma
volume.

It is our conviction that extremes of sodium withdrawal or supple-
mentation almost always modify the resting blood pressure of hypertensives. Comparable diets have no effect on the arterial tension of
normotensives. The changes, with a sodium chloride intake of just
under 1 gm., are of small magnitude (about 20 mm. Hg systolic and
15 diastolic), though somewhat greater when the restriction approximates that of the so-called rice diet. To our minds, perhaps those who
fail to demonstrate these changes do not employ such rigorously controlled conditions or they measure the blood pressure by some casual
or more variable method. Those who claim more extravagant results
generally ignore the effects of psychotherapeutic influences or omit an
adequate base line period. Preliminary studies in our clinic suggest
that thiocyanates increase the excretion of sodium, particularly when
administered to hypertensives. One might speculate that the depressor
action of thiocyanates involves sodium mechanisms. By our method
of study, thiocyanates have showed a small but consistent effect of
lowering the blood pressure in all the hypertensive cases we have
observed. Of perhaps greater import is the fact that the rigid restric-

tion of salt masks the pressor response of hypertensives to desoxycorticosterone.

There is considerable evidence of a salt and water disturbance in hypertensive vascular disease. You are aware, no doubt, that many patients can remain on diets containing practically no salt for periods of weeks or months—with maintenance of serum sodium values and of well-being and no apparent difficulties except distaste for the diet. Normal persons, on the other hand, are more prone to develop one or more symptoms of sodium depletion and dehydration, and demonstrate a reduced ability to maintain their sodium concentrations and plasma volume. The difference can be brought out by a single day of rigid salt restriction; hypertensives hold to their weight and fluid balance, whereas normotensives lose weight and have a more pronounced diuresis.

What is the mechanism of the alterations in the blood pressure which follow modification of the sodium intake? I wish I knew. However, the following story gives rise to the strong suggestion of adrenal cortical participation.* We recently observed a woman with both established essential hypertension and Addison's disease (who also had diabetes mellitus, rheumatoid arthritis, and a few other less important conditions). On two separate occasions it was noted that a high sodium chloride intake failed to modify the blood pressure. When she was maintained on either 1 or 4 mg. of desoxycorticosterone acetate daily, the blood pressure rose with an increased intake and fell when the salt dosage was reduced. One could not account for this response on the basis of hemodilution alone. In other words, this patient, with no clinical or laboratory evidence of significant residual adrenal function, with a marked reduction in neutral reducing lipid values, and no eosinophile response to administered adrenocorticotrophic hormone, exhibited a pressor response only when some exogenous steroid source was provided. As a result, I would suggest that the action of sodium is mediated through an adrenal mechanism rather than through direct vasopressor action or the intervention of some independent renal pressor substance.

Returning to the effects of steroid administration, we first administered desoxycorticosterone acetate to 3 normotensive patients without adrenal disease. This was associated with a gradual increase in the blood pressure over a period of weeks which bore no relation to

---

* G. A. Perera and C. Ragan: Hypoadrenalism: Steroidal mediation of sodium action on blood pressure; modification of antiarthritic response to cortisone. Submitted for publication.

salt or water retention. The response of hypertensive patients was considered next, and in this group definite increases in the arterial tension were obtained within a few days. A single study employing Compound S of Reichstein gave rise to similar pressor effects. Again this could not be ascribed to alterations in the plasma volume, transient retention of comparable degrees being observed here but also in normal controls in whom no immediate changes in the blood pressure could be detected. If one continued the desoxycorticosterone by means of daily injections, a transient but at times a sustained increase in pressure could be produced. Up to the present time we have studied 2 patients with both documented hypertensive and Addison's disease. In both instances the elevation of the blood pressure disappeared with the advent of hypoadrenalism, even when the electrolyte balance was restored and maintained, but returned to abnormal levels while the patients were receiving steroid therapy.

Hoping to disclose the existence of some counteracting hormone or to depress existing adrenal cortical function, we subsequently demonstrated that whole extracts of the adrenal cortex gave rise to small decreases in the resting blood pressure in 3 of 4 hypertensive subjects. In addition, the simultaneous use of adrenal cortical extract appeared to block the pressor effect of desoxycorticosterone.

Finally, we have had the opportunity to employ cortisone (Merck) and the adrenocorticotrophic hormone (Armour) in a small series of patients with essential hypertension. While having no demonstrable effect in normotensives, and associated with a rise in tension in 2 persons with Addison's disease (and in adrenalectomized animals), cortisone has resulted in small but definite decreases in the resting blood pressure in 5 hypertensive patients. The adrenocorticotrophic hormone, on the other hand, may have little action or may be definitely pressor in both those with a normal and those with an elevated arterial tension, even to the point of being responsible for the development of hypertensive encephalopathy. We are now engaged in preliminary studies suggesting that the responses of hypertensives to certain steroids differ, depending on whether they have essential hypertension or hypertension of renal origin. If further cases continue to conform, the results may provide a further clue separating these two groups rather than bringing them together under one etiological classification.

It is now clear that at least some forms of hypertension can exist in the absence of intact adrenals. It is now clear that steroidal responses are probably not on a primary humoral basis, as they occur only after lags and delays of many hours and days. By varying techniques, it is still difficult to demonstrate any adrenocortical dysfunction in hypertensive vascular disease. It should be emphasized that the data that have been presented do not justify the view that the adrenals cause the hypertensive state, but they do imply that both sodium and the adrenal cortex are related very definitely to the regulation of the blood pressure. Possibly this approach may give rise to methods whereby we can gain further insight into the mechanisms.

Questions and Discussion

DR. HANS SELYE: I think Dr. Perera's observations are certainly of the greatest importance in evaluating the nature of the role of the adrenals in hypertension. I might add that in rats in which we have produced hypertension by the endocrine kidney technique, removal of the adrenals usually causes a very considerable drop in the blood pressure, but if such adrenalectomized animals (which bear an endocrine kidney) are treated with maintenance doses of an adrenal extract, the blood pressure rises again to hypertensive levels. Treatment with such threshold doses of adrenal extract in itself causes no hypertension. We conclude that probably the drop in the blood pressure in adrenalectomized rats bearing an endocrine kidney occurs largely because these animals are in poor physical condition and hence tend to develop the hypotension of "shock" and nonspecific damage.

The fact that sodium deprivation also tends to decrease the blood pressure of hypertensive patients and completely prevents the pressor effect of DCA in animals, also suggests some close pathogenetic correlation between the clinical and the experimental types of hypertensive disease.

As regards the relation between the hypertensive and vasotoxic actions of DCA and the relationship of DCA to rheumatic changes, I should like to say the following: When in 1944 we first pointed out the relationship between the adrenal cortex and the pathogenesis of rheumatic diseases, we had to base our theory exclusively on the experimental observation that arthritis and rheumatic-like cardiovascular changes can be elicited in animals by DCA overdosage. Such changes were always considerably more common and more intense in adrenalectomized than in intact animals, which suggested the production of some "anti-DCA factor" by the adrenal cortex. However, it was only thanks to the more recent observations of Kendall, Hench, and their co-workers that this effect could be traced to gluco-corticoids, particularly cortisone.

More recently we have developed a simple test which permits us to study with special ease this antagonistic effect between gluco- and mineralo-corticoids, particularly as regards the production and prevention of arthritis. Adrenalectomized animals are injected with a small amount of formaldehyde, mustard powder, or any other irritant in the periarticular region of the metatarsal joints in one of their hind legs. If such animals are previously given DCA the resulting arthritis is considerably aggravated, while gluco-corticoids (e.g., cortisone, dehydrocorticosterone) effectively inhibit the formation of a periarticular inflammatory granuloma. ACTH also inhibits the formation of this experimental "topical irritation arthritis," but only in the presence of the adrenals—presumably through the production of endogenous gluco-corticoids.

Some time ago we noted that rats treated with an impure anterior pituitary preparation, for instance, lyophilized anterior pituitary (LAP), respond with the development of pronounced nephrosclerosis and exhibit a great tendency to develop a spontaneous arthritis.* In this respect the LAP exhibits actions which appear to be diametrically opposed to those of purified ACTH. We have not yet succeeded in identifying the active principle in LAP, but it is certainly not identical with ACTH. It may be a new hormone, but there is nothing to prove that it is not identical with one of the already identified anterior pituitary principles.

If LAP and ACTH are injected simultaneously into rats, the nephrosclerosis-producing action of the former is greatly enhanced by the latter. LAP given concurrently with cortisone likewise causes pronounced nephrosclerosis in rats. It appears that the nephrotoxic action of the "LAP factor" is greatly enhanced in its effect by the simultaneous administration of ACTH (which is predominantly glucocorticotrophic) or cortisone (which is itself a gluco-corticoid hormone). This is all the more noteworthy since neither pure ACTH nor cortisone causes such renal damage at any dose level even if fatal amounts are injected into rats. The mechanism of this phenomenon has not yet been explained, but it appears to me that it could have considerable bearing on the interpretation of renal diseases as "diseases of adaptation." Perhaps the LAP factor so alters the metabolism of gluco-corticoids that they are transformed into mineralo-corticoids. It is also conceivable that the LAP factor acts directly upon the target organs (for instance, the kidney) in such a manner as to change their responsiveness to gluco-corticoids and to cause the latter to become

*Hans Selye: J. Clin. Endocrinol., Feb. 1946.

toxic. All these observations have been described in more detail else-where,* but I wanted to mention them here because of their probable bearing upon the role of the adrenals in the production of renal and hypertensive disease. I should much appreciate it if Dr. Perera would comment on these remarks.

DR. EDUARDO BRAUN-MENENDEZ: I should like Dr. Perera to give us further evidence of the statement that hypertension induced by de-soxycorticosterone in hypertensive and normotensive patients is not caused by an increase in the cardiac output but is only due to an in-crease in the peripheral resistance.

DR. PERERA: I am afraid I have no additional comment to make about Dr. Selye's remarks except to reveal features about which I am confused.

Are there other pathways in response to stress? Are the adrenals essential? After all, the adrenalectomized animal is still capable of developing and forming antibodies. We have seen a patient, about whom I spoke, who has several metabolic disturbances in addition to hypoadrenalism. The entire role of the adrenal cortex in the develop-ment or accentuation of various disorders is still a matter of pure speculation.

With reference to Dr. Braun-Menendez's remarks, I think he raised an important question yesterday. Although small blood pressure changes occur in response to the administration of certain steroids, rather than interpreting these changes as evidence of disease modifica-tion, we must bear in mind that the hypertensive may respond in a different way. These changes, I agree, cannot be used as evidence that the adrenal participates in or causes the hypertensive state.

Dr. Braun-Menendez raised another question yesterday that de-serves a great deal of study—what is the role of the interstitial com-partment as an index and as a messenger to invoke hemodynamic re-sponses? Because there is a demonstrable change in peripheral resist-ance, it does not tell us the various mechanisms and pathways involved. I am always reminded of the problem that when we stop taking salt by mouth, we stop putting out urine that contains a great deal of sodium. Something must tell the kidneys, and that messenger is not the serum concentration of sodium as far as we can determine. For there are many situations in which the serum concentration is reduced without modification of the renal "faucet" to sodium. The interstitial compartment's place in electrolyte regulation is worthy of a great deal more study.

* Hans Selye: Stress, Montreal, Acta Inc. Medical Publishers, 1950.

· · · · · · · · · · · · · · · · · *by* EPHRAIM SHORR

Hepatorenal Factors in Essential Hypertension in Man

IN MY initial presentation I summarized the evidence for the participation of the vasoactive factors, VEM and VDM, of renal and hepatic origin respectively, in experimental renal hypertension induced in dogs and rats (1). Specific derangements were observed in the metabolism of both humoral principles, as well as in the structure and function of the capillary bed with whose regulation they are concerned. These observations have provided the basis for a concept relating these humoral and peripheral vascular changes to the development and maintenance of hypertension. They also furnished a set of criteria by which the relation of different hypertensive syndromes to experimental renal hypertension could be specifically evaluated.

The relevance of these observations for human essential hypertension is, of course, dependent upon the extent to which they also occur in the latter syndrome. The relation of essential hypertension to that produced by the Goldblatt clamp or perinephric wrapping remains controversial. The importance of establishing or excluding such a relationship is obvious. If the validity of experimental renal hypertension can be established as an experimental condition comparable to essential hypertension, then the continuation of such studies can be justified as directly pertinent to the problem.

The development of new and highly specific yardsticks provided such an opportunity, at least with respect to the humoral factors and vascular structures with which we have been concerned. My discussion today will be devoted to the results of such a comparative study.

NOTE. This paper is based on experiments carried out with Drs. Benjamin W. Zweifach, Abraham Mazur, Silvio Baez, Richard E. Lee, and Maurice M. Black, under grants from the National Institutes of Health, U.S. Public Health Service, the Josiah Macy, Jr., Foundation, the New York Heart Association, Eli Lilly and Company, and the Postley Hypertension Fund.

The first criterion explored with patients having well-documented, essential hypertension was the bio-assay of blood samples for the presence of VEM and VDM. Approximately 30 subjects have been studied in this manner (2). Representative bio-assays are given in Tables 1 and 2. The data were identical with those obtained in animals with experimental renal hypertension. Unfractionated bloods were either neutral or showed a slight predominance of VEM, as was found in the chronic stage of experimental renal hypertension. In the patients described in these tables, the fractionation procedure consisted of the inactivation of VEM by aerobic incubation with normal kidney slices, a measure which unmasks the VDM content in mixtures of both humoral factors. In every instance the presence of VDM was established, and, by inference, of VEM. The neutral blood samples, as in chronic experimental renal hypertension, therefore, consisted of mixtures of both VEM and VDM in concentrations which neutralized each other in the rat mesoappendix test. In other cases not illustrated here, complete fractionations were carried out, VDM being inactivated with antiferritin serum and VEM by aerobic kidney slices; these provided a direct demonstration of the presence of both factors.

Attention is called to several cases of particular interest which have been included in Table 1. Patient A. P. had Cushing's syndrome, with a malignant adrenal cortical tumor. Her humoral pattern was typical of chronic essential hypertension. Two other subjects with Cushing's syndrome, one aged 9, the other aged 12, not included in this table, showed a similar picture. Three patients with unilateral or bilateral sympathectomies and persistent hypertension also showed the typical picture (Table 2). Of special interest is patient R. P. (Table 1), who had hypertension of 7 years' duration, associated with an aneurysm of the left renal artery. Prior to operative removal of that kidney, she showed VEM predominance, as well as high titers of VDM in the fractionated blood sample. The nephrectomy was followed by a return to normotensive levels and the disappearance of these humoral factors from the blood stream. A series of normotensive subjects served to establish the absence of these humoral factors in the normotensive state.

In a small series of normotensive and hypertensive subjects, the renal and hepatic veins were catheterized and bio-assays carried out on blood coming directly from the kidney and liver, in order to test another criterion, namely, the *in vivo* elaboration of these factors by their tissues of origin (unpublished observations, Shorr and Zweifach). In the normotensive subjects neither VEM nor VDM could be de-

TABLE 1. A Bio-Assay of the Blood of Patients with Essential Hypertension
(Adapted from Shorr and Zweifach: Tr. A. Am. Physicians 61:356, 1948)

Patient (Sex, Age)	Duration of Hyper. in Years	Blood Pressure (mm. Hg)	Renal Impairment (0-3+)	Retinopathy (0-4+)	Cereb. Phenom.	Rat Test of Plasma	
						Un-treated (min.)	After Kidney Incubation (min.)
MK (f, 52)	?	172/92	0	0	0	Neutral	Tr. VDM
ET (f, 25)	2	180/110	0	0	H	Neutral	VDM-31
RP (f, 26)	5	182/110	0	1+	H-D	Tr. VEM	VDM-21
AP (f, 49)	11*	250/135	1+	1+	0	Neutral	VDM-29
RC (m, 45)	7	172/104	0	2+	H	Neutral	VDM-24
EM (f, 37)	3	230/130	0	2+	H-D	Tr. VEM	VDM-36
EA (m, 39)	6	190/120	1+	2+	0	Neutral	VDM-21
CT (f, 41)	1½+	220/135	1+	2+	H-D-En	Neutral	VDM-33
RP (f, 32)	7†	180/106	1+	2+	H	VEM-27	VDM-24
RP (f, 32)	7‡	116/76	1+	2+	0	Neutral	Neutral

*Cushing's syndrome with malignant adrenal cortical tumor.

†Aneurysm of the left renal artery.

‡Three months after left nephrectomy.

NOTE. In this table and the following one the letters H, D, En, and S in the column Cerebral Phenomena stand for headache, dizziness, encephalopathy, and cerebral accident.

TABLE 2. A Bio-Assay of the Blood of Patients with Essential Hypertension
(Adapted from Shorr and Zweifach: Tr. A. Am. Physicians 61:356, 1948)

Patient (Sex, Age)	Duration of Hyper. in Years	Blood Pressure (mm. Hg)	Renal Impairment (0-3+)	Retinopathy (0-4+)	Cereb. Phenom.	Rat Test of Plasma	
						Untreated* (min.)	After Kidney Incubation (min.)
HS (f, 48) ....28†		210/140	0	3+	H-S	Neutral	VDM-30
MF (f, 76) 22		194/90	1+	3+	0	Neutral	VDM-30
MS (f, 45) ....8‡		260/130	1+	3+	H	Neutral	VDM-26
TE (m, 30) 1		180/120	1+	3+	H	Tr. VEM	VDM-21
MK (f, 41) ....20‡		172/132	1+	3+	H-En	Tr. VEM	VDM-21
MK (f, 43) ....22†		164/112	1+	3+	0	Neutral	VDM-32
SC (m, 50) 4		228/190	2+	3+	0	Tr. VEM	VDM-19
FH (f, 48) 5		240/110	2+	3+	H-D-En	VEM-21	VDM-27
AG (m, 53) 4		238/148	3+	4+	0	VEM-21	VDM-36

* Plasma incubated in 95% O_2 + 5% CO_2 but without the kidney gave the same reaction as untreated plasma.
† Bilateral sympathectomy.
‡ Unilateral sympathectomy.

268

tected except for traces in 3 of 13 subjects, attributable to the conditions of the experiment. In contrast, the hypertensive subjects showed very high titers of VEM in the renal vein blood and high concentrations of VDM in the blood from the hepatic vein; in the mixed peripheral blood, neutral reactions or slight VEM predominance was the rule, the resultant of the admixtures of VEM and VDM issuing from the kidney and liver, respectively.

For a similar exploration of the acute stage of hypertension, patients were selected with acute hypertension due to the toxemia of pregnancy, normal pregnancies serving as controls (unpublished observations, Shorr and Zweifach). In several of the normal pregnant women, minimal amounts of both principles were detected. Of the 9 cases of toxemia, all showed high titers of VEM and VDM during the hypertensive phase prior to delivery. Two cases were restudied post partum, on the ninth and thirteenth days respectively, when the blood pressure had returned to normotensive levels. In one, both factors had

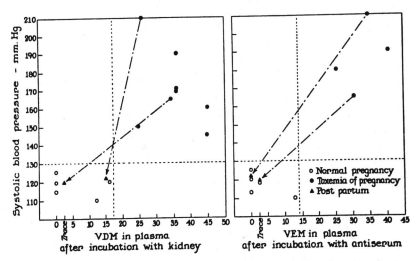

FIGURE 1. Amounts of VDM and VEM present in the blood in normal pregnancy and in toxemia. (Shorr and Zweifach, unpublished.)

disappeared; in the other, there was still a residual trace of VDM (Figure 1). In this connection it may be recalled that renin also has been found in measurable amounts in the blood during the toxemia of pregnancy.

The next criterion investigated was the *in vitro* VEM metabolism of the renal cortex in normotensive and hypertensive subjects (3). To date kidney biopsies have been obtained on 4 normotensive and 4 hypertensive subjects at operation for urological conditions or at sympathectomy in the latter group. The same defect in renal VEM metabolism observed in animals with experimental renal hypertension was exhibited by kidney slices from hypertensive patients; VEM appeared following both aerobic and anaerobic incubation, whereas kidney slices from normotensive subjects behaved as do those from normal dog and rat kidneys, forming VEM only under anaerobic conditions.

We then turned our attention to the structural and functional changes previously noted in the mesenteric capillary bed of the renal hypertensive dog and rat. We have not as yet been able to study the identical capillary beds in the human subject. However, Dr. Richard E. Lee of our laboratory (4, also unpublished data) has made observations on the conjunctival vessels of normal and hypertensive human subjects and has observed analogous phenomena to those previously noted in the mesenteric capillary bed of animals. In the normal subject, the pathway of a conjunctival metarteriole is relatively straight. The true capillaries arise from the precapillary sphincters of this metarteriole and usually follow a relatively straight course, to become confluent with the metarteriole and form the collecting venules (Figure 2, Left). The precapillary sphincters display a threshold constriction upon the topical application of epinephrine in concentrations of between 1:20,000 and 1:50,000. These concentrations are much higher than those required to produce a constrictor response in the delicate mesentery of the rat, a circumstance which may be attributable to the less rapid absorption of epinephrine through the corneal epithelium. In sharp contrast to the conjunctival vessels of the normotensive subject, whose architecture incidentally is comparable to that of the mesenteric capillary bed of the rat and dog, those of hypertensive patients show a sinuous pathway of the metarteriole, which is usually greatly narrowed, and a tremendous elongation and tortuosity of the true capillaries, with frequent complete loops and coilings (Figure 2, Right). This feature is analogous to the hyperplasia noted in the mesenteric capillaries of the renal hypertensive dog and rat. There was, in addition, a striking enhancement of the sensitivity of the constrictor response of the precapillary sphincters to topically applied epinephrine, these vessels reacting to approximately $\frac{1}{10}$ the concentration which elicits a constrictor response in the normotensive subject. Thus the capillary vessels of the orbital conjunctiva in the patient with essential hypertension exhibit an increased vascular re-

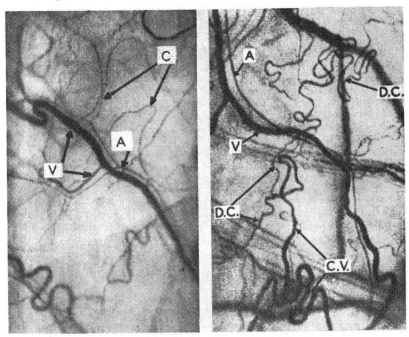

FIGURE 2, Left. The capillary bed in the left temporal conjunctiva of normotensive subject E. H. (× 150). The terminal arteriole (A) gives off true
capillaries (C), which cross the conjunctiva in a moderately uniform manner
to enter the collecting venules (V). The capillaries are smooth, without coiling
or looping or elongation. Threshold closure of the precapillary sphincters in
this area occurred routinely after topical applications of epinephrine 1:50,000.
(This figure is reproduced, by permission of the copyright owner, from R. E.
Lee and E. A. Holze: J. Clin. Investigation 29:147, 1950.) FIGURE 2, Right.
The capillary bed in the left temporal conjunctiva of hypertensive patient
M. C. (× 150). The terminal arteriole (A) follows a more sinuous pathway
than that seen in the normotensive subject. In addition the true capillaries
(D.C.) are tremendously looped and coiled, and elongated to more than three
times the usual length. This coiling and tortuosity may also be found in the
collecting venules (C.V.). Threshold precapillary closure in this field occurred
following topical applications of epinephrine 1:400,000.
(Lee and Holze, unpublished.)

activity and hyperplasia comparable to that of the mesenteric vessels.
of the renal hypertensive dog and rat.

In Table 3 are assembled the several criteria, metabolic, vascular,
and humoral, which characterize the renal hypertensive dog and rat
as compared with the data presently available for human essential
hypertension. The conclusion is amply justified that experimental

TABLE 3. The Criteria for Evaluating the Hypertensive Syndrome

	Rat (Perineph.)	Dog (R. A. Clamp)	Human (Essential)
Aerobic formation of VEM by the kidney in vivo	...	+	+
Aerobic formation of VEM by the kidney in vitro	+	+	+
VEM in the blood during the acute stage ..	+	+	+
VEM and VDM in the blood during the chronic stage	+	+	+
Vascular hyperreactivity to epinephrine ...	+	+	+
Vascular hyperreactivity to VEM	+	...	...
Hyperplasia of the capillary bed	+	+	+
Renal histochemistry (tetrazolium pattern) .	+	+	+

renal and human essential hypertension share in common the same metabolic defects in the hepatorenal vasotropic mechanisms, an identical reflection of these defects in the blood; and there is some indication that both exhibit similar alterations in the behavior and structure of the terminal vascular bed.

One additional criterion has recently been added to this list, namely, the tetrazolium pattern in the kidney tubule. The presentation of the data may be prefaced with a description of this new histochemical tool. The 2-, 3-, 5-triphenyl tetrazolium chloride (TTC), is a colorless, water-soluble substance which, on reduction, yields a deep red, water-insoluble formazan. The incubation of living tissue slices with this compound leads to its intracellular reduction by virtue of its ability to act as a hydrogen acceptor with tissue reductases, such as dehydrogenases (Figure 3). The insoluble formazan is deposited in the cell, presumably at the sites of its enzymatic reduction, yielding patterns which are characteristic for different tissues. This property of TTC serves as an excellent indicator, not only of the extent of the enzymatic activity of a cell, but also of the pattern of the intracellular distribution of the enzymes for which TTC acts as a hydrogen acceptor.

The technique, in brief, is as follows: The tissue to be studied is kept chilled in physiological saline from the moment of its excision. Sections are made as for microrespiration studies and incubated at 37.5° C. for an hour in a solution of TTC. The tissue slices are then fixed in 10 per cent formalin and frozen sections are made and mounted in glycerin for microscopic study. The deposits of formazan are readily recognizable by their brilliant red. Cellular detail also emerges after a counterstaining with appropriate reagents, such as methylene blue.

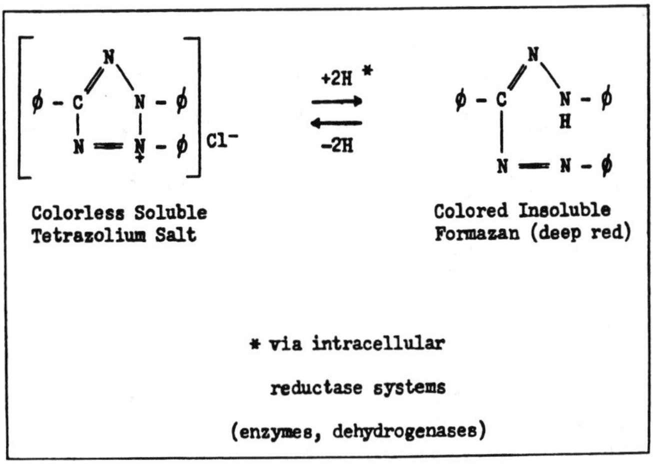

Colorless Soluble
Tetrazolium Salt

+2H *
⇌
-2H

Colored Insoluble
Formazan (deep red)

* via intracellular

reductase systems

(enzymes, dehydrogenases)

FIGURE 3

We were struck with the potentialities of this method for testing our concept that the derangement in VEM metabolism in the kidney cortex might be related to an underlying enzymatic disturbance in the cellular metabolism. Were this the case, there might be a parallel distortion in the tetrazolium pattern in the kidney. In collaboration with Dr. Maurice M. Black (3), we proceeded to establish the tetrazolium pattern in normal kidney slices (Figure 4, Left). The normal kidney slice exposed to TTC showed a characteristic histologic picture. The greatest deposition of formazan occurred in the cells of the proximal convoluted tubules, which were seen to be filled with finely dispersed, dustlike granules of formazan throughout the cytoplasm. The deposition of these granules was less marked in the distal tubules.

The first experimental variation introduced was to incubate normal kidney slices in nitrogen for 1 hour and then restore them to aerobic conditions. As pointed out in my initial presentation, this procedure leads to the development of the typical hypertensive pattern of VEM formation in oxygen as well as in nitrogen, as contrasted with the normal restriction of the appearance of VEM to anaerobiosis. Exposure of these kidney slices, after anaerobic incubation, to TTC revealed that a profound change had also occurred in the pattern of formazan deposition in the proximal convoluted tubules (Figure 4, Right). Formazan was now deposited as coarse needles and plaques, predominantly toward the borders of the cell and to some extent extracellularly. This was in sharp contrast to the diffuse, finely granu-

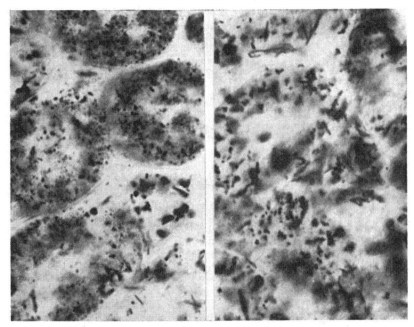

FIGURE 4. The TTC pattern of the kidney cortex of a dog (× 320), (left) under aerobic control and (right) after preincubation in nitrogen. (Figures 4, 5, and 6 are reproduced, by permission of the copyright owner, from B. N. Zweifach, M. M. Black, and E. Shorr: Proc. Soc. Exper. Biol. & Med. 74:850–853, 1950.)

lar distribution of the formazan in the normal proximal tubule. It would seem that as a result of the preincubation in nitrogen for an hour, there were parallel derangements both in the character of the renal VEM metabolism and in the intracellular distribution of the enzymes reacting to tetrazolium. The latter derangement was confined to the proximal convoluted tubules, no appreciable change being recognizable in the distal tubules.

It was now of interest to observe the tetrazolium pattern in the proximal convoluted tubules of animals with experimental renal hypertension. Biopsies were made of the renal cortex of dogs and rats and immediately incubated with TTC in the manner described above. The formazan pattern of the proximal convoluted tubules showed the same distortion in its arrangement (Figure 5) as observed in the normal kidney slice which had been preincubated in nitrogen and then re-exposed to aerobic conditions. In each instance slices from the same biopsy specimen were incubated in nitrogen and oxygen and

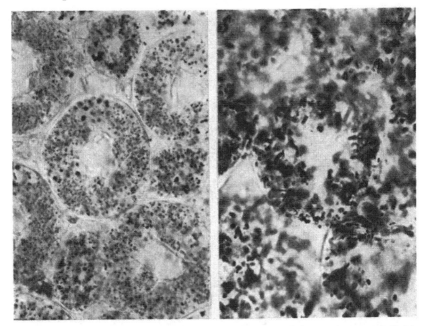

Figure 5. The TTC pattern of the kidney cortex of a dog (× 320), (left) normal and (right) hypertensive.

found to have the typical hypertensive pattern of VEM formation in oxygen as well as in nitrogen.

It would appear that for the first time a well-defined histochemical lesion has been demonstrated in experimental renal hypertension which involves a specific portion of the nephron, namely, the proximal convoluted tubule. Furthermore, this lesion would seem to reflect some type of enzymatic derangement, the enzymes being now distributed in "disorderly" fashion in the proximal tubular cells. Of particular pertinence to our own concept is the parallel appearance of a metabolic derangement in the renal VEM mechanism, of such a nature as to suggest that it is enzymatically conditioned.

Once this new criterion was available, it was applied to a study of renal biopsies from patients with essential hypertension. The tetrazolium pattern (Figure 6) was indistinguishable from that seen in kidney slices of animals with experimental renal hypertension, whereas kidney slices from normotensive subjects showed the same uniform dispersion of dustlike formazan granules in the proximal convoluted tubules as in normal dogs and rats.

This tool was also utilized to complete our assessment of desoxy-

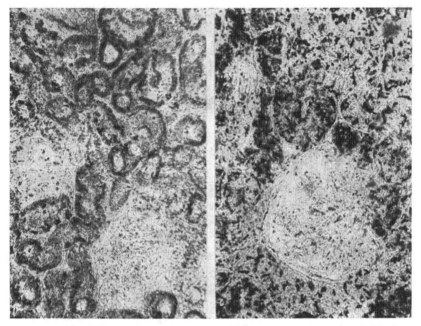

FIGURE 6. The TTC pattern of a human kidney cortex (× 80), (left) in a normal subject and (right) in a hypertensive subject.

corticosterone hypertension in the rat (Zweifach, Black, and Shorr, unpublished observations). The results bore out our previous evaluation of this syndrome as differing from experimental renal and human essential hypertension. Except for the small percentage of animals (approximately 20 per cent) which sustained extensive vascular damage in the course of the development of this syndrome, the kidneys from rats made hypertensive by DCA showed an entirely normal tetrazolium pattern in the proximal convoluted tubules.

We are now in a position to summarize our present data bearing on the participation of VEM and VDM in essential hypertension in man. Utilizing a variety of specific criteria—metabolic derangements of the renal VEM and hepatic VDM mechanisms, in vitro and in vivo, the appearance of VEM and VDM in the blood stream, the alterations in the reactivity and structure of the capillary bed, and the tetrazolium pattern of the proximal convoluted tubules—it has been shown that the findings in human essential hypertension are essentially the same as those in experimental renal hypertension in the dog and rat.

In closing, certain implications of these findings may be re-emphasized. They suggest an essential similarity between experimental renal and human essential hypertension with respect to the participation of the hepatorenal principles VEM and VDM in both conditions, as well as a similarity in the involvement of the peripheral vascular bed upon which these vasoactive principles exert their effects. They reinforce the validity of the experimental approach to essential hypertension, an approach that utilizes animals made hypertensive by the Goldblatt clamp or perinephric wrapping and that permits a more detailed analysis of humoral and vascular mechanisms than has hitherto been possible in the human subject. While these studies do not exclude the existence of certain differences between experimental renal and human essential hypertension, they do demonstrate unequivocally the many aspects which are common to both. Finally, the observations on the tetrazolium pattern make it clear that there is, as part of the picture of both experimental renal and essential hypertension, a lesion of an enzymatic character in the proximal convoluted tubules and that this lesion may be related to the metabolic alterations in renal VEM metabolism which occur parallel with it.

Questions and Discussion

DR. GEORGE W. PICKERING: I have been much interested in these observations of Dr. Shorr on VEM and VDM, and obviously the disturbance of equilibrium which he describes must be accounted for in any hypothesis which tries to explain the vascular changes in hypertension. What I should like to ask him is this: whether he thinks it is conceivable or likely that this system plays a major part in the mechanism of essential hypertension in man. I ask that because it seems to me very doubtful that it can do so for these reasons: first, as I understand it, it hasn't been possible to show that VDM injected intravenously produces a depressor response or that VEM injected intravenously produces a pressor response. What you can show is that the vasomotor response of the capillaries and arterioles is altered in the sense that there is an alteration in response to the application of adrenaline. Now, if that kind of mechanism were involved in hypertension, I think one would expect an alteration in the sensitivity of the vascular system to adrenaline or perhaps noradrenaline.

Some years ago Hülse, one of Volhard's assistants, claimed that patients with essential hypertension show a normal sensitivity to adrenaline, but patients with Volhard's pale hypertension, that is, malignant and nephritic hypertension, show an increased sensitivity to this substance. Kissin and I repeated those observations, but we were unable to demonstrate any alteration in the sensitivity to adrenaline in patients either with benign, malignant, or nephritic hypertension. We used, of course, quite crude methods at the time, and it might be possible with better methods now to show whether or not there is an alteration in the sensitivity to these substances.

But I am always a little doubtful whether adrenaline or noradrenaline can play any significant part in the pathogenesis of essential hypertension because one of the most striking and constant things you see when you inject adrenaline or noradrenaline into men, either as a single injection or as a continuous infusion, is blanching of the face, and you are all familiar with the fact that the average patient with essential hypertension has a red face.

You can show that in patients with essential hypertension a small dose of adrenaline, such as blanches the face of a normal subject, also will blanch the faces of the patients. Therefore, it seems to me very unlikely that they can have enough circulating adrenaline or nor-adrenaline to alter their vessels in a way that is different from the normal.

DR. R. W. GOEN (TULSA): I am a complete newcomer to this field, and I am simply coming up here and asking a simple question. We have heard that the changes that we see in the arteries and the arterioles of the kidneys are seen even in the absence of hypertension. We have seen hypertension in the absence of these changes. We have seen hypertension with the kidneys damaged and with normal kidneys.

We have seen hypertension persist when the kidneys are removed, or develop when they are removed; likewise with the adrenal. It seems to me that the studies of Dr. Shorr are the most fundamental of all that we have heard to date; namely, we are getting at the fundamental, pathological physiology here when we say that alterations in these cells themselves—something that we haven't paid very much attention to, the actual tubules, the cells of the proximal convoluted tubules —may actually be producing the substances which cause the hyper-reactivity we have seen so often in these cases of essential hypertension.

Furthermore, I should like that Dr. Shorr be given the opportunity to philosophize; so rather than ask him a question, I should like to ask Dr. Shorr to please go ahead and devote the rest of his allotted time to philosophizing. I think it would be worth listening to.

DR. SHORR: What the rest of the audience does not know is that Dr. Pickering's question is actually the continuation of a discussion we had last night, which was interrupted at 12:30 this morning through sheer cerebral exhaustion.

I am glad that Dr. Pickering has asked this question because it provides me with another opportunity to try to clear up what has been a common misunderstanding of our point of view. The use of topical epinephrine in the rat mesoappendix assay has merely been a convenient device to bring out the reactivity of the capillary mesenteric vessels as it is affected by the presence of VEM or VDM in the circulation, whether naturally occurring or intravenously administered. This should not be taken to mean that the influence of VEM and

VDM on capillary vasomotion involves circulating epinephrine. On the contrary, in our view it is much more likely that the sympathomimetic agent involved is locally produced and is something of the nature of sympathin.

In point of fact, I believe it is questionable whether any constrictor effects of epinephrine have been shown to be exerted on the peripheral vascular bed with the usual pressor concentrations given intravenously. The recent experiments of Goldenberg, comparing the action of epinephrine and norepinephrine, show that the effects of epinephrine on the blood pressure are largely, if not entirely, attributable to its action in increasing the heart rate and cardiac output, and not to its peripheral vasoconstrictive effects. Indeed, whatever action it has on the peripheral vascular bed is predominantly of a vasodilator character.

For these reasons, the experiments cited by Dr. Pickering showing no difference in the pressor effects of epinephrine in normotensive and hypertensive subjects, cannot be used as evidence against the participation of humoral factors such as VEM in the genesis and maintenance of the increased peripheral resistance in hypertension.

In response to the request by Dr. Goen that I philosophize a bit about our concept as to the relation of VEM and VDM to hypertension, I should like first to thank him for his generous comments on the significance of our studies.

It has only been a matter of five years or less that we have been aware of the existence of these humoral principles. We appreciate fully that there are many gaps in our knowledge of their role in vascular homeostasis, particularly with respect to their causal relationship in the regulation of the blood pressure. We have always in the past been careful to refrain from what would be a premature consideration of causality and have preferred to limit our discussion of these principles to a descriptive level. However, it is desirable to set up a working hypothesis in order to provide a logical basis for our experimental program.

In such a working hypothesis, we must clearly differentiate between factual data and inference. The facts about which we are certain are as follows: The peripheral vascular bed, and specifically the capillary unit with which we are concerned, has a characteristic architecture and pattern of behavior. It consists of a muscular thoroughfare channel, the metarterioles, precapillary sphincters, and endothelial capillaries. These muscular components exhibit a periodic constriction and dilatation, which we term vasomotion, by which adjustments can be brought about between hydrostatic and osmotic pressures; these in turn influence the exchange of fluids between the blood stream and the extracellular tissue spaces to maintain the constancy of the internal environment. This vasomotion is regulated by humoral factors which may be produced locally or in special organs, such as the kidney and liver. Two such humoral principles with opposite effects on the vasomotion and reactivity of the capillary muscular vessels have been recognized. The first of these, the hepatic vasodepressor VDM, which has been identified as ferritin, depresses vasomotion and reduces the reactivity of these vessels. The second principle, VEM, not yet isolated, has the opposite effect. These opposite effects suggest that VDM and VEM may constitute a homeostatic system which participates in the regulation of the peripheral vascular bed.

Both of these principles normally arise under specific conditions, namely, hypoxia, and are inactivated by their tissues of origin under aerobic conditions. They are therefore to be considered physiological principles whose appearance in excessive amounts in circulatory derangements is the result of metabolic alterations in the organ systems in which they arise.

Derangements in their metabolism arise in a variety of circulatory disturbances, such as shock and hypertension. In these conditions, the nature of the metabolic derangements responsible for their appearance in the circulation in abnormal amounts has been demonstrated. Their presence in the blood stream in shock and in hypertension is associated with characteristic alterations in the behavior of the capillary bed which are consistent with the mode of action of these principles on this unit of the vascular system. What these derangements are in hypertension I have already described and need not repeat here. The metabolic lesion in hypertension which occurs in the kidney and leads to the appearance of VEM under both aerobic and anaerobic conditions has been correlated, by means of the tetrazolium technique, with enzymatic derangements in the proximal convoluted tubule. The secondary derangements in the hepatic ferritin mechanisms occur apparently as a response to the excessive concentrations of VEM in the blood stream. The findings with respect to VEM and VDM in hypertension are not limited by species but are consistently observed in the several species studied, which include the rat, the dog, and man. They must therefore be considered an integral part of the hypertensive syndrome.

The problem now arises as to what may be their causal relationship to the genesis and maintenance of hypertension. Here our evidence is at present largely circumstantial but also, in some measure, factual as well. It is experimentally demonstrable that no changes occur in capillary behavior without appropriate readjustments of the arterioles proximal to the capillary bed. It is also demonstrable that changes which occur in the behavior of the arterioles are accompanied by appropriate readjustments in the capillary bed. Were this not so, circulatory homeostasis would break down and tissue dehydration or edema formation inevitably result. It is one of the essential functions of the vascular system to prevent such alterations in the composition of the internal environment; and it is only with the breakdown of the vascular compensatory mechanisms that we observe the development of either of these two abnormal situations. In this broader sense, the capillary bed is the unit which the rest of the vascular system serves; and it is this key position which points to the importance of VEM and VDM in circulatory homeostasis and persuades us that they will be found to play a significant role in the genesis of hypertension.

This does not mean, however, that they must play an exclusive role. On the contrary, they represent, in our opinion, only one of a number of factors, humoral, neurogenic, etc., all of which cooperate in the regulation of the blood pressure. Thus the larger blood vessels are largely under the control of the sympathetic nervous system, and the smaller arterioles, while partially so, are predominantly responsive to humoral factors, such as the renin-hypertensin system. Any complete concept of hypertension would therefore of necessity involve an integration of all the vasotropic factors which can be shown to be regularly deranged in the hypertensive syndrome. We are all too prone to exclude this or that factor because it fails to provide the complete explanation for hypertension. Such a rigid point of view is unwarranted, for it represents an over-simplification of a highly subtle and complicated regulatory mechanism.

In this final picture, it is our expectation that VEM and VDM will be assigned an essential role, and we shall continue in our efforts to provide more evidence as to what this role may be.

· · · · · · · · · · · · · · · · *by* RICHARD V. EBERT

Pulmonary Hypertension

THE term arterial hypertension is commonly used to refer to elevated pressure in the systemic arteries. This usage implies a certain lack of interest in arterial hypertension of the pulmonary vascular system. In the past this was due to the absence of methods for measuring the pressure in the pulmonary arteries in human beings. The introduction of cardiac catheterization has rendered this measurement possible, and information is gradually being accumulated regarding pulmonary arterial hypertension.

In considering the subject of pulmonary hypertension, it is important to emphasize certain characteristics of the pulmonary vascular system. The normal pressure in the pulmonary arterial system is low. The diastolic pressure is relatively constant, being approximately 9 mm. Hg, whereas the systolic pressure is more variable, ranging from 11 to 30 mm. Hg (1, 2, 3). It is of interest that the pulmonary arterial pressure is much the same in the reptile, bird, and mammal, although the systemic arterial pressure differs greatly among these species (4). An unusual feature of the pulmonary arterial system is that the pressure changes at birth. In the fetus the pulmonary and systemic arterial pressures are approximately the same, thus allowing for flow from the pulmonary artery to the aorta through the patent ductus arteriosus. At birth, upon expansion of the lungs, the pulmonary arterial pressure falls (5).

Pulmonary arterial hypertension is almost always related to obvious disease of the heart or lungs. Essential hypertension of the systemic arterial system is not associated with an elevation of pressure in the pulmonary arteries unless heart failure is present (6). Although the pressure in the pulmonary arteries never rises to the levels observed in the systemic arteries in systemic arterial hypertension, the relative increase in pressure is much greater. The diastolic pressure may increase to seven or eight times its normal value in pulmonary hypertension.

In considering the etiology of pulmonary arterial hypertension, three factors are important, namely, the pulmonary vascular resistance, the pulmonary blood flow, and the pulmonary venous pressure. Diseases of the lung may lead to pulmonary hypertension by increasing the vascular resistance, but only if the involvement of the lungs is diffuse and bilateral. The commonest diseases of the lung producing pulmonary hypertension are pulmonary emphysema and silicosis (1, 7, 8). Unilateral pulmonary disease may produce a marked diminution in the flow of blood to one lung, but the pulmonary arterial pressure remains normal (Fig. 1). Pneumonectomy will not produce pulmonary

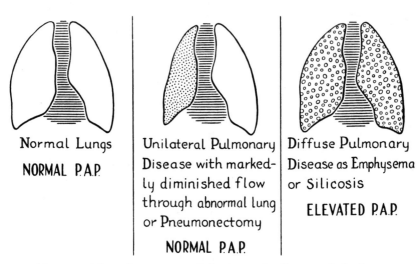

Normal Lungs	Unilateral Pulmonary	Diffuse Pulmonary
NORMAL P.A.P.	Disease with marked-ly diminished flow through abnormal lung or Pneumonectomy	Disease as Emphysema or Silicosis
		ELEVATED P.A.P.
	NORMAL P.A.P.	

FIGURE 1. The pulmonary arterial pressure in diseases of the lung.

hypertension if the opposite lung is normal (9). Primary pulmonary hypertension is excessively rare, but does occur (10). Whether the arteriosclerotic lesions in the small vessels are the cause or effect of the hypertension is not established.

An increased blood flow through the lungs would produce pulmonary hypertension if the vascular resistance remained the same. In normal human beings the increase in the pulmonary blood flow due to exercise is accompanied by a decrease in the pulmonary vascular resistance, the pulmonary arterial pressure remaining unaltered. In pulmonary emphysema the increase in the cardiac output due to exercise does increase the pulmonary arterial pressure (11, 12). Congenital heart disease with left to right shunts, such as interauricular septal defect, interventricular septal defect, and patent ductus arteriosus, may produce a tremendous increase in the pulmonary blood flow. This is most frequently accompanied by only a slight increase in the pulmonary arterial pressure (13, 14, 15). Occasional patients with this type of congenital defect will have a marked increase in the pulmonary arterial pressure (16, 17, 18). It is apparent that in these patients the pulmonary vascular bed has been altered. A similar change in the pulmonary vascular bed accompanies Eisenmenger's complex, as marked pulmonary hypertension invariably occurs in this congenital defect (19, 20, 13).

Pulmonary arterial hypertension is commonly observed in heart disease and is usually attributed to elevation in the pulmonary venous pressure. In contrast to the systemic circulation, an elevation of the venous pressure in the pulmonary circulation causes a rise in the arterial pressure (21). This is due to the small gradient of pressure between the arteries and veins. As might be expected on clinical grounds, the most severe degree of pulmonary hypertension occurs in patients with mitral stenosis and dyspnea at rest or on slight exertion (22). Those patients with dyspnea only on moderate exertion have a lesser degree of hypertension, and patients with mitral stenosis who are asymptomatic may have a normal pulmonary arterial pressure. Patients with left ventricular failure due to systemic hypertension or aortic valvular disease usually exhibit a mild or moderate pulmonary hypertension.

As mentioned previously, pulmonary arterial hypertension occurring in the common types of heart disease is usually attributed to pulmonary venous hypertension. Some recent observations would indicate that under certain circumstances there may also be an alteration in the pulmonary vascular resistance. Certain patients with mitral stenosis exhibit a severe grade of pulmonary hypertension, the level of pressure often approaching that in the systemic circulation. Yet these patients may exhibit none of the signs of frank pulmonary edema, although they are usually incapacitated by exertional dyspnea. It would be difficult to explain the absence of overt pulmonary edema if we assume the gradient of pressure in the pulmonary vascular system to be normal. For if this were true, the pulmonary capillary pressure would be well above the colloid osmotic pressure of the plasma. A likely explanation is an increase in resistance in the pulmonary arterioles. Recent studies of Dexter (23) have offered proof for this hypothesis. He has been able to measure the pulmonary capillary pressure by an ingenious technique and has found the gradient of pressure between the pulmonary artery and pulmonary capillaries to be increased in certain cases of mitral stenosis and left ventricular failure.

Much work remains to be done on the mechanism by which the pulmonary vascular resistance is increased. Neurogenic factors do not appear to play an important role in the increase, but there is some evidence that anoxia may have a part (24, 25, 26). The significance of the arteriosclerotic lesions of the small pulmonary arteries which often accompany pulmonary hypertension has been a controversial subject. On the one hand, these lesions have been implicated as the primary etiologic factor in the production of hypertension. On the other hand, the vascular changes have been ascribed to the effect of prolonged pulmonary hypertension on the vascular system. The solution of this problem would appear to await further knowledge of the pathogenesis of arteriosclerosis.

Questions and Discussion

DR. MAURICE B. VISSCHER: I have been very much interested in Dr. Ebert's excellent work on this problem. I just want to ask him one question—whether in the type of case that he referred to last, in which there was no histological morphological evidence of damage to the pulmonary vessels and yet there was great pulmonary hypertension—whether in such cases, he has measured the cardiac output and calculated the pulmonary resistance?

DR. EBERT: The cardiac output in the patient that Dr. Visscher mentioned was decreased to about half the normal value. Therefore the vascular resistance was markedly increased.

· · · · · · · · · · · · · · · · · · · *by* STEWART WOLF
and HAROLD G. WOLFF

A Summary of Experimental Evidence Relating Life Stress to the Pathogenesis of Essential Hypertension in Man

Introduction

SINCE the introduction of the sphygmomanometer for routine use in the examination of patients, there has been a lively and increasing interest in the occurrence of pressure readings in the brachial artery elevated beyond the average range. Although the significance of such deviations in terms of sickness and death has not been established, its occurrence from time to time has led to the recognition of a disease, essential hypertension, the diagnosis of which may depend entirely upon the consistent finding of an elevated arterial pressure in the absence of evidence of vascular or other anomaly or primary renal disease. Recently investigators have been re-evaluating the concept of "essential hypertension." In the words of Perera: "The evidence points strongly toward a group of independent processes related to or augmented by hypertensive vascular disease, not necessarily related to each other, and so variable in the degree and role of their appearance that a direct correlation with the level of blood pressure is conspicuously absent. Rather than look upon the blood pressure as responsible for other complications it would be preferable to regard it as one of a group of effects all stemming from the same underlying disorder." (1)

A study of essential hypertension, therefore, involves a consideration not only of blood pressure levels, but of the whole hemodynamic

NOTE. This paper is based on studies carried out with the collaboration of Drs. George A. Wolf, John Pfeiffer, Ian P. Stevenson, Charles H. Duncan, Robert A. Schneider, John T. Flynn, and Herbert S. Ripley.

The study was aided by grants from the Commonwealth and the U.S. Public Health Service, National Institutes of Health.

288

process, of the destructive arteriolar changes in the brain, heart, and kidney, and ultimately of the hypertensive person himself.

There has been a gradually accumulating body of evidence to indicate that a consideration of the hypertensive himself, of his attitudes and reaction pattern, may be basic to the understanding of the disease essential hypertension. Since the earliest investigations, data have been accumulating linking elevations in the blood pressure and the accompanying changes of the hypertensive syndrome with stressful life situations (1). The concept that the body may react to "the slings and arrows of outrageous fortune" much as it does to actual slings and arrows has become fairly well established for the respiratory passages (2), the gastrointestinal tract (3, 4), and elsewhere (5, 6, 7). The morbid process involves the unduly intense or sustained use of normal homeostatic adaptive patterns designed for phasic or short-term needs. The "misuse" of such adaptive patterns has thus contributed to the pathogenesis of troublesome symptoms and disease states (8). The present communication attempts to pull together evidence relating life stress and the consequent reactions of adaptation to the pathogenesis of essential hypertension.

Experimental subjects. One hundred and three persons with the usual signs of essential hypertension were followed from day to day over a period of from one to five years. Data on most of them have been reported in detail elsewhere (9). The evidences of essential hypertension included repeatedly finding the arterial pressure in the arms at 160/95 mm. Hg or higher, in the absence of evidence of primary renal disease, endocrine disorder, or congenital anomaly. The ages of the subjects ranged from 28 to 58 years; the duration of known hypertension varied greatly, but in one instance was 23 years. A careful life history and personality study was made by methods already described elsewhere (10). Data concerning these patients were gathered from discussion, questioning, associative procedures, dream analysis, social service case study, and psychologic tests. Moreover, the attitudes and motivations of the subjects were assessed by observation of their behavior and reactions, especially during the discussion of difficult life experiences, by things said and left unsaid, and by statements from other members of their families and from others. The severity of the hypertensive process in most of these subjects was classified as mild or moderate. Very few had advanced retinopathy or evidence of severe cardiac or renal damage. Less than one third of them displayed minimal retinal change or slight cardiac enlargement or EKG abnormality. In only 18 did clearance and concentration tests show any impairment of renal function.

Most of these persons became subjects for one or more of the various experimental procedures outlined below. Twelve were studied both before and after lumbodorsal sympathectomy and 4 before and after complete sympathectomy.

In the day-to-day records of these subjects special note was made of the circumstances surrounding a sudden transitory rise or fall of striking proportions in the blood pressure. A sustained lowering of the blood pressure also became a subject for special attention. Finally, short-term observations were made in the experimental setting during the discussion of significant personal conflicts. The effects of discussing a troublesome topic were observed directly by recording the words of the patient and by noting his reactions, gestures, facial expressions, and general behavior; inferences concerning the significance of the interview situation were drawn with due consideration of these and earlier observations.

Control subjects were selected from a variety of sources. In an attempt to highlight the characteristic features of the hypertensive person and his responses, comparisons were made with a group of 150 patients with vasomotor rhinitis or bronchial asthma. Twenty healthy adult persons of both sexes (12 women, 8 men) from the laboratory and hospital staff also served as controls, and, finally, control studies were made on 61 patients with a variety of disorders, but without hypertension.

The Over-All Attitudes and Reactions of Hypertensive Subjects

In agreement with the findings of Sheldon, we found that hypertensive subjects were more square and muscular than average (11). They were nonreflective and displayed a taste for dealing with problems by action. Many of them exhibited signs and symptoms of excessive skeletal muscle tension. From the standpoint of attitudes as well as of circulatory physiology, they were mobilized for combat, but did not engage in it against the pertinent adversary. Under a facade often affable and easygoing, they were tense, wary, and suspicious, afraid of committing themselves. They were poised to strike, but withheld their punch with a guilty fear of its consequences. At the same time they displayed a strong need to conform and keep peace. This, coupled with an inability to throw themselves wholeheartedly into things because of fear and suspicion, made it difficult for them to believe strongly in anything or to derive real satisfaction from their accomplishments. They felt a need to show prowess without exhibiting aggression and continually feared that they would not succeed in doing so.

Hypertensive persons were found to take out their aggression in some vicarious way, by excelling in sports or merely by an excess of general activity or excessive eating. They were prominently preoccupied with appearances and saving face. As children they had all been unduly shy. They blushed easily and were rarely able to admit they were wrong. Most of the married ones selected domineering mates.

In the background of the subjects we studied were the following common circumstances, which may have provided conditioning situations. Many of their mothers were stiff and domineering. They were inclined to demand compliance and withheld approval if it was not given. They especially refused to tolerate outbursts of anger. Their children felt themselves forced to compete for affection and approval by being "good." Many of our hypertensives dealt fairly successfully with this challenge and managed for a time, at least, to consider themselves "closest" to the mother. This accomplishment inevitably involved the development of strong hostility toward the mother, which was suppressed with varying degrees of success, but was associated with guilt.

In brief, our hypertensive subjects, often gentle, poised, and apparently easygoing, were filled with aggressive drive, which was tightly restrained by a need to please (10). These findings are in general agreement with those reported by earlier observers (12, 13, 14, 15).

Changes in the Blood Pressure during Periods of Stress

An analysis of changes in the blood pressure was made in a group of 23 hypertensive and 32 control subjects who during a period of relative tranquillity and security were abruptly subjected to discussions of significant personal problems while the blood pressure was measured at as frequent intervals as possible. In "stimulus strength" the interviews could be grouped into three general categories: (1) those in which the subject felt threatened by the discussion of his important personal conflicts; (2) those in which the subject did not feel threatened by the examiner, but in whom the recollections of pertinent matters evoked such painful associations as to constitute a reliving of the situation discussed; (3) those in which the positive benefit of being able to talk over problems with a sympathetic and detached person predominated so that the interview was more re-assuring than stressful.

The effects on the patients of interviews in the first two categories were variable, but fell generally into one of two groupings: (a) they considered themselves menaced or trapped; (b) they considered themselves defeated or overwhelmed. None of the interview situations was so startling as to evoke sudden fright or alarm.

When the subject considered himself, as in the first group, menaced or trapped, he might or might not give open evidence of his feeling. When he responded, as in the second, with a feeling of being overwhelmed, however, his accompanying feelings of terror or abject despair were usually evident.

Generally speaking, reactions of the first type were accompanied by conscious or unconscious emotions of anxiety, resentment, or hostility and were associated with a rise in the blood pressure, while reactions of the second type were associated with a fall in the blood pressure or no change.

RISE IN THE ARTERIAL PRESSURE

Twenty-one of the hypertensive and 16 of the control subjects displayed the first type of response and with it a rise in the blood pressure. The data are reported in detail elsewhere (16).

The 16 normotensive subjects exhibited an over-all average control blood pressure of 119/76, while the average control blood pressure of the hypertensive group was 165/103 mm. Hg. The average mean pressure in the normotensive group was 90 mm. Hg and in the hypertensive group 124 mm. Hg (Table 1). During the stressful interviews the blood pressure of the control group rose to an average figure of 131/81, of the hypertensive group to 189/117. There was an average increase in the mean blood pressure of 8 mm. in the normotensive group and an increase of 17 in the hypertensive group.

Comment. It is evident that during certain types of emotional conflict all of the subjects, hypertensives and normotensives alike, responded with increases in the blood pressure, indicating that such a reaction is not peculiar to those with vascular hypertension, but is part of a widely shared reaction to stress.

FALL IN THE ARTERIAL PRESSURE

Two persons in the hypertensive group and 6 among the controls showed during interview a response of the second type, with an attitude of being overwhelmed. In each instance the blood pressure fell

TABLE 1. Changes in the Blood Pressure and in Other Hemodynamic Indicators in Hypertensive and Normotensive Persons during Periods of Anxiety

	Hypertensive Group*				Non-Hypertensive Group			
	Relaxed†	Anxious	Absolute Change	Per Cent Change	Relaxed	Anxious	Absolute Change	Per Cent Change
Systolic blood pressure	165	189	24	14.5	119	131	12	10.1
Diastolic blood pressure	103	117	14	13.6	76	81	5	6.6
Mean blood pressure	124	141	17	13.7	90	98	8	8.9
Heart rate	74	80	6	8	79	89	10	12
Stroke volume	66	83	17	26	79	105	26	33
Cardiac index	2.6	3.7	1.1	42	3.6	5.5	1.9	53
Peripheral resistance	55	44	—11	20	29	20	—9	32
Increase in mean blood pressure, mm. Hg/1.0 liter increase in cardiac index	16				4			

* The hypertensive group includes subjects recently showing diastolic hypertension—i.e., /100 mm. Hg and above. The non-hypertensive group includes other patients and therefore includes 1 subject who was formerly hypertensive.

There are 16 subjects in the non-hypertensive group and 21 in the hypertensive group. Mean figures are given and adjusted for the proportion of males to females. Mean blood pressure = diastolic + ⅓ pulse pressure.

† The word relaxation does not imply complete relaxation, but merely that the subject was more relaxed on that occasion than when he was judged to be emotionally disturbed.

293

below the initial levels. In one person during a period of feeling over-whelmed, even a cold-pressor test induced a precipitous drop in the blood pressure rather than the sharp rise this patient usually dis-played (Fig. 1).

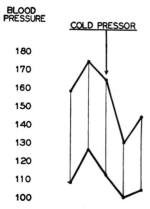

FIGURE 1. The fall in the systolic and diastolic pressures during a cold-pressor test in a hyper-tensive subject during feelings of being over-whelmed. Under usual circumstances this subject displayed a brisk rise in the blood pressure.

Changes in Other Indicators of Cardiovascular Dynamics

Earlier students of the subject have shown that the elevation of the arterial pressure in essential hypertension is largely accomplished by an increase in the peripheral resistance. Thus only limited inferences can be drawn from measurement of the blood pressure alone, since thereby one cannot distinguish the underlying mechanism responsible. It thus becomes pertinent to inquire into the factors which control and modify the peripheral resistance as well as those which evoke and modify the blood pressure response.

In an attempt to gather data on this point, 39 of the hypertensive subjects and 36 of the control subjects were observed on one or more occasions while lying on a critically damped ballistocardiographic table constructed according to the specifications of Nickerson and Warren (17). Six of these subjects were studied before and after bilateral lumbodorsal sympathectomy, and 2 before and after total sympathectomy.

The ballistocardiographic observations were usually made with the subject in the "basal" state, although for special reasons observations were recorded at various times throughout the day, but never less than 2 hours after meals. In each instance recordings were begun after 20 minutes' rest on a comfortable bed in the laboratory. The blood pressure was ascertained by the auscultatory method approximately every minute; ballistocardiographic recordings were made almost con-tinuously in some experiments and at approximately 5-minute intervals in others. Stroke volume, cardiac output, and peripheral resistance were calculated by the methods of Nickerson in a manner described elsewhere (18).

Since one of the simplest ways of inducing an elevation in the blood pressure is by undertaking vigorous muscular exercise, observations were made during the performance of the Standard Master Step Test; they are reported in detail elsewhere (16).

REACTION FOLLOWING EXERCISE

Average measurements at rest and following exercise during relaxation in 20 hypertensive and 28 non-hypertensive (and healthy) subjects are given in Table 2 and graphically in Figure 2. Although the

TABLE 2. Changes in the Blood Pressure and in Other Hemodynamic Indicators in Hypertensive and Normotensive Persons Immediately after a Standard Exercise

Group	Resting	After a Standard Exercise			
		2 Minutes	3 Minutes	5 Minutes	10 Minutes
Normotensive (28)					
Blood pressure, S/D	108/67	118/65	114/65	111/64	107/67
Heart rate	67	69	68	67	67
Stroke volume (cc.)	83	107	100	91	83
Cardiac index					
(l/min sq m)	3.1	4.1	3.8	3.5	3.0
Peripheral resistance					
(mm/Hg, l/min sq m)	28	22	24	26	28
Hypertensive (20)					
Blood pressure, S/D	175/110	188/108	179/107	172/108	174/110
Heart rate	71	76	74	74	73
Stroke volume (cc.)	67	87	79	73	66
Cardiac index					
(l/min sq m)	2.7	3.8	3.3	3.1	2.7
Peripheral resistance					
(mm/Hg, l/min sq m)	54	39	44	48	51

average heart rate was higher and the average stroke volume lower in the hypertensive group, the significant difference between the two sets of measurements was the high peripheral resistance and the elevation of the blood pressure in the hypertensive group. The response to the stress of exercise as judged by rates of the return of the heart rate and cardiac index to resting values was essentially similar in the two groups. Peripheral resistance was considerably lower rather than higher following exercise in both groups.

Comment. These results confirm those of Taylor *et al.* (19) by demonstrating the failure of exercise to elevate the blood pressure

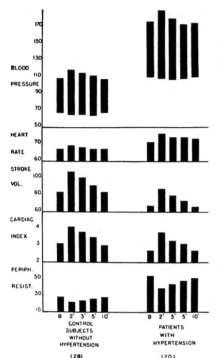

FIGURE 2. A graphic representation of the average figures from Table 2. Note the similarity of the responses in the two groups, but the consistently higher peripheral resistance of the hypertensive subjects.

more in hypertensive than in non-hypertensive subjects. They do not support the notion that exercise is a form of stress unfavorable to the hypertensive process, an idea which is often implied in the frequent restrictions placed on these subjects with respect to exercise.

CHANGES DURING STRESS

1. With relatively free expression. In contrast to the responses of the subjects to physical exercise, a difference was noted in the circulatory reactions of the hypertensive and normotensive subjects during stress. Measurements were made on subjects of both groups during periods of life stress associated with feeling states of anxiety and resentment. The averages of all the measurements made in both groups are given in Table 3 and shown graphically in Figure 3. The usual, almost invariable, observations in both groups during the periods of disturbance were an elevation in the blood pressure, heart rate, stroke volume, and cardiac output and a fall in the peripheral resistance. In a few instances in both groups the peripheral resistance rose. The average increase in the blood pressure both in millimeters of mercury and percentage was greater in the hypertensive than in the normotensive subjects. The average increase in the cardiac output was somewhat less in the hypertensive than in the normotensive subjects. In Figure 4 is shown graphically the prototype of this response.

Comment. It is apparent that in both groups the increase in the cardiac output during the stressful period was somewhat compensated

TABLE 3. A Comparison of Control Values and Changes in Clearances, Blood Pressures, and Vascular Resistances in the Normotensive and Hypertensive Groups. (Reproduced, by permission of the copyright owner, from J. B. Pfeiffer, Jr., and H. G. Wolff: J. Clin. Investigation 29:1227–1242, 1950.)

Average Values	Normotensive	Hypertensive	"P"
Average, Control Periods			
Mean blood pressure (*mm. Hg*)	93.5 ± 9.9	137.3 ± 19.4	<0.01
Effective plasma flow (*cc./min.*)	509.0 ±94.2	460.4 - ±110.3	<0.3
Glomerular filtration rate (*cc./min.*)	89.1 ±11.9	102.5 ± 23.4	<0.05
Filtration fraction	0.176± 0.021	0.225± 0.035	<0.001
Peripheral resistance (*mm. Hg/cc./min.*)	0.098± 0.034	0.171± 0.054	<0.001
Average, Discussion Periods			
Mean blood pressure (*mm. Hg*)	102.6 ±12.8	151.4 ± 20.7	<0.001
Effective plasma flow (*cc./min.*)	482.3 ±77.3	418.0 ± 99.1	<0.05
Glomerular filtration rate (*cc./min.*)	88.8 ± 13.2	102.6 ± 26.8	<0.1
Filtration fraction	0.186± 0.023	0.247± 0.030	<0.001
Peripheral resistance (*mm. Hg/cc./min.*)	0.122± 0.022	0.212± 0.066	<0.001
Average, Post-discussion Periods			
Mean blood pressure (*mm. Hg*)	97.8 ±10.4	137.5 + 16.9	<0.001
Effective plasma flow (*cc./min.*)	493.2 ±84.8	414.2 + 81.6	<0.01
Glomerular filtration rate (*cc./min.*)	88.3 ±18.1	99.9 + 26.2	<0.2
Filtration fraction	0.180± 0.022	0.241+ 0.038	<0.001
Peripheral resistance (*mm. Hg/cc./min.*)	0.112± 0.021	0.186+ 0.048	<0.001

Average Changes	Normotensive	Hypertensive	"P"
Discussion—Control Periods			
Mean blood pressure (*mm. Hg*)	+9.3±5.7 (<0.01)	+17.3±10.8 (<0.001)	<0.02
Effective plasma flow (*cc./min.*)	−26.5±30.1 (<0.01)	−42.4±52.6 (<0.001)	—
Glomerular filtration rate (*cc./min.*)	−0.8±5.7 (——)	+0.0±6.9 (——)	—
Filtration fraction	+0.011±0.009 (0.001)	+0.022±0.018 (0.001)	<0.05
Peripheral resistance (*mm. Hg/cc./min.*)	+0.014±0.012 (<0.001)	+0.041±0.026 (<0.001)	<0.01
Post-discussion—Control Periods			
Mean blood pressure (*mm. Hg*)	+2.7±6.4 (<0.2)	+3.0±7.1 (<0.1)	—
Effective plasma flow (*cc./min.*)	−22.7±30.4 (<0.02)	−34.5±49.6 (<0.01)	—
Glomerular filtration rate (*cc./min.*)	−0.6±2.3 (——)	−0.2±6.6 (——)	—
Filtration fraction	+0.005±0.013 (<0.2)	+0.015±0.021 (<0.01)	<0.2
Peripheral resistance (*mm. Hg/cc./min.*)	+0.005±0.010 (<0.1)	+0.017±0.026 (<0.01)	<0.2

a) The normotensive group consisted of 13 subjects. The hypertensive group consisted of 20 to 22 subjects. This variation was taken into consideration in the calculation of "t". Each figure is followed by its standard deviation.

b) "P" represents the degree of probability that the two figures on the same horizontal row are not significant, and was obtained from the tables of distribution after calculation of "t". The omissions signified by dashes indicate that "P" was greater than 0.2. Levels of 0.01 or less are to be considered significant.

$$t = (\bar{X}_1 - \bar{X}_2) \cdot \sqrt{\frac{n_1 - n_2 (n_1 + n_2 - 2)}{(n_1 + n_2) (\Sigma x_1 + \Sigma x_2)}}$$

$$\Sigma x = \Sigma X^2 - \frac{(\Sigma X)^2}{n}$$

c) The figures in parentheses beneath each value represent "P" with the same significance as under (b), regarding the respective average differences immediately above. "t" was calculated as follows:

$$t = \frac{\bar{X}}{S.D./\sqrt{n}} \qquad S.D. = \sqrt{\frac{X^2 - \frac{(\Sigma X)^2}{n}}{n - 1}}$$

by vascular dilatation with a resultant over-all fall in the peripheral resistance. In the normotensive group this vasodilatation was sufficiently great to prevent more than a slight rise in the blood pressure. In the hypertensive subjects, however, either there was less general vasodilatation, or the vasodilatation in some areas was offset by vaso-

Figure 3. Changes in the blood pressure and other hemodynamic indicators in normotensive and hypertensive persons during more or less overt anxiety and conflict. Note the similarity of the responses in the two groups, but the relative preponderance of the peripheral resistance over the stroke volume in the hypertensive group.

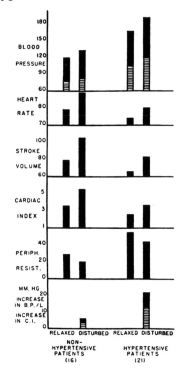

constriction in others. The net result was a considerably greater increase in the blood pressure in proportion to the increase in the cardiac output among the hypertensive than among the normotensive subjects.

2. "Reined In." It was more characteristic for hypertensive subjects reacting to the interviews by feeling menaced or trapped not to show obvious affective change but to display a calm and unruffled exterior. Often

the reaction was altogether unconscious, but it invariably was associated with a brisk rise in the blood pressure. On 21 occasions Flynn (20) observed hypertensive subjects in such a situation and normotensives in 17. The hemody-

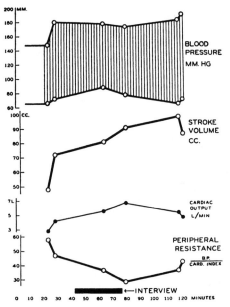

Figure 4. Elevation of the blood pressure attributable to an increased cardiac output, with a fall in the peripheral resistance, during an interview which evoked overt manifestations of anxiety and conflict.

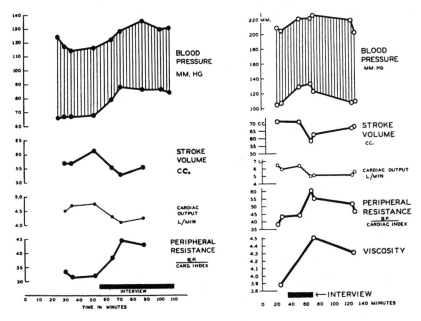

FIGURE 5. Elevation of the blood pressure attributable to an increased peripheral resistance with a fall in the cardiac output in a normotensive subject
during an interview concerning significant personal conflicts to which the
subject reacted by consciously or unconsciously "reining in" his feelings
so that he displayed an attitude of unruffled calm.

FIGURE 6. Changes similar to those in Figure 5 observed in a hypertensive
subject during suppressed or repressed conflicts. In this experiment
measurements of the blood viscosity were also made.

namic reaction which characterized this type of response included
mainly an increase in the peripheral resistance with no change in the
stroke volume or a slight fall. A typical example of such a reaction in
a normotensive subject is shown in Figure 5. Figure 6 shows graphically the same type of response in the hypertensive subject described
below.

The patient, a 47-year-old unmarried woman, first came to the clinic
in December 1946 complaining of headaches and easy fatigability.
Hypertension had been discovered two years before. Her blood pressure was usually in the neighborhood of 200/110. During the experimental procedure she lay quietly, smiled frequently, and seemed
superficially composed, even during a discussion of her relations with
her mother, toward whom she felt intense hostility. An underlying
truculence was evident in her attitude, however, as manifested by

laconic replies, irony, and understatement. During the period of interview her blood pressure rose briskly, a rise associated with a marked
increase in the peripheral resistance but none in the stroke volume.

Two of the hypertensive subjects and 2 of the controls who displayed
a fall in the blood pressure during interview with the characteristic

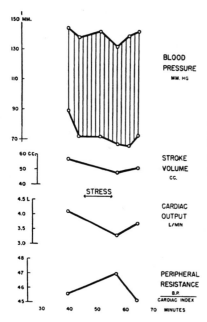

FIGURE 7. A hypodynamic response during feelings of being overwhelmed. The
subject was a hypertensive who usually
displayed a pattern of reaction similar
to that described in Figure 6.

reaction of being overwhelmed were observed on the ballistocardiograph. In each instance there occurred a pronounced drop in the stroke
volume with a relative increase in the peripheral resistance (Fig. 7).

Comment

It is evident from these observations that the cardiovascular apparatus is capable of various hemodynamic responses to situational
stimuli. The blood pressure level is merely the resultant of some of
these adaptive changes. Thus, in seeking a formulation of essential
hypertension, if one focused only on the blood pressure elevation, it
would be necessary to consider and explore all the many factors
which contribute to the establishment of the blood pressure level.
The problem might be simplified, however, if one could view essential
hypertension as a complex in which the cardiovascular changes, including the blood pressure elevation, were of a particular type. For
example, in clinical essential hypertension one is able to identify not

only that the systolic and diastolic blood pressures are more or less persistently elevated but that the pulse rate is not accelerated and the stroke volume is not increased. The cutaneous blood flow is not altered, but the visceral blood flow, notably the renal blood flow, is more or less reduced. The hemodynamic changes, then, fall into a pattern which may be distinguished from at least one other cardiovascular pattern involving blood pressure elevation.

In the course of earlier studies, and as mentioned briefly above, several more or less distinct patterns of cardiovascular reaction in response to stress have been identified. One is a hypodynamic pattern which may be accompanied by fainting or near fainting and is characterized by a sharp decrease in the cardiac output or peripheral resistance or both with a consequent fall in the blood pressure. Such a pattern was identified when persons found themselves in situations in which they felt overwhelmed and was encountered occasionally even among hypertensives. A second pattern, a hyperdynamic one, appeared to occur in adaptation to the demands of muscular exertion; it increased the heat loss and enhanced the peripheral blood flow, and was encountered most characteristically during or immediately after vigorous exercise as well as in association with more or less overt anxiety and resentment. This pattern was found to be characterized by an increased cardiac output and a decreased peripheral resistance, often with an elevation in the blood pressure. The increase in the cardiac output was attributable either to tachycardia or an increased stroke volume. According to Stevenson et al. (18) the former mechanism was more often encountered among normal subjects during transitory apprehension, while the latter mechanism predominated among neurotic subjects with so-called neurocirculatory asthenia.

Another pattern, also a hyperdynamic one, apparently directed toward conservation of the blood volume and maintenance of the blood pressure, was the one which most closely fitted the observation of the hypertensive state. It was identified in persons who were tightly restraining conscious and unconscious feelings of anxiety and hostility. A study of hypertensive subjects indicated they were frequently and chronically in that state. In this pattern the blood pressure was elevated, chiefly on account of an increase in the peripheral vascular resistance without significant change in the cardiac output either in terms of rate or stroke volume. As noted below, it was found that hypertensive subjects did not display exclusively this latter pattern, but under certain circumstances of stress reacted with the first hyperdynamic response. The distinction is important, chiefly because of the

302 A Symposium on Hypertension

fact that in terms of energy expenditure for work done the latter pattern was found to be far more costly than the former. Reference to Poussieu's formula (36)

$$\text{Blood pressure} = \frac{\text{length of arteries} \times \text{viscosity} \times 8\Pi \times \text{co}}{(\text{cross section area})^2}$$

makes this point evident and suggests that recourse to one or the other pattern for elevating the blood pressure may have some prognostic significance for the hypertensive. Athletes and others who continually evoke the former have demonstrated that frequent use of that pattern is not incompatible with good health and long life.

Changes in the Physical Characteristics of the Blood

In the formula quoted the factor of blood viscosity equals in weight that of cardiac output and is therefore not inconsiderable. Up to the present, investigators have assumed that the blood viscosity remains constant over a short period of observation. In view of the importance of the viscosity factor, however, in determining the efficiency of the heart pump mechanism, it seemed worth while to explore the possibility of changes in the viscosity and other physical characteristics of the blood. Such studies on 16 healthy adult volunteers, 9 normotensive, and 12 hypertensive patients were carried out by Schneider (21), who found that a pressor response, however induced, was accompanied in both normotensive and hypertensive subjects by an increase in the blood viscosity and a shortening of the clotting time.

The viscosity of the blood was measured by use of the apparatus described by T'ang and Wang (22).

The blood clotting time was determined by using the siliconized tube method as described by Barker and Margulies (23).

STANDARDIZATION

To attempt to ascertain the reliability of the method, three experiments were carried out on 3 subjects, in which four specimens (at approximately 9:30 and 11:00 A.M., 2:00 and 4:00 P.M.) were drawn within a single day while each subject went about his usual duties. The clotting time in each case remained remarkably constant, with a range of deviation of 1 minute in one subject, 5 minutes in the second, and 4 minutes in the third subject. In approximately one third of the tests the commonly used Lee-White Method (chemically clean dry tubes of the same size and depth at 37° C.) was carried out simultaneously with the silicone tube method of measurement. The two methods corresponded well, but the spread of values was much greater with the silicone tube.

It was concluded that the silicone method was the better suited to detecting shortened clotting times. Arbitrarily the mean clotting time of 54 minutes, obtained in testing 48 relaxed normotensive control subjects, was accepted as the "normal" clotting time; a clotting time less than 44 minutes was considered "accelerated"; and a clotting time in excess of 64 minutes was considered "prolonged."

RELAXED NORMOTENSIVE VOLUNTEERS

Samples of blood were drawn from apparently relaxed, healthy volunteers over a 6-month period to determine the mean value of the clotting time for both males and females, by use of the silicone tube method. Thirty-seven specimens from 25 women (non-menstruating) showed a range of from 44 to 69 minutes, with a mean value of 54 minutes. Six specimens were obtained from 5 women during the first day of menstruation and showed a range of from 30 to 38 minutes, with a mean value of 34 minutes. Twenty-one samples were obtained from 18 males, and the clotting times ranged from 47 to 65 minutes, with again a mean value of 54 minutes.

EFFECTS OF NOXIOUS STIMULATION

Noxious stimulation was accomplished by use of a modified cold-pressor procedure. Nine relaxed normotensive volunteers immersed the left hand in ice water for a 5-minute period. The first blood sample was obtained prior to the immersion of the hand after the blood pressure had stabilized. The next specimen was obtained 2 minutes after the hand was withdrawn from the water, and a final specimen of blood was obtained 1 hour later. The subjects were recumbent throughout the experiment. Four of the 9 subjects failed to get a rise in the blood pressure in excess of 20 mm. systolic or 15 mm. diastolic after 30 or 60 seconds of the immersion, and according to Brown and Hines (24) would be classified as normal reactors. Five of the 9 subjects had a rise in the blood pressure exceeding 20 mm. systolic and 15 mm. diastolic after the 30- or 60-second interval of immersion and could therefore be classified as hyperreactors.

The non-reactors failed to show any significant changes in any of the blood measurements. The hyperreactors, however, showed an average shortening of the clotting time by 25 per cent in the specimen obtained following the cold-pain experience, with a return to the original values in 1 hour, without changes in the other indicators. In

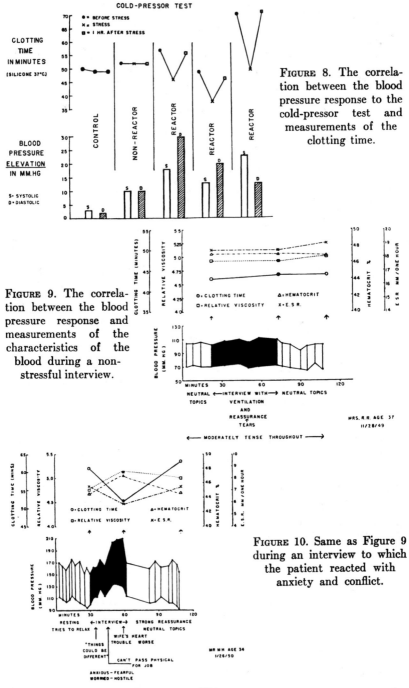

FIGURE 8. The correlation between the blood pressure response to the cold-pressor test and measurements of the clotting time.

FIGURE 9. The correlation between the blood pressure response and measurements of the characteristics of the blood during a non-stressful interview.

FIGURE 10. Same as Figure 9 during an interview to which the patient reacted with anxiety and conflict.

304

all, 8 of the 9 subjects experienced varying degrees of pain, but the clotting time was shortened only in those subjects who had a pressor response with the pain (Fig. 8).

Comment. From an earlier study (25) it was postulated that the elevation in the arterial pressure which often accompanies the cold-pressor test is a part of the pain reaction. It would appear that the changes in the clotting time observed in these experiments constitute also a reaction to noxious stimulation.

EFFECTS OF STRESSFUL INTERVIEWS

Schneider has reported in detail the changes observed in short-term experiments when his subjects were exposed briefly to a discussion of personal conflicts (26). When the interviews were predominantly reassuring and unassociated with a rise in the blood pressure, no significant change in the measured characteristics of the blood was observed (Fig. 9). When the interviews aroused conflict, however, with conscious or unconscious anxiety and resentment, there occurred in association with the elevated arterial pressure a shortening of the clotting time (and sedimentation rate) and an increase in the blood viscosity (with a rise in hematocrit), as shown in Figure 10.

DAY-TO-DAY OBSERVATIONS

Day-to-day observations were conducted on both normotensive and hypertensive subjects. The blood pressure was ascertained and the clotting time and relative blood viscosity were measured two or three times a week. In the day-to-day observations carried out in the manner already described, a close correlation was observed between the feeling state, the level of the blood pressure, and the measured value of the clotting time and blood viscosity.

Figure 11 illustrates representative measurements of the clotting time, the blood viscosity, the blood pressure, and the feeling state and life situation in 2 young adult males, one with essential hypertension and one with normal blood pressure.

The hypertensive subject. A 35-year-old office worker was first discovered to have essential hypertension at the age of 29 while a noncombatant in the army. He was a conscientious, rigid person, with marked feelings of inadequacy, who had a great need to do well and to please others. He was found to be extremely tense and hostile underneath a pleasant and calm facade. He had not made an adult sexual adjustment and was in strong rivalry with his two siblings. The hypertension developed following the death of his father and the marriage of his younger brother. He was unable to work when first seen because of marked anxiety. Living at home with his aged mother, supported by his spinster sister, he had made several unsuccessful attempts to emancipate himself from his family.

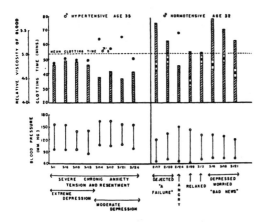

FIGURE 11. The day-to-day correlation between the blood pressure, the clotting time, and the blood viscosity in a hypertensive and a normotensive subject.

He was followed over a 4-month period, during the first 3 months of which his blood pressure was nearly always in the hypertensive range. He was examined 5 days a week during this period, and the clotting time and relative viscosity of the blood were measured on Tuesdays and Fridays of each week. The left half of Figure 11 gives representative measurements of the clotting time, relative viscosity, and blood pressure levels on the days indicated, and note is made of the relation between these values and the patient's emotional status and life situation. On March 1, 6, 10, and 13 the clotting times (46 to 49 minutes) were just slightly shorter than the average for the relaxed male, and the viscosity values (4.80 to 4.90) were within the average range for males. The blood pressures ranged from 142/95 to 154/98. On all four of these occasions, which were during the first 2 weeks, he was depressed, tense, preoccupied, and anxious. Dreams during this period indicated hostility directed at both the brother and the father. On March 14, 17, 21, and 24 clotting times were distinctly shortened (36 to 44 minutes), and the blood viscosity values were decidedly elevated (4.90 to 5.36). The blood pressures during this period ranged from 155/98 to 164/108. During this 2-week period the depression had lessened appreciably, as noted by clinical observation and by projective psychometric tests. However, the anxiety, resentment, and hostility had increased, as evidenced clinically and by such statements on the part of the patient as "I'm feeling very tense and anxious," "I'm angry with myself at home," "I feel frustrated and resentful toward my family." His sleep was disturbed by vivid, fearful dreams that showed sexual anxiety, rivalry with, and resentment toward his brother and anxiety and fear in connection with his father. Note that throughout the period of observation the clotting time and relative viscosity of the blood roughly paralleled the changes in the arterial pressure.

Further measurements and observations made on this patient over the subsequent 4 months are shown in Figure 12. There was a gradual return to a nearly normal blood pressure, with the clotting times returning to an average value of 50 minutes and the blood viscosity to

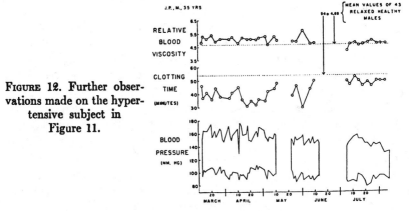

FIGURE 12. Further observations made on the hypertensive subject in Figure 11.

values of from 4.6 to 4.8, as he was able to express himself more freely and talk about his resentments and anxieties more directly and frankly. Coincident with these changes the patient had shown less evidence of depression, and the anxiety had decreased enough to permit his return to gainful employment.

The normotensive subject. The right half of Figure 11 gives representative measurements, over a 10-week period of study, of the clotting time and blood viscosity of a healthy 32-year-old physician, together with blood pressure readings and data on his emotional state and life situation. On February 17 and February 20, during a period of frustration and lack of progress in his work, the subject felt dejected and depressed. The blood pressures were normal, the clotting times were prolonged (78 and 64 minutes), and the viscosity of the blood was relatively low. On February 24, while acting as a volunteer for an experimental procedure, he became anxious and openly angry with a technician who had wrongly prepared the equipment. Note that the blood pressure at that time rose to 150 mm. systolic, the clotting time was short (44 minutes), and the viscosity of the blood was high (5.4). On February 28 and again on March 3 the subject felt in "optimum spirits." The blood pressures were normal and the clotting times were nearly exactly those of the mean value in the relaxed male. On March 6, 15, and 21, following the receipt of several letters bearing "bad news from home," the subject felt overwhelmed and depressed. Note the normal blood pressures, but the prolongation of the clotting times (as long as 80 minutes). This correlation between feelings of depression and long clotting times was commonly observed.

Comment. In the present investigation it was found that viscosity was increased whenever the clotting time was shortened. Likewise, whenever the hematocrit rose, the blood viscosity increased.

Cannon (27) considered that the acceleration of blood clotting was one of several responses in the organism in time of danger designed to prepare for fight or flight and, more specifically, to "be regarded as an adaptive process—useful to the organism—in conserving the blood, especially in the struggles of mortal combat."

It is conceivable that these changes in the blood, which are most generally accompanied by a pressor response, represent a protective reaction pattern in man, used during short transient periods of stress, which is beneficial in that the likelihood of excessive blood loss is reduced (shortened clotting time) and added oxygen demands are satisfied (increased hematocrit and increased blood viscosity). However, it is also conceivable that if such a protective reaction pattern is used for a very long period, perhaps inappropriately, then it may no longer be useful, but actually become detrimental in that a shortened clotting time and an increased blood viscosity may predispose to intravascular thrombosis.

Moreover, it appears that there occurs in the hypertensive subject a significant increase in the over-all peripheral resistance, especially when his arterial pressure is made to rise further under a stress which he feels called upon to meet with a tightly restrained attitude and an avoidance of overt hostility and aggression, and that changes in the blood viscosity form a not inconsiderable part of that change in the peripheral resistance. The mechanism whereby these changes are brought about, however, remains obscure. Earlier students of the hypertensive process have shown the importance of changes in the renal blood flow. Therefore, measurements of the renal blood flow were included in the investigation of these subjects.

Correlation between Hemodynamics and Measurements of the Physical Characteristics of the Blood

Hypertensive and normotensive subjects were studied simultaneously by the ballistocardiographic and the blood viscosity and clotting time techniques before, during, and after stressful interviews. The prototype of the response is shown in Figure 6. It will be noted that whether the hypertensive response was accomplished chiefly by the cardiac output or the peripheral resistance, the blood viscosity increased and the clotting time shortened (not shown on the graph). Thus, when a rise in the calculated peripheral resistance was observed, it was clear that it represented a predominantly arterial vasoconstriction.

Changes in the Renal Circulatory Dynamics

Thirty-five of the hypertensive subjects and 13 of the control subjects were observed during measurement of the effective renal plasma flow and glomerular filtration by the para-aminohippurate and inulin-clearance methods of Homer Smith (28).

The details of these studies have been reported elsewhere (10, 29), but the prototype of the response is shown in Figure 13. Both hypertensive and control subjects whose blood pressures rose during the interview situation displayed evidence of renal vasoconstriction, with

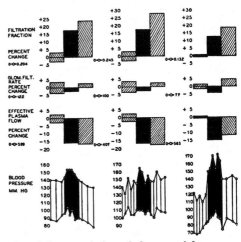

FIGURE 13. The changes in the blood pressure and renal hemodynamics in 4 representative subjects of the 21 tested. The first section of cross-hatching represents the range of variation of three separate control periods. The mean value in each instance is shown at the left of the scale as 0⟳. The solid black column represents the average change during the periods of traumatic interview, and the last cross-hatched column shows the average change in the post-interview periods. (This figure and the one that follows are reproduced, by permission of the copyright owner, from J. B. Pfeiffer, Jr., and H. G. Wolff: J. Clin. Investigation 29:1227–1242, 1950.)

a sharp reduction in the effective renal plasma flow and an increased filtration fraction.

THE EFFECTIVE PLASMA FLOW, GLOMERULAR FILTRATION RATE,
AND RENAL VASCULAR RESISTANCE

The average effective plasma flow when corrected for body surface area was 509 ± 94.2 cc/min. (This is low when compared to the figures given by Goldring and Chasis, 697 ± 151 cc/min for males and 594 ± 102 cc/min for females.) During the discussion periods there was an average decrease of -26.5 ± 30.1 cc/min in the effective plasma flow in the normotensive group. The hypertensive group had a still lower renal plasma flow, 460 ± 110 cc/min, and exhibited a decrease of -42.4 ± 52.6 cc/min during the period of stress.

In general during the period of stress and in some cases for a considerable time thereafter, there was a change in the renal hemodynamics characterized by a fall in the effective plasma flow, insignificant changes in the glomerular filtration rate, and a rise in the filtration fraction. When the individual cases are examined and the standard deviations are consulted, it is seen that there was more uniformity in this change than in the others; the variations in the renal plasma flow and glomerular filtration rate operated more consistently to produce a rise in the filtration fraction. In addition, it can be seen that the variations did not necessarily parallel the blood pressure response, the renal hemodynamics being disturbed long after the latter had returned to normal.

Utilizing the ratio of mean blood pressure to effective blood flow (corrected for body surface area) as a crude indication of the vascular resistance of the kidney, other inferences were made possible. In both groups there were large increases in the renal vascular resistance; 0.014 ± 0.012 units in the normotensive and 0.041 ± 0.026 units in the hypertensive group (Fig. 14). As might be expected, the control values in the latter group were considerably higher to begin with. The prolongation of the increase in the renal vascular resistance is indicated by the length of time required for the figures to return to control values (Table 3 and Fig. 15). Thus in both normotensives and hypertensives the kidney adjusted itself by means of vasoconstriction to the rise in the systemic blood pressure, preventing an increase of the blood flow through it. There is suggestive evidence that the hypertensive kidney overcompensates so that it exhibits both a more intensive and more prolonged constriction, even after the blood pressure has returned to near control levels.

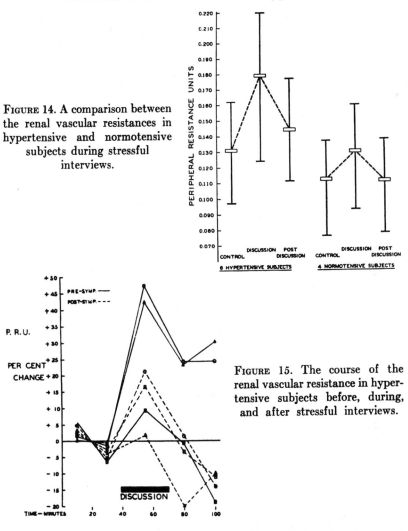

FIGURE 14. A comparison between the renal vascular resistances in hypertensive and normotensive subjects during stressful interviews.

FIGURE 15. The course of the renal vascular resistance in hypertensive subjects before, during, and after stressful interviews.

VARIATIONS IN THE BLOOD PRESSURE, EFFECTIVE PLASMA FLOW,
GLOMERULAR FILTRATION RATE, AND RENAL VASCULAR
RESISTANCE DURING RELAXATION

The converse of the above experiments was exhibited when, in attempting to restrict the sphere of attention by the use of sodium amytal, one hypertensive subject became very relaxed and indulged in pleasurable phantasies before the interview was started. An effort was then made to promote and maintain this relaxation. The blood pressure fell from an average control level of 197/109 to 152/92 during the period of relaxation. During the fall in the blood pressure there was a rise in the effective plasma flow of 24 per cent and in the glomerular filtration rate of 19 per cent, with a resultant fall in the filtration fraction (Fig. 16). At the end of the clearance period the subject was aroused from his pleasurable relaxation, and the blood pressure returned sharply to control levels, as did the other values.

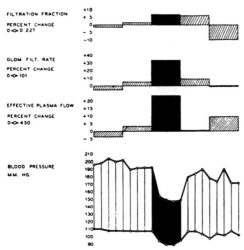

FIGURE 16. Changes in the renal hemodynamics associated with a fall in the blood pressure in a hypertensive person during relaxation induced by intravenously injected sodium amytal.

Comment. The observation that the arterial pressure and renal clearance may change toward normal during relaxation supports the view that the rise in pressure and the fall in clearances during the interview situation are truly a reaction to stress and suggests, in addition, that the subject with essential hypertension may well be living in a sustained state of overreaction to the minor stresses of daily life. The mechanism producing the increased blood pressure in responses of this type and in essential hypertension has been the subject of intensive investigation. Evidence has been adduced both to implicate the kidney in the genesis of the elevated pressure (20) and, on the other hand, to indicate that the kidney is a passive sufferer from systemic vascular disease (31). Our studies shed no light upon this problem except insofar as they indicate a more intense renal vascular activity in the hypertensive which may in itself be damaging to the kidney.

Simultaneous Measurement of the Renal and General Hemodynamics

In order to correlate the above data with studies of general hemodynamics and to ascertain whether or not the decrease observed in the renal blood flow actually represented vasoconstriction rather than reflected a fall in the cardiac output, measurements of the renal hemodynamics were made in 2 subjects while they lay on the ballistocardiographic table before, during, and after a stressful interview.

Case 1. A 45-year-old Swedish housewife was referred to the clinic because of dizziness and headaches related to hypertension, which had been first noted 16 years earlier during her first pregnancy. Episodes of dizziness were closely correlated with stressful incidents in her life, chiefly concerning her alcoholic husband. At her first visit to the clinic her blood pressure was 236/148. The physical examination showed her heart to be moderately enlarged, and there was a faint basal systolic murmur. The radiological examination of the chest also showed enlargement of the left heart, and the electrocardiogram showed left axis deviation.

The results of observations on this patient during an interview are shown in Figure 17. After a preliminary period of rest and relaxation

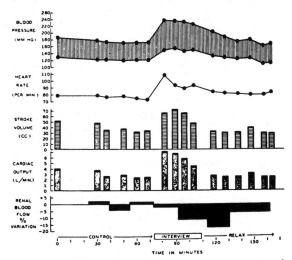

FIGURE 17. The correlation between measurements of the renal blood flow and general hemodynamics during a stressful interview.

in which there was no conversation, the patient was engaged in a discussion of her marital life by one of the physicians. She described the alcoholism of her husband, its effect on her son, who was nervous like herself, and her own feelings about her husband's behavior. Talking of these matters, she showed anxiety mingled with resentment. Her blood pressure rose from 186/128 to 242/168, and there were

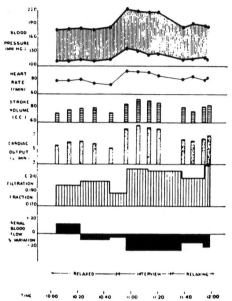

FIGURE 18. Same as Figure 17 in another patient prior to lumbodorsal sympathectomy.

concomitant elevations in the heart rate, stroke volume, and cardiac output. During this period the peripheral resistance (not shown on the figure) fell from 89 units to 43. There were a decrease in the renal blood flow and an increase in the filtration fraction. At the end of the interview the patient became quiet and apparently calm. The stroke volume and pulse fell, but there was a persistent elevation of the blood pressure, associated with a sharp rise in the peripheral resistance to 98 units. During this period the renal blood flow remained decreased. Finally the blood pressure, peripheral resistance, and renal blood flow all returned to essentially their original values.

Case 2. A 42-year-old woman came to the clinic because of repeated episodes of dizziness. She was found to have hypertension, with readings around 180/110. Physical and laboratory studies failed to reveal any evidence of heart disease or other structural abnormality. Observations of the systemic and renal circulatory dynamics in this patient during an interview are shown in Figure 18. After an initial period of relaxation, during which control observations were made, a physician talked to the patient about some of her current conflicts, such as her preoccupation with the behavior of her adolescent daughters. In this instance the physician adopted a tone of noncommittal interest, which was interpreted by the patient as unfavorably judicial. She became tense and irritated. During the period of the interview her blood pressure rose from 180/110 to 220/136. At the same time the heart rate and stroke volume increased, and the peripheral resistance (not shown on the figure) fell from 36 to 30 units. There were a fall in the renal blood flow and an increase in the filtration fraction, indicative of renal vasoconstriction. At the close of the discussion the physician

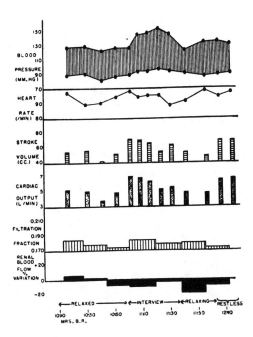

FIGURE 19. Same as Figure 18 following lumbodorsal sympathectomy. Note the consistently lowered filtration fraction and the failure of the renal blood flow to decrease significantly except during a period of lowered cardiac output.

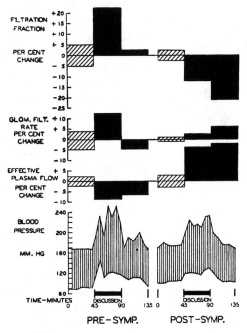

FIGURE 20. Changes in the blood pressure and renal hemodynamics before and after bilateral thoracolumbar sympathectomy. (Reproduced, by permission of the copyright owner, from J. B. Pfeiffer, Jr., and H. G. Wolff: J. Clin. Investigation 29:1227–1242, 1950.)

315

offered friendly reassurance to the patient, and she was encouraged to relax while further observations were made. The blood pressure and cardiac output declined somewhat, and the peripheral resistance again rose, although these values did not return to their original levels before the close of the experimental period. During this period the renal blood flow increased slightly and the filtration fraction fell slightly, indicating a persistence of renal vasoconstriction.

Modifications of Effects by Sympathectomy

The 2 patients described were observed according to the same technique following bilateral dorsolumbar sympathectomy. In the first patient the interview was accompanied by a rise in the blood pressure, as shown in Figure 19. There was noted a preliminary increase in the cardiac output without a change in the blood pressure. Later, when the blood pressure rose, the peripheral resistance increased significantly. Following the interview the patient was encouraged and became more relaxed. At this point the measured indicators fell again toward control levels, until at the end of the experimental period she became restless once more and the cardiac output rose again. There was no significant change in the renal hemodynamics during this interview, a result duplicated by other observations on sympathectomized patients (10, 29). The second patient's reactions after sympathectomy were so similar as to be almost identical. In other persons, however, the pressor response to stress after lumbodorsal sympathectomy was dependent chiefly upon an increased peripheral resistance. For example, in one sympathectomized patient who displayed during the interview a rise in the blood pressure from 142/88 to 184/138, there was a negligible increase in the cardiac index but a marked increase in the peripheral resistance, which must be presumed to have arisen from vasoconstriction in areas of the body other than those denervated of efferent sympathetic nerves.

The Effect of Lumbodorsal Sympathectomy and Splanchnicectomy on the Renal Vascular Function during Stress

Six of the subjects with essential hypertension who had undergone lumbodorsal sympathectomy and splanchnicectomy nevertheless displayed a considerable rise in the blood pressure during the discussion of disturbing topics, but not an increase in the renal vascular resistance. In 2 of these subjects (Fig. 20) the changes in the renal vascular function were the complete reverse of those observed before the operation, i.e., with the rise in the blood pressure, there was a rise instead of a fall in the effective plasma flow and a fall instead of a rise in the filtration fraction. In the others, there was a partial inversion of the pattern, consisting either in a failure of the filtration fraction to rise or of the effective plasma flow to fall. The formulae of Lamport (32) for the calculation of efferent and afferent arteriolar resistance were applied to the data available from all the subjects with and without sympathectomy.

TABLE 4. A Summary of the Afferent and Efferent Arteriolar Resistance before and after Sympathectomy.* (Reproduced, by permission of the copyright owner, from J. B. Pfeiffer, Jr., and H. G. Wolff: J. Clin. Investigation 29:1227–1242, 1950.)

Pt.		Aver. MBP	Calculations by Lamport's Formulae						by Gomez' Formulae	
			1000×Ra	1000×Re	1000×Rt	Δ% Ra	Δ% Re	Δ% Rt	Re×K	Δ% Re×K
17 R. W.	C	119	42.0	17.9	59.9	—	—	—	0.116	—
	D	142	77.9	25.8	103.7	+85.5	+44.1	+73.0	0.148	+27.6
Pre	PD	115	46.1	29.1	75.2	+ 9.8	+62.6	+25.5	0.160	+37.9
Post	C	123	53.9	25.7	79.6	—	—	—	0.157	—
	D	141	79.3	25.8	105.1	+47.2	+ 0.4	+35.0	0.155	− 1.3
	PD	124	55.7	22.1	77.8	+ 3.3	−14.0	− 2.3	0.124	−22.0
20 M. G.	C	122	57.7	18.2	75.9	—	—	—	0.110	—
Pre	D	160	109.0	22.6	131.6	+88.8	+24.2	+73.4	0.140	+27.3
	PD	145	87.1	19.7	106.8	+33.6	+ 8.2	+40.7	0.115	+ 4.5
Post	C	135	112.4	49.1	116.5	—	—	—	0.185	—
	D	158	147.0	38.6	184.6	+30.8	+21.4	+14.3	0.160	−13.5
	PD	134	103.0	34.2	137.2	− 8.4	−30.4	−15.0	0.142	−23.2
21 H. W.	C	129	85.3	27.9	113.2	—	—	—	0.127	—
Pre	D	146	103.1	30.9	134.0	+20.9	+10.8	+18.4	0.133	+ 4.7
	PD	131	84.4	25.9	110.3	− 1.1	− 7.2	− 2.6	0.121	− 4.7
Post	C	139	103.1	27.1	130.2	—	—	—	0.131	—
	D	151	122.0	27.7	149.7	+18.3	+ 2.2	+15.0	0.143	+ 9.2
	PD	141	100.3	25.2	125.5	− 2.7	− 7.0	− 3.6	0.127	− 3.1
27 B. R.	C	140	77.6	19.4	97.0	—	—	—	0.134	—
	D	163	123.0	31.8	154.8	+58.5	+63.9	+59.5	0.155	+18.7
	PD	145	96.5	25.0	121.5	+24.4	+28.9	+25.3	0.153	+14.2
Post	C	103	31.6	16.9	48.5	—	—	—	0.119	—
	D	116	48.2	18.8	67.0	+52.5	+11.2	+38.2	0.123	+ 3.4
	PD	108	41.1	19.3	60.4	+30.1	+14.2	+24.6	0.117	− 1.7
30 E. W.	C	143	125.6	35.2	160.8	—	—	—	0.133	—
Pre	D	184	218.0	44.5	262.5	+74.4	+26.4	+63.2	0.163	+22.3
	PD	154	153.9	42.0	195.9	+22.6	+19.3	+21.8	0.148	+11.6
Post	C	159	166.1	36.1	202.2	—	—	—	0.136	—
	D	180	187.3	33.8	221.1	+12.8	− 6.4	+ 9.4	0.144	+ 5.9
	PD	160	153.4	34.7	188.1	− 7.7	− 3.9	− 7.0	0.139	+ 2.2
32 R. L.	C	160	148.8	40.8	189.6	—	—	—	0.142	—
Pre	D	174	175.3	44.3	219.6	+17.8	+ 8.6	+15.8	0.152	+ 7.0
	PD	158	136.3	35.1	171.4	− 8.4	−14.0	− 9.6	0.134	− 7.0
Post	C	152	107.2	26.4	133.6	—	—	—	0.115	—
	D	164	133.2	27.4	160.6	+23.3	+ 3.8	+20.2	0.112	− 2.6
	PD	159	113.0	25.1	138.1	+ 5.4	+ 4.9	+ 3.4	0.115	± 0.0

* Definition of Symbols

MBP—mean blood pressure
Ra   —afferent arteriolar resistance
Re   —efferent arteriolar resistance
Rt   —total renal resistance (equals Ra plus Re)
C   —control period

D   —discussion period
PD —post-discussion period
Pre —before sympathectomy
Post—after sympathectomy
Δ% —change in per cent

The results of these calculations (Table 4) indicated that there was a rise in both the afferent and efferent arteriolar resistance in all 35 subjects without sympathectomy. Following the operative procedure in 5 of the 6 subjects, however, although the afferent arterioles continued to constrict during the rise in the blood pressure induced by stress, the efferent arteriolar resistance was definitely inhibited. It is of interest that the subject in whom this phenomenon was not successfully demonstrated had a partial sympathectomy; the lower portion of the sympathetic chain, L-2, was not identified in the specimen examined postoperatively and presumably had not been removed as intended. For comparison, because Gomez (33) has developed a different mathematical treatment of renal hemodynamics, the efferent arteriolar resistance was calculated by his method. The results are also shown in Table 4 and are comparable to those obtained with Lamport's formulae, both in magnitude and direction of change.

Comment. It is suggested by these experiments that during the response to stress both the afferent and efferent arterioles constrict but that the action of the latter is diminished or abolished after removal of the renal nerve supply by sympathectomy. However, even though the efferent arteriole ceases to function, the afferent arteriole has a certain autonomy of control which enables the kidney to "protect" itself against a systemic rise in the blood pressure.

The relation between a susceptibility to transitory hypertensive episodes during stress and the pathogenesis of sustained "essential" hypertension is still not altogether clear, but the data recorded suggest that the two are related as reactions of different degree and intensity to a similar set of circumstances in an appropriately susceptible person. An important connection between genetic and cultural background or "stock" and susceptibility to hypertension has long been recognized, since certain persons and families are more likely to exhibit hypertension than others. Indeed, experience with others of man's protective reaction patterns would indicate that they are deeply ingrained since they occur in many persons of the same stock under analogous conditions. It seems likely that they are "stock bound," analogous to the retriever pattern in dogs, the running pattern in horses, hoarding in squirrels, building and space orientation in birds and insects, and sham death in opossums. The implication is that the individual and his clan meet life in a particular way, and in a different way from the members of other stocks. An individual may have been a potential "nose reactor" or "colon reactor" all his life without ever actually having called upon the protective pattern for sustained periods because he did not need to. Thus a given protective pattern may during long periods of relative security remain inconspicuous and then during stress become evident as a disorder involving the gut, the heart and vascular system, the nasorespiratory apparatus, the skin, or the general metabolism.

With the accumulation of data, interest has shifted to focus upon the constellation of bodily changes, feelings, and attitudes that a given individual experiences and exhibits in reaction to stress. Thus Graham (6) indicates that the person with hives is characteristically preoccupied more with his resentments than with what to do about them. Grace (4) suggests that the constipated person exhibits "grim holding on," reactions and feelings in contrast to those of the same or another person with diarrhea, who develops this "riddance" pattern when he feels overwhelmed, has "lost face," been humiliated, or is faced by circumstances calling for aggressive assertive action which he fears to exhibit.

Concerning stock proclivities for the development of the hypertensive reaction pattern, the observations of Flynn and Wolf (34) and Sheldon and Ball (35) made on twin girls aged 20 are illuminating. These girls, identical as far as can be ascertained from the evidence provided by birth history, early photographs, dominant handedness, finger prints, palm prints, blood groups, somato-types, hair structure, and skeletal structure as studied by X-ray, nevertheless exhibit important differences. One has had arterial hypertension for about 8 years; the other is normotensive. One of the pair at birth, during infancy, through childhood and adolescence, and even at the time of writing is "behind" the other. Lighter in weight at birth, somewhat slower in growth, less well-developed, burdened with more frequent and severe infections, less outgiving emotionally, less able to learn, less capable of evoking love, less imaginative in work, and less hopeful of success in pursuit of a mate, she has been indeed since infancy, in relation to her sister, truly in the position of an "also-ran." It is this relatively lesser one who has developed hypertension.

Flynn and Wolf were able to show that both girls vigorously react as regards blood pressure elevation and increase in peripheral resistance during interviews in which pertinent personal data are brought into focus. These changes are shown graphically in Figures 21 and 22. It will be noted that during the period of stress the hemodynamic changes of both girls were of the same order, although one began the experiment at a hypertensive and the other at a normotensive level. It thus appears that not only were they poured out of the same mold

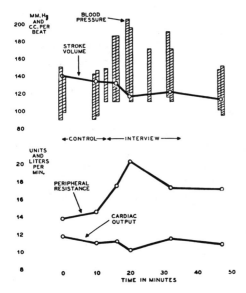

FIGURE 21. The hemodynamic changes in the hypertensive twin during a stressful interview.

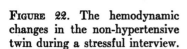

FIGURE 22. The hemodynamic changes in the non-hypertensive twin during a stressful interview.

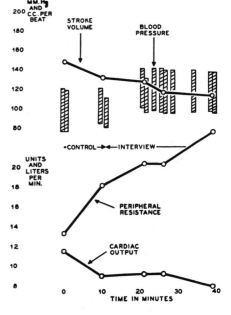

as to their structure, but they both respond similarly during stress. They exhibit those protective reaction patterns having to do with mobilization for action. Notwithstanding, only one has felt obliged to strive almost continuously from birth. It may be that the difference between the hypertensive and normotensive is one of congenital defect, but it is hardly likely to be specific in terms of a deranged apparatus for regulating the blood pressure. It is simpler to postulate that the hypertensive girl is exhibiting in her cardiovascular apparatus the effects of sustained attempts to compensate for her inadequacies, made especially apparent to her by the achievements of her better-endowed sister. In all events these twins demonstrate the nature of the inherited stock factor. Both possess a lively vasomotor reactivity— only one to date because of life experience has used it excessively.

Conclusion

From the experimental data summarized in this communication it is apparent that variations in the systolic and diastolic blood pressure levels in normal as well as hypertensive subjects correspond closely to variations in the individual's attitude toward his life situation. In general, when the subject considered himself menaced or trapped, elevations in the arterial pressure were observed. When, on the other hand, he felt overwhelmed and utterly defeated, for the time being his blood pressure fell below normal levels.

In producing elevations in the blood pressure a variety of hemodynamic mechanisms were concerned. Among these could be distinguished two more or less distinct patterns. In the first, the blood pressure elevation was attributable predominantly to an increased cardiac output. In the other, it was due chiefly to peripheral vasoconstriction. In both reactions the blood viscosity was increased and the clotting time shortened, and associated with both these there was observed a decrease in the renal blood flow. The first response, that characterized by an increased cardiac output without an increase in the peripheral resistance, occurred regularly in association with physical exertion and was typical of reactions in which anxiety and conflict were evident and mainly overt. The second response, that characterized by peripheral vasoconstriction with an increased cardiac output, was typical of reactions in which restraint was prominent and in which the subject displayed a striking need to suppress the recognition or repress the manifestations of his conflict.

Applying the formula of Poussieu which relates energy expenditure to blood pressure, cardiac output, and peripheral resistance, it is evident that the second pattern is far more costly to the organism than is the first for the same quantity of work done. The first pattern is usually invoked by athletes in adapting to the demands of unusual exertion. The second pattern appears to be that characteristically invoked by those with essential hypertension as part of their attempt to adapt to stressful life experiences. A study of these hypertensive subjects revealed that they were chronically in a state of conflict in which they felt a strong need to repress their aggressive drives and to gain approval by maintaining peace. They differed from normotensive subjects, many of whom displayed a similar reactive capacity, by invoking more or less continuously the pressor pattern referred to. The studies of Heinbecker, Selye, and Green indicate that such responses involve the pituitary-adrenal mechanism. This study does not illuminate the middle steps whereby the alterations are brought about, but it suggests that the adaptive reaction characterized by increased peripheral arteriolar constriction when unduly intense and sustained may lead to irrevocable vascular changes and ultimately impair the integrity of brain, heart, and kidneys.

Questions and Discussion

DR. BENJAMIN J. CLAWSON: This very interesting paper is now open for discussion. Do we have any psychiatrists here?

DR. SIBLEY W. HOOBLER (ANN ARBOR): I don't answer to being a psychiatrist, but the work of Dr. Wolff and his associates has been very interesting and stimulating to me.

I should like to point out a central problem that we often forget in studying the hypertensive person, which is that we study him at rest and not under the conditions of stress and the impact of life situations such as are described in this report.

It may well be, as Dr. Smithwick has pointed out, that psychogenic influences are essential initiating factors in hypertensive disease. We also have been interested in the effect of neurogenic influences on the renal circulation, and hoping to get a renal vasoconstrictor response, we have elected another type stimulus which might suggest that the kidney of the hypertensive patient was exposed to periods of ischemia during stress.

Our stimulus was the inhalation of carbon dioxide, which raises the blood pressure and causes a generalized sympatho-adrenal discharge. It was early shown in the study that about the same number of hypertensive and normotensive patients underwent marked renal vasoconstriction in response to the stimulus, so that the response is not peculiar to hypertension. It was also shown that after splanchnicectomy this constrictor response is abolished, so that we have confirmed by another technique Dr. Wolff's observations that a neural pathway for an important renal vasoconstrictor mechanism is present in the human subject.

DR. ROBERT W. WILKINS: The only comment I can make that might be pertinent to the work of Dr. Wolff and his associates has to do with an incidental observation that we made some years ago in a woman with very labile hypertension. This patient, as far as we could make out with our inexpert psychiatric methods, had very marked emotionally exciting factors involved in the rises in her blood pressure. She felt she had always been discriminated against by her mother in favor of her brother. Her mother had recently died, leaving the estate to her brother; whereupon the patient transferred her feelings of resentment and hostility to her brother, who, she said, didn't really appreciate all she had done for the family.

Completely unaware of this background, I happened to enter the laboratory while Dr. Stanley E. Bradley, then associated with me, was doing a renal blood flow study on her. (Incidentally, Dr. Bradley was following up the experiments that Dr. Chasis reported this morning with respect to pyrogens increasing the renal blood flow and lowering the blood pressure in hypertensive patients.) At the time that I entered the laboratory, the patient had been given a pyrogen, blocked, so far as the fever was concerned, with aminopyrine, and had had a very striking lowering of the blood pressure. Dr. Bradley remarked to me that he had lowered the blood pressure in this woman, though, of course, he didn't know what had happened to the renal blood flow. (It had gone up very markedly, as was shown later.) I then innocently asked the patient a question that completely ruined Dr. Bradley's experiment. I said, "What do you think caused your high blood pressure?" She immediately burst into tears and said that it all began with the death of her mother. That was her explanation at the moment, although Dr. Bradley assured me later that her trouble had not begun with the death of her mother but long before, and that she had found her mother's death to be an acceptable explanation for her feelings, since it was always understood by others that these feelings were of grief rather than of resentment or hostility.

Now the most interesting thing was that during the emotional outburst her hypotensive response to the pyrogen was completely abolished. Her blood pressure returned to its original level and the renal blood flow measurements also reverted. This experience made us aware of the very marked effect of the emotions on renal physiology, even during the action of a very potent vasodilating agent like intravenous pyrogen.

I have followed with great interest the work of Drs. Stewart Wolf and Harold Wolff, as well as of others, on this subject. I am sure that when we learn to study patients accurately under such conditions of emotional stress we are going to know more about the dynamics of essential hypertension.

DR. HARRY GOLDBLATT: Because the high incidence of hypertension in the American Negro is frequently attributed to emotional disturbance, resulting from competition with the white man, I thought it might interest you to hear about the great incidence of hypertension in a Negro population that is definitely not in competition with the white man. Several years ago Dr. Sanders, a former colleague at the School of Medicine, Western Reserve University, made a health survey of the population of the Virgin Islands. Fully 95 per cent of the population is black. Emotionally, Dr. Sanders found that these Negroes are unusually stable. They have no worries because they have absolute security. They are a happy-go-lucky kind of people, as he put it, "singing while they work, and singing most of the time." Yet he found that the incidence of hypertension among them was far greater than among the whites and even greater than in the Negro population in the United States. I had an opportunity to examine the kidneys of 2 hypertensive Negroes from these islands, and, although in the gross the kidneys were smooth and large, yet microscopically they were the seat of profound diffuse arteriolosclerosis. Certainly, in those people, the significance of any emotional disturbance appears to have been at a minimum, and, in my opinion at least, the cause of the hypertension was probably the vascular disease of the kidneys.

DR. WOLFF: It is very gratifying indeed to find that the observations on renal circulation that Dr. Pfeiffer and I have made are supported by two such distinguished groups of investigators. The effects of carbon dioxide described by Dr. Hoobler are in every regard like those evoked by stresses of the type I described, and it is most interesting to establish that there is a renal vasoconstrictor effect which is diminished by the renal sympathectomy. I wish to express my appreciation to Dr. Hoobler for the suggestions, observations, and comments.

Dr. Wilkins' observations are of the greatest interest and importance. I am surprised and delighted to know that even the potent vasodilator effects of pyrogens can be neutralized by the vasoconstrictor response during an incident of mounting resentment. This indicates even further to me the potency of these contributing factors and their importance in the management, if not the genesis, of the hypertensive reaction.

I am extremely grateful to Dr. Wilkins for bringing these observations into the discussion at this time. In my opening remarks I alluded to the observations of workers in different centers regarding the occurrence of hypertension.

Important evidence on the relationship of essential hypertension to the attitudes and goals of the individual and to the general functioning of his personality have accumulated from various studies involving lobotomy procedures.

Support for the point of view that pressor reaction patterns involve the cerebral cortex as well as lower neural structures derives from the work of Tibbetts (37), Freeman and Watts (41), Chapman et al. (38), Spiegel (39), and Pool (40) and his associates, who performed bilateral topectomy on 2 psychotic subjects with essential hypertension, removing the medial portion of Brodman areas 9 and 10. Prior to operation the blood pressure of the first subject ranged between 200 and 220 systolic and 120 and 130 diastolic. For 2 years after operation the average range was 170 to 180 systolic and 100 diastolic. The continued moderate hypertension in this subject suggests that part of the hypertensive mechanism at least is not reversible by the interruption of cortical pathways. The second subject has only been followed for 5 months postoperatively, but coincidentally with clinical improvement characterized by a lessening of depression and a decreased preoccupation with problems and conflicts, the blood pressure fell from an average range of 180–200 systolic and 110–120 diastolic to 120/80.

Tibbetts studied a hypertensive patient before and over a period of 1½ years after leucotomy. Prior to operation the patient, a 54-year-old woman, displayed evidences of serious hypertensive disease. Her blood pressure varied between 170/100 and 260/160. Headaches were incapacitating, retinal arterioles were spastic, and a hemorrhage was observed. The blood pressure range immediately after operation was 140/80–160/90. One and a half years later the patient was having no troublesome headaches. The retinae were clear of hemorrhage, and the range of the blood pressure was from 140/95 to 160/100.

Freeman and Watts described one lobotomized patient studied by them. A woman (Case 13) 66 years of age with agitated depression had had a blood pressure of 220/110 for an undefined period. During operation under local anesthesia supplemented by morphine and scopolamine medication, the blood pressure ranged from 172/80 to 185/100. At the conclusion of the lobotomy it was 194/95. During the postoperative course in the hospital the blood pressure ranged between 130/70 and 155/80. Later it was 195/75, and according to the incomplete case reports has remained about at this level for approximately 3 years. Freeman and Watts summarize their experience with lobotomized patients by saying that although the level of the blood pressure was not appreciably lowered in the group of patients after they resumed their usual activities (attitudes not mentioned), it never again reached the highest peaks recorded before the time of the brain damage.

Another patient was very carefully studied by J. Groen of Amsterdam. With his kind permission, I will give you the details of his observations.

A 45-year-old plumber was admitted to the Wilhelmina Gasthuis, 2d Medical Service, in December 1948 in a semicomatose condition, complaining of severe headaches with spells of vomiting. He was a pale, well-nourished man. His heart was enlarged to the left with markedly accentuated second aortic sounds. His blood pressure on admission was +250/160. The eyegrounds revealed choked discs bilaterally, with bilateral hypertensive retinopathy with hemorrhages and exudates, and irregular caliber of the vessels with nicking and arterial venous crossings. The urine contained 2+ albumin, numerous red blood cells and white blood cells, and a few casts. The blood urea nitrogen was elevated. He was treated with a diet of rice, salt-free butter, and sugar. On this regimen his blood urea nitrogen dropped to normal, and later kidney function tests revealed a 70 per cent urea clearance. However, the blood pressure remained elevated, 210–230/135–150, and the eyegrounds remained unchanged. Electrocardiograms showed marked left preponderance and ST depression, indicating left ventricular strain.

During the war he had been sent to a concentration camp—by error, the patient said, because he had been mistaken for a Jew. His father said that he had some suspicion that it was because of black marketeering and perhaps because of illegal liquor manufacturing. When he was released after "liberation," he found his wife cold, independent, and vindictive and the children estranged. At about this time headaches developed, hypertension was discovered, and a salt-free diet was prescribed. His wife, however, was negligent in preparing his diet. "She tried to poison me," he said, "by putting extra salt in my food."

Ultimately, because of the discovery of an episode of infidelity in which he acquired syphilis, his wife put him out of the house and began divorce proceedings. He refused to cooperate, however, and feeling too ill to work, he was obliged to live with his parents, who did not support his position on the divorce. Moreover, he felt that because he was unable to pay for his room and board he was a burden to them. An attempt was made by the physician to help him to see his situation, hoping that after a divorce he could make a new start, but he was not receptive. He insisted on remaining united to his wife.

Once he succeeded in inducing the head nurse to persuade his wife to come to see him because of the critical nature of his state, but when she came with the children and found that he was not dying, she did not conceal her disappointment, and he felt worse than ever. Even this incident, however, failed to induce him to let his wife divorce him.

At this point the possibility of recourse to frontal lobotomy was first considered and ultimately decided upon.

Bilateral lobotomy was performed by Dr. Lenshoek through burr holes in the temporal region in early February 1949. The operation and convalescence were uneventful, except for the usual postoperative period of drowsiness, incontinence, and impairment of memory. He remained on the rice diet for 10 days postoperatively. Thereafter he was given a salt-free diet containing about 2 gm. of NaCl per day. Presumably he has continued to limit his salt intake. The week after the operation his blood pressure dropped slightly to 200–210 systolic and 140 diastolic. Nurses noted that he was now more cooperative and tractable. He became very dependent on his physician and especially on his mother, who promised to take care of him.

A month after discharge from the hospital his blood pressure, it was found, dropped gradually to a level of 180/120. Only on one or two occasions did it rise to 200/130. His EKG improved. The papilledema disappeared completely, as did the hemorrhages and exudates in the eyegrounds, so that only small scars were left, as shown in the photographs in Figure 23. Visual acuity improved strikingly in both eyes.

After a convalescence of 8 months the patient expressed a desire to resume his work. He was encouraged to do so for half days only. But since he couldn't find a half-time job, he took on full-time work. He has performed adequately and steadily at his work for 12 months (September 1950).

Following operation stressful interviews no longer raised his blood pressure as they formerly had. It appeared that the lobotomy had, per se, not affected the blood pressure, as it was not found to be significantly lowered immediately after the operation, but the patient became much more amenable to interviews, in which he let himself freely discuss his former stressful situations, and it was this malleability of personality that led to the relief of his tensions and the improvement in his condition.

In September 1950, 20 months after the lobotomy, although the blood pressure was still elevated (145/100), it was strikingly lower

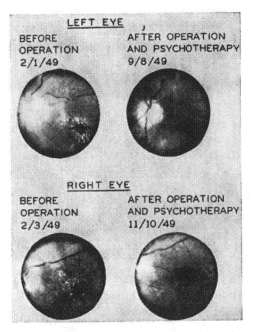

LEFT EYE
BEFORE   AFTER OPERATION
OPERATION   AND PSYCHOTHERAPY
2/1/49   9/8/49

RIGHT EYE
BEFORE   AFTER OPERATION
OPERATION   AND PSYCHOTHERAPY
2/3/49   11/10/49

FIGURE 23. Changes in the eyegrounds of Groen's patient, observed prior to and following lobotomy.

than before the operation (230–210/150–135), and under comparable conditions at the time of taking the reading.

Dr. Groen's notes on September 12, 1950, state that "he has had sundry emotional difficulties but it has always been possible to help him over them. He has lost his personality rigidity and has become an easygoing individual who is happy to come to the hospital whenever he is in trouble. He has confidence in the physician's judgment and when a situation seems threatening to him it is possible to make him laugh it off by a pat on the back, a joke, or the assurance that 'together we will manage the situation'."

Since the operative procedure of lobotomy is not always the same and the amount of brain damage is not uniform, variable results would be expected. They may be striking, as in this case of Groen's patient; or they may be less dramatic, though in some instances not negligible, as in the patient of Chapman. The subsequent change in the level of the blood pressure seems to be more dependent upon the better contact gained with the patient and the greater malleability of his attitude than upon the destruction of brain tissue having specific functional significance in relation to hypertension.

Unfortunately, as Dr. Goldblatt has pointed out, the evidence concerning the incidence of disease in various cultures is difficult to evaluate. Rarely have the stresses created by cultures and the body changes and dysfunctions that accompany the effort to adjust and adapt to them or to other noxious factors introduced by the environment been equally well studied. However, though not established— any more than that our own Western culture is, in mounting incidence, the setting for stress disorders or hypertension—the facts, such as they are, are suggestive and should evoke workers to collect more evidence rather than to consider the relationships of no significance. I should also like to remind Dr. Goldblatt, apropos of his remarks on the Virgin Islanders with hypertension, that the hypertensive person in our society is outwardly not one ruffled or disturbed and dissatisfied. Certainly, in our culture, he often is the exemplar of the poised, successful, "stable," and well-adjusted.

I cannot follow Dr. Goldblatt's next line of thought, if I understood him correctly. It is to be expected that a Virgin Islander who had hypertension of years' duration and died ultimately either directly from renal disease or from other causes should exhibit at autopsy kidneys showing evidence of renal disease. I cannot see how just vascular disease in the kidney helps us to understand whether it preceded the hypertension, is an accompaniment thereof, or resulted from prolonged renal vasoconstriction. I cannot follow the argument as to how such vascular disease militates against my thesis. I should expect that if the hypertensive reaction is part of an adaptive or protective arrangement, the prolonged existence of such a response would be associated with visible change in the kidneys whether or not the primary incident was renal vasoconstriction. I am grateful to Dr. Goldblatt for bringing out these points, but I cannot see how we basically differ. I must emphasize that the noxious factors bringing about hypertension, including the changes in the kidney (whether primary or secondary), may be these I have brought to your attention this afternoon. I should also like to emphasize in conclusion that there are myriads of stresses to which the human organism must adjust. A feature of the manner in which some persons will react will be hypertension.

My thesis is that although a man often reacts in a similar way to a number of different noxious stimuli, the threats created for him by man are among the most severe. In discussing the various assaults and threats to which he is exposed, it becomes very important, therefore, and especially in a symposium on hypertension, to consider the effect of man upon man.

· · · · · · · · · · · · · · · · *by* EDGAR A. HINES, JR.

Vascular Reactivity and Hypertensive Disease

QUICK rises in the blood pressure unassociated with a significant cardiac acceleration or an increased cardiac output are considered to result from vasoconstriction, which produces an increase in the peripheral resistance. "Vascular reactivity" refers to this type of change in the blood pressure—the change, that is, produced by peripheral vasoconstriction. Strictly speaking, the reactivity is largely in the arteriolar and small artery component of the vascular system, and a more limiting term denoting the part of the vascular system mainly involved would be desirable.

Vascular reactivity can be estimated by determining the range of the diastolic blood pressure from a curve of hourly or half-hourly blood pressure readings for from 24 to 48 hours during periods in which the subject is active and during periods of rest. Another method of determining vascular reactivity is by use of a test which measures the reaction of the diastolic blood pressure to a standard stimulus after a basal level of the blood pressure has been established.

Several methods of determining vascular reactivity have been devised. I have had more experience with the cold-pressor test than with others and shall confine my remarks largely to my experience with this test as a measure of vascular reactivity. It should be emphasized that all such methods so far devised for determining vascular reactivity are indirect and should be considered as giving only an estimation of the degree of vascular reactivity. Clinically the cold-pressor test might be compared in accuracy to the clinical determination of the basal metabolic rate. The method of carrying out the test is a standard procedure, but difficulties in obtaining a purely basal blood pressure and of eliminating all other stimuli which might be causing peripheral vasoconstriction result in some variation of the range of response on repeated tests (1). However, in my experience, if care is taken to reproduce the same basal conditions and to carry

331

out the test in exactly the same manner on each occasion, the results will be reasonably consistent on repeated tests.

In presenting the subject of vascular reactivity and hypertensive disease, I shall consider it within the framework of the usually normal diastolic blood pressure and the following tentative and perhaps over-simplified classification of diastolic hypertension.

Diastolic Hypertension (temporary or persistent increased peripheral resistance)

    I. Vascular hyperreactor
   II. Latent hypertension
  III. Essential hypertension (diffuse arteriolar disease)
       Groups 1, 2, 3, 4
  IV. Secondary hypertension
       Coarctation of the aorta
       Pheochromocytoma
       Glomerulonephritis
       Atrophic pyelonephritis
       Polycystic disease of the kidney
       Cushing's syndrome

Vascular Reactivity and Usually Normal Blood Pressure

In persons with a normal blood pressure the range of vascular reactivity may be small, as indicated by little variability in the diastolic blood pressure or by a slight rise from the basal level in response to an external stimulation such as is used in the cold-pressor test. Such a response in the blood pressure may be considered to indicate *vascular hypoactivity*. The majority of people with a normal blood pressure will have a moderate variation in the diastolic blood pressure and a moderate pressor response to strong stimuli; they may be called *normoreactors*. A small but undetermined number of persons with a usually normal blood pressure will have marked reactions of the diastolic blood pressure to various internal and to strong external stimuli. These may be called *vascular hyperreactors*. The expression "person with a usually normal blood pressure" means one who does not have persistent hypertension—that is, one whose blood pressure remains within normal limits unless caused to rise by a stimulus.

In relation to hypertensive disease, the importance of vascular reactivity in persons with a normal blood pressure hinges upon the problem of whether or not the degree of vascular reactivity is related to the eventual development of significant and persistent diastolic hypertension.

Some evidence that vascular hyporeactors do not, and that many vascular hyperreactors do, subsequently have hypertension has been accumulated from follow-up studies of persons subjected to the cold-pressor test, and from the study of a group of patients in whom the significance of elevation of the blood pressure in the upper ranges of normal as the result of the stimulus of nervous stress was evaluated in regard to the subsequent development of hypertension (2, 3).

TABLE 1. The Reaction of the Diastolic Blood Pressure to the Cold-Pressor Test, Correlated with the Subsequent Development of Hypertension

Classification (Blood Pressure Normal) *	Cases	Hypertension 15 Years Later	
		Cases	Per Cent
Hyporeactors 36		0	0
Normoreactors 48		8	17
Hyperreactors 57		31	54

*By normal blood pressure is meant a diastolic blood pressure always less than 100 mm. Hg except during the cold-pressor test.
Hyporeactors: those showing a rise of less than 10 mm. Hg.
Normoreactors: those showing a rise of 10–20 mm. Hg.
Hyperreactors: those showing a rise of more than 20 mm. Hg.

TABLE 2. The Incidence of Subsequent Hypertension according to the Original Diastolic Blood Pressure in a Group under the Stimulus of Nervous Stress

Classification (Blood Pressure Normal) *	Cases	Hypertension 10 or 20 Years Later	
		Cases	Per Cent
Hyporeactors 198		0	0
Normoreactors 878		31	4
Hyperreactors 446		254	57

*By normal blood pressure is meant a diastolic blood pressure of always less than 100 mm. Hg.
Hyporeactors: those having a maximal diastolic pressure of less than 70 mm. Hg.
Normoreactors: those having a maximal diastolic pressure of 70–84 mm. Hg.
Hyperreactors: those having a maximal diastolic pressure of 85–99 mm. Hg.

Unfortunately the group of persons with a usually normal blood pressure who have been subjected to the cold-pressor test and whose condition has been followed for a number of years is still small. A follow-up of from 15 to 20 years is now under way on a large group and should be completed within another year. The data on this group up to the present time are shown in Table 1. The data on the group with the stimulus of nervous stress are given in Table 2. These data indicate that vascular hyporeactors are unlikely to have subsequent hypertension; that a small number of normoreactors have subsequent hypertension; and that the majority of vascular hyperreactors have subsequent hypertension. The importance of the response of the diastolic blood pressure as an indication of the subsequent development of hypertension, as compared to the significance of the response of the systolic blood pressure alone, is indicated by the fact that none of 148 patients who had a systolic blood pressure of more than 140 mm. Hg, but a diastolic blood pressure of less than 80 mm., had subsequent hypertension.

Other investigators (4–6) have found that the incidence of sustained hypertension tended to be great among those who had transient elevations of the blood pressure at an earlier age. Unfortunately most of these workers did not make any analysis of their data on the basis of a transient elevation of the diastolic blood pressure alone.

Further evidence of the significance of vascular reactivity in persons with a usually normal blood pressure may be obtained from studies of the blood pressure reactions in families and among twins. Studies (7, 8) have shown that among twins and in family groups the response of the blood pressure to the cold-pressor test follows an inherited pattern as a dominant characteristic and that vascular hyperreactors occur more frequently in families with a high incidence of hypertensive disease. There is great need for further studies of the hereditary aspect of vascular reactivity, especially among large numbers of twins.

Vascular Reactivity and Latent Hypertension

I have observed more than 150 patients in the mid and later decades of life (from 40 to 60 years of age) who had hypertensive changes in the retinal arterioles, but whose blood pressure was usually normal and who gave no history of hypertension. The blood pressure of many of these patients was observed over a number of years, and they are known not to have had any persistent hypertension. All of these patients were vascular hyperreactors. I have designated these patients as having "latent hypertension" and have attributed the vascular changes to the vascular hyperreactivity and not to hypertension earlier in life.

The condition of a small number of patients from this group has been followed for from 10 to 15 years since the diagnosis of latent hypertension was made. About one third have subsequently had vascular complications commonly seen in essential hypertension, such as coronary occlusion, cerebral thrombosis, cerebral hemorrhage, and occlusions of the retinal artery and vein, without having any persistent or progressing hypertension. About one fourth have subsequently had persistent hypertension, which could now be diagnosed as essential hypertension. The significance of this type of vascular hyperreactivity is still uncertain and cannot be determined until a much larger group has been carefully observed for many years. However, it does suggest that organic vascular changes may result from the type of vascular hyperreactivity which we are discussing, in which persistent intra-arterial hypertension is absent.

There is another group of patients who may be said to have temporarily latent hypertension. These are persons who are known to have had persistent hypertension and who have hypertensive changes in the retinal arterioles, but whose blood pressure is now usually normal. This situation may occur as a result of cardiac failure or from a surgical procedure which temporarily lowers the blood pressure, such as sympathectomy or removal of a kidney affected by atrophic pyelonephritis. Such patients almost always are vascular hyperreactors during the period when their blood pressure is normal. This suggests that they retain the mechanism for rapid changes in the diastolic blood pressure, but that the mechanism for sustaining the diastolic blood pressure at high levels has been at least temporarily altered and that in these patients the hyperreaction to the cold-pressor test is evidence of previous hypertension which is temporarily latent.

Vascular Reactivity and the Prehypertensive State

A statistical study of vascular reactivity as measured by the cold-pressor test, and a consideration of vascular reactivity in persons with a normal blood pressure or latent hypertension, indicate that those of the group with a usually normal blood pressure who are vascular hyperreactors include many who will eventually have essential hypertension. However, it is important to point out that there is no test which will measure vascular reactivity accurately enough or consistently enough to use it as a measure of determining the probability of future hypertension in an individual case. The general use of the cold-pressor test to predict the future development of hypertension has not been advocated by me. Furthermore, the exact significance of vascular hyperreactivity in persons with a usually normal blood pressure is still unknown, but thinking of it and discussing it may help in attempting an explanation of the mechanism and perhaps the cause of essential hypertension.

I have found it useful to classify as vascular hyperreactors patients who usually have a normal blood pressure, who have little or no hypertensive changes in the ocular fundi, and who are hyperreactors in respect to the diastolic blood pressure. This avoids the temptation to make a diagnosis of essential hypertension or to attempt a prognosis as to the significance of the patient's blood pressure variability until the condition of the patient has been followed long enough to determine if a progressing hypertensive disease is developing.

Vascular Reactivity and Essential Hypertension

The vascular reactivity, estimated by methods described in the foregoing part of the paper, has been determined in a large group of patients with essential hypertension by a number of different workers (8–13). The combined data indicate that the majority of patients with essential hypertension are vascular hyperreactors, with the response of the diastolic blood pressure to a standard stimulus being from two to six times greater in them than in a control group with a usually normal blood pressure. The range of variation of the diastolic blood pressure in a group of patients with essential hypertension will be from 15 to 60 mm. Hg. In my experience with the cold-pressor test, 95 per cent of patients with essential hypertension for whom a satisfactory basal level of the blood pressure could be determined have had a rise of 15 mm. Hg or more in the diastolic blood pressure as compared with a similar rise in only 18 per cent of a large group with a usually normal blood pressure. A summary of data on the mean rise in the diastolic blood pressure of patients with essential hypertension and of those with a normal blood pressure is given in Table 3.

Vascular reactivity as measured by the cold-pressor test is decreased in most patients with essential hypertension by heavy sedation or drugs that produce vasodilatation. It is also decreased in most

TABLE 3. A Summary of Data on the Reaction of the Diastolic
Blood Pressure to the Cold-Pressor Test

Subjects	Number	Mean Rise (mm. Hg)
Group with essential hypertension 841		30.9
Group with a normal or usually normal blood pressure 1015		13.2

patients following extensive sympathectomy, but rarely is it completely eliminated. High spinal anesthesia and tetraethylammonium
chloride or priscoline (benzazoline hydrochloride) will almost always
abolish vascular reactivity as measured by the cold-pressor test. As
pointed out by Reiser and Ferris (14), this indicates that the immediate rise in the blood pressure produced by the cold-pressor test is
the work of a neurogenic mechanism. Their studies, however, showed
an interesting difference in the effect of tetraethylammonium chloride
on the delayed cold-pressor response sometimes observed in patients
with essential hypertension, in that this response was not abolished by
tetraethylammonium chloride. They interpreted this as indicating
that the immediate response to the cold-pressor test was mediated by
a neurogenic mechanism, but that the delayed response was mediated
through a humoral mechanism. Benzodioxane (933F) does not abolish
the response of the blood pressure to the cold-pressor test in essential
hypertension. All of these findings and my own experience would indicate that vascular reactivity is largely controlled by neurogenic
mechanisms.

There seems little doubt that vascular hyperreactivity is almost always present in essential hypertension except when high fixed levels
of the blood pressure are present, and that it is largely controlled by
a neurogenic and not a humoral mechanism. The significance of the
vascular hyperreactivity in essential hypertension is uncertain at the
present time. Although at first I thought the blood pressure reaction
to the cold-pressor test tended to be maximal in almost all subjects,
I have since found that in some patients with essential hypertension
the vascular hyperreactivity seems to be of the same degree at different levels of the blood pressure in the same individual. For example, the reaction to the cold-pressor test when performed with the
diastolic blood pressure at a level of 80 mm. Hg may produce a rise
to 100 mm. Hg, or a change of 20 mm.; if the test is performed with the
diastolic level at 100 mm., the pressure may rise to 120 mm., which is
equivalent to the 20 mm. rise that occurred at a lower level. Such a
constancy in the range of the reaction at different levels of the blood
pressure may be demonstrated in some patients by performing cold-
pressor tests under different degrees of narcosis produced with thio-
pental sodium (pentothal sodium) given intravenously. This observation and observations on the blood pressure responses of patients with
orthostatic hypotension, together with the observations of Reiser and
Ferris (14) and others, have led me to believe that there may be two
mechanisms for regulating the systemic blood pressure: one mecha-

nism for changing the diastolic blood pressure quickly (a neurogenic mechanism), and the other for maintaining the blood pressure at sustained levels or for changing the blood pressure over longer periods of time (perhaps a humoral mechanism).

That vascular hyperreactivity has something to do with the development of the clinical picture which we call essential hypertension is suggested by the finding that of 206 patients who recently had essential hypertension, 86 per cent had, from 10 to 20 years previously, given evidence of a hyperreaction of this probably neurogenic mechanism for regulating the blood pressure, although they had a usually normal blood pressure at that time and did not present the clinical picture of essential hypertension until a number of years had elapsed. Whether this vascular hyperreactivity is a coincidental finding in patients with essential hypertension, or whether it supplies a necessary background for the development or persistent hypertension, or whether it in itself eventually produces the circulatory changes initiating a pressor mechanism which maintains more persistent and serious hypertension is still a subject for speculation. As I have already stated, the evidence is reasonably good that a person with vascular hyporeactivity (a low maximal diastolic blood pressure under stress) will not have essential hypertension within 10 or 20 years. On the other hand, it is purely speculative whether a person who is a vascular hyperreactor (one having a high maximal diastolic blood pressure under stress) will have essential hypertension later in life, although his chances seem considerably greater than those of the hyporeactor.

Vascular Reactivity and Secondary Hypertension

A small number of diseases, such as adrenal tumors, glomerular nephritis, and coarctation of the aorta, clearly can produce arterial hypertension. There is a much larger group of diseases of which it is still not known whether they produce arterial hypertension, are just one of the factors producing it, or are coincidentally associated with it. In the group of diseases generally conceded to produce arterial hypertension, with the exception of pheochromocytoma, the mechanism of its production is still undetermined, although it is thought that a humoral pressor mechanism plays a predominant and perhaps exclusive role.

Except for patients with pheochromocytoma, all those whose diastolic hypertension has been thought almost certainly to be secondary to some disease and who have undergone the cold-pressor test, have showed vascular reactivity of the same type and of the same degree as the group of patients with essential hypertension. One group of patients with hypertension due to pheochromocytoma have been hyporeactors, while another group have been hyperreactors. There has been some overlapping of the two groups, but largely the patients with paroxysmal hypertension have been vascular hyporeactors and the patients with persistent hypertension have been vascular hyperreactors. The significance of this is not clear, although it may be concerned with differences in the epinephrine or norepinephrine factor in the production of the hypertension. That this may not be the predominant factor is indicated by the fact that benzodioxane does not eliminate vascular reactivity as measured by the cold-pressor test, whereas benzodioxane will depress the blood-pressure-raising effect of tumors containing a predominance of epinephrine or of norepinephrine.

It is of interest that in a follow-up study of a group of patients who had various types of renal diseases, including many who had diseases that are considered to produce arterial hypertension, the subsequent development of hypertension was correlated with their original vascular reactivity, much as had been observed in a control group who did not have any diseases which might have eventually produced hypertension (15). The data on this group are shown in Table 4. It is espe-

TABLE 4. The Incidence of Subsequent Hypertension according to the Original Diastolic Blood Pressure among Patients with Renal Disease

Classification (Blood Pressure Normal) *	Cases	Hypertension 10 to 20 Years Later	
		Cases	Per Cent
Hyporeactors 30		2	7
Normoreactors 129		18	14
Hyperreactors 105		72	69

* By normal blood pressure is meant a diastolic blood pressure of always less than 100 mm. Hg.
Hyporeactors: those having a maximal diastolic pressure of less than 70 mm. Hg.
Normoreactors: those having a maximal diastolic pressure of 70–84 mm. Hg.
Hyperreactors: those having a maximal diastolic pressure of 85–99 mm. Hg.

cially noteworthy that the vascular hyporeactors, including several who eventually had bilateral atrophic pyelonephritis, almost never had hypertension subsequently regardless of the type of renal disease.

I have followed for five years or longer the condition of a number of patients in whom surgical procedures performed for the amelioration or cure of hypertension, such as removal of an atrophic kidney or a pheochromocytoma, or sympathectomy, did not remove their vascular hyperreactivity as determined by the cold-pressor test. None of these patients has remained "cured," but all have had a recurrence of hypertension after several months or years; and I should predict that if they are observed long enough, many of them will eventually be found to die of the effects of hypertensive disease.

The few patients who had a normal blood pressure and low vascular reactivity as measured by the cold-pressor test following their surgical procedure for the relief of hypertension have not had a recurrence of hypertension. One of these is a patient who had a pheochromocytoma removed and whose condition has been followed for 16 years, and one was a patient with severe hypertension who had an atrophic kidney removed and whose condition has been followed for 12 years.

Summary

Vascular reactivity refers to quick rises in the blood pressure resulting from intermittent increases in the peripheral resistance produced by vasoconstriction. The change in the diastolic blood pressure as the result of strong emotional or external stimulation is a measure of vascular reactivity. Persons may be grouped as hyporeactors, normoreactors, and hyperreactors.

Some evidence that vascular hyporeactors do not and that many vascular hyperreactors do subsequently have hypertension has been accumulated from follow-up studies of persons without hypertensive changes in the retinal arterioles and with a normal or usually normal blood pressure.

A group of patients with hypertensive changes in the retinal arterioles and with a usually normal blood pressure who are vascular hyperreactors but do not and have not had persistent hypertension has been described. The findings in this group suggest that organic vascular changes such as are seen in essential hypertension may result from vascular hyperreactivity without the necessity of persistent intra-arterial hypertension.

Almost all patients with essential hypertension, except those in the late and fixed stages, are vascular hyperreactors and have been for some time before developing the clinical picture of essential hypertension. The significance and role of vascular hyperreactivity in essential hypertension is not well understood. However, it is probable that vascular hyperreactivity is importantly concerned with the development of persistent diastolic hypertension in essential hypertension.

Vascular reactivity in patients with secondary hypertension, with some exceptions in cases of hypertension caused by pheochromocytoma, is of the same type and of about the same degree as in essential hypertension. Vascular hyperreactivity may be of the same significance in the development of hypertension in patients with various types of renal disease as it is in essential hypertension.

If marked vascular hyperreactivity persists during the period of normal or usually normal blood pressure after procedures for the amelioration or cure of hypertension, there is usually a recurrence of persistent hypertension after a few months or years.

Questions and Discussion

DR. R. W. GOEN (TULSA) : We have recently completed a study of the cold-pressor reactions in 256 persons in which we attempted to correlate this response with the whole family of psychological tests. We were attempting to find, if possible, a simple procedure for relating personality patterns to hyporeactive response.

We were totally unable to do this in our data, and oddly this further points up the work of Dr. Wolff. The patterns of hypertensives are not simple ones. They require extensive study and cannot be restrained by such simple procedures.

I should like to call your attention particularly to the fact that although we talk freely about repressions, intervention in life situations, etc., as yet we have no evidence which helps us to distinguish which individual in a given situation will develop hypertension, which will develop peptic ulcers or colitis, or which will become an alcoholic or, in Minneapolis evidently, join the church.

• • • • • • • • • • • • • • • *by* GEORGE W. PICKERING

Cerebral Attacks in Hypertension

I SUPPOSE that you have asked me to talk on this subject because you know that my views differ from those which have been expressed in most papers and textbooks on neurology and cardiology published in the last 20 years. The chief point in dispute is the extent to which local vasoconstriction or spasm of the cerebral arteries or arterioles is concerned in producing the cerebral attacks that occur in hypertensive disease. Most contemporary writers believe that cerebral vasoconstriction is an important factor in producing the transient cerebral attacks, termed pseudo-uremia by Volhard (1) and hypertensive encephalopathy by Oppenheimer and Fishberg (2). Others even go so far as to claim that localized vasoconstriction or spasm may be an important factor in producing the more permanent lesions in which evidence of cerebral arterial thrombosis or hemorrhage is found. To quote a recent textbook on neurology: "It has been pointed out, however, that though exact knowledge on the subject is far from complete there are reasons for thinking that cerebral softening may follow transient spasm of arterioles and that this may be the mechanism in many of the cases that in the past we have been content to regard as cerebral thrombosis from clot formation within the vessel" (3).

It is usual in the contemporary world to seek the source of a minority view in a psychological injury sustained in childhood. As I look back, I can see clearly the incidents in my youth which led me to hold the view that I now have. I received my early training in medical science and the biological scientific method in the Cambridge School of Physiology. Sixty years ago one of the most eminent products of that school, happily still alive, Sir Charles Sherrington, working with Roy (4), came to the conclusion that there were three factors regulating the cerebral blood supply: first, the arterial pressure, second, a local chemical mechanism, and third, the general venous pressure.

They could find no evidence of vasomotor nervous control of the cerebral vessels. To quote their paper, "We conclude then that the chemical products of cerebral metabolism contained in the lymph which bathes the walls of the arterioles of the brain can cause variations in the calibre of the cerebral vessels; that in this reaction the brain possesses an intrinsic mechanism by which its vascular supply can be varied locally in correspondence with local variations of functional activity." Twenty years later, Leonard Hill and J. J. R. MacLeod, destined, like Sherrington, to win a Nobel prize, were unable to demonstrate any action of the vasomotor nerves on the cerebral vessels (5).

Twenty-five years ago, when I was an undergraduate at Cambridge, Florey, a pupil of Sherrington's, later also to win a Nobel prize, was engaged at Sherrington's suggestion on a direct study of the reactions of the cerebral vessels. Like Sherrington, Florey was unable to demonstrate that the sympathetic nerves had any effect on the diameter of the cerebral vessels (6). And, in fact, it was left to H. S. Forbes of Boston and Harold Wolff to demonstrate that the cerebral vessels are indeed under vasomotor nervous control (7). Forbes and Wolff inserted a glass window into a trephine hole in the skull of a cat. The conditions in the cranial cavity were thus restored approximately to normal. Direct inspection of the cerebral vessels showed that they constricted definitely though very slightly to stimulation of the cervical sympathetic nerves. They also constricted definitely though very slightly to the local application of adrenaline. If, however, adrenaline was injected intravenously, the pial vessels dilated, presumably because the constrictor effect of the drug was outweighed by the rise of intra-arterial pressure. The diagram in Forbes *et al.* (8) shows how feeble are the reactions of the cerebral vessels in comparison to those of the skin. In fact, the failure of Sherrington and Florey to demonstrate the existence of cerebral vasomotor nerves may be regarded simply as testimony to the feeble reactivity of the cerebral vessels. This feeble reactivity is no doubt the expression of their peculiar structure. For the cerebral arteries are thin-walled, and in the media muscle is sparse and in places absent. You will understand, then, that I should require a great deal of evidence before I could accept the view that the cerebral arteries constrict more fiercely than other arteries in the body in hypertension or that a cerebral artery or arteriole can suddenly and without apparent cause constrict so fiercely that the tissues it supplies may die, while the other cerebral vessels remain widely patent. Yet these are the two components of the hypothesis that is generally held to explain the attacks currently designated as acute and chronic hypertensive encephalopathy.

Before proceeding to a detailed consideration of the cerebral attacks of hypertension, we must consider three rather fundamental questions, namely, (1) the effects on the nerve cell of ischemia, (2) the extent to which the cerebral arteries and arterioles anastomose with one another, and (3) the vascular response to an interrupted blood supply. The effects of ischemia on the peripheral nerves are known in great detail (9). In the upper arm the larger fibers cease to conduct after from about 20 to 30 minutes. This loss of function is not permanent and is regained a few minutes after the restoration of the circulation to the limbs. A permanent paralysis occurs after ischemia lasting some hours. In the central nervous system the tissues are much more sensitive, as is shown by the effects of breathing nitrogen or of a sudden arrest of the heart. It is clear that at least certain nerve cells cease to function after the interruption of their oxygen supply for a few seconds or less. It is also certain that some cells lose their function permanently after the interruption of their oxygen supply for only a few minutes, as is shown by the permanent dementia that sometimes occurs following ventricular arrest of a few minutes' duration. It would seem extremely probable that different nerve cells are paralyzed at different rates, as are the different-sized fibers constituting the mixed nerves of a limb.

In the circle of Willis the anastomoses between the arteries of the brain are so free that an occlusion of one carotid in the neck by digital pressure usually produces no cerebral manifestations whatsoever. Beevor (10) showed that injections made into one of the three main arteries supplying the convexity of the brain passed freely into the territory of the other. It is now known that free anastomoses exist at the arterial and arteriolar level through at any rate most of the substance of the brain. Cohnheim's conception of end arteries has been largely abandoned.

The technical difficulties of investigating the speed with which the collateral circulation is re-established in the brain when a large artery is occluded are so great that this experiment has never been performed. The experiments of Roy and Sherrington 60 years ago showed the importance of local metabolites, or a vasodilator nature, in the regulation of the cerebral circulation. Quite recently Shepherd (11) has studied the development of the collateral circulation in the leg. When the femoral artery is suddenly occluded, the blood flow through the calf falls from about 4 cc. a minute to a negligible value. The blood flow is re-established within about 30 seconds and rises to its original level at about the fourth minute, after which it remains normal. This finding corresponds with the observation of Lewis, Rothschild, and me that an occlusion of the femoral artery in the groin maintained for 30 minutes produced no paralysis of the nerves of the leg (9). It would seem highly probable, therefore, that with healthy vessels the sudden occlusion of an artery or arteriole produces only transient ischemia in the territory it supplies.

There is quite general agreement that certain attacks occurring in subjects with hypertension are due to hemorrhage from or thrombosis of one of the cerebral arteries. In these attacks the onset is usually sudden, consciousness is frequently lost, and when regained is accompanied by a local loss of cerebral function which frequently leaves a permanent residuum. This is not the place to discuss either whether hemorrhage is always preceded by thrombosis or the differential diagnosis between cerebral hemorrhage and cerebral thrombosis. It is to be noted, however, that in such attacks the loss of cerebral function is greatest at the beginning or near the beginning and gradually recedes over days or weeks. Some of this recession may be due to the assumption of these functions by intact nervous tissues, but some at least is probably due to the recession of ischemia and to the recovery of neurones only temporarily paralyzed by a transient loss of the blood supply.

Much more controversial are attacks in which there is a focal loss of function that is entirely transient in nature. These attacks are termed chronic hypertensive encephalopathy and are commonly ascribed to transient spasm or constriction of the relevant cerebral artery or arteriole. Typically, when the patient is in good health and engaged in his usual, varied occupations, paralysis of the limb or of half of the body, aphasia, sensory loss, or blindness of an eye or loss of half the field of vision abruptly supervenes. Consciousness is usually not lost, but the patient may be confused or excited. The condition may last a few minutes or a few hours, and then gradually passes off, leaving the patient apprehensive or tired, but without signs of any focal disturbance of the central nervous system. Such is the typical attack as it has been described, but while such attacks by their dramatic character focus the attention of the investigator, it is a mistake to think that there is an abrupt dividing line between these brief and evanescent paralyses, those which clear more slowly, and those which may leave residual symptoms and signs of a permanent lesion of the central nervous system. In fact, in my own experience, fully diversified in an earlier paper (12), there is a continuous series from attacks in which paralysis is brief and totally reversible to those in which paralysis persists for months or years to leave some permanent residuum. By general consent the latter are regarded as due to cerebral arterial thrombosis. The contention here presented is that the former are due to the same lesion. The following report presents an example of a patient who experienced a paralysis of long and one of brief duration.

Case 3. J. C., an intelligent clerk of 41, was standing in a crowded underground train on December 29, 1933, when his left arm and leg suddenly became weak. He did not lose consciousness or fall, but managed to stagger out of the train and walk 100 yards (91.4 meters) to a friend's office, whence he was taken home to bed. During his walk he tended to fall to the left. After this attack he noticed difficulty in articulation, in managing his dentures, and in using his left arm and leg. He had slowly been recovering from these disabilities when he was first examined by me on January 2, 1934. He showed the typical picture of severe essential hypertension (arterial pressure 220 systolic and 150 diastolic, normal urine and urea concentration to 2.5 per cent, and moderate retinal arteriosclerosis). He had slight but definite weakness of the left side of the face, the left arm and the left leg of the upper motor neuron type, deviation of the tongue to the left, exaggerated tendon jerks in the left upper and lower limbs, and a left extensor plantar response. Sensation and fields of vision were normal. By January 26, only weakness of the left side of the face remained. Ten months later, while at work, he suddenly felt dazed, and a severe headache developed lasting 5 minutes only. At the same time his left hand suddenly felt numb and weak, recovering in about 5 minutes. But for the next half-hour he kept hitting the wrong keys on the typewriter. For the rest of the day he was excited and walked about as if in a dream. He was discharged the next day for his behavior. Three years later, on September 6, 1937, he woke with severe bilateral frontal headache. When he reached his office he found himself unable to speak intelligently, though he knew what he wanted to say and understood what was said to him. He was sent home, and said that his speech had recovered an hour from the onset. Seen by me later that afternoon, he showed some slight residual difficulty in speaking; he was slow and hesitant, but presented no other signs in the central nervous system. In December 1937, cardiac asthma, Cheyne-Stokes respiration, and early albuminuric retinitis developed. He died of acute pulmonary edema, having maintained a severe hypertension throughout.

Necropsy showed changes characteristic of malignant hypertension. The arteries of the circle of Willis showed moderately severe atheroma. A lesion of the cerebral substance characterized by pigmentation and irregular linear and punctate pits was found extending inferiorly from the junction of the middle and posterior thirds of the putamen into the internal capsule superiorly, and having a maximum area of 9 x 7 mm. No other focal cerebral lesion was found.

The only other case which need be cited is the following, in which coronary thrombosis, proved at necropsy, was followed four years later by a spectacular attack of transient paralysis lasting 20 minutes and leaving no clinical sequelae; but a small cyst was found in the putamen at necropsy four months later.

Case 1. J. T., then a 32-year-old sergeant in the 8th Army, had a sudden attack of severe pain over the lower part of the sternum while at a Christmas party in North Africa in 1942. He had to lie down, and the pain passed off after 20 minutes. He felt easily tired subsequently. In August 1943, while he was on a march in Palestine, pain developed over the sternum and spread across his chest and down the left arm. It gradually reached a maximum, at which it remained during the last hour of the march; he was short of breath and sweated profusely. At the end of the march he lay down, and the pain passed off in about 15 minutes. Subsequently he often experienced sternal pain on exercise; the pain was relieved by rest, and he was discharged from the army in December 1943. He eventually obtained a clerical post, and apart from angina and occipital headache on waking, remained in fair health until December 20, 1946, when at 10 A.M., while sitting at his office desk, he noticed that his lower lip on the right side was numb. He bit his lip to confirm this. Then the fingers of his right hand became numb, and he found that he could no longer write. He could neither form the letters nor put the words on paper in their correct order, though he knew what he wanted to say. He thought that there was no weakness of the right hand, but it was clumsy and movements were difficult. He went into the next office and found that he could not speak; he knew what he wanted to say, but the words were jumbled, and his colleagues accused him of being drunk. All these disturbances cleared up completely in about 20 minutes, and he was able to continue his work for the rest of the day. Shortly afterward his eyesight began to fail, and he went to the hospital. Examined on February 3, 1947 (now aged 36), he showed gross hypertension (230 systolic and 144 diastolic) in the malignant phase (bilateral albuminuric retinitis), gross enlargement of the heart with gallop rhythm, normal urine and renal function, and no abnormal signs in the nervous system. He died of acute pulmonary edema on April 7, 1947, after adrenalectomy.

At post mortem the heart was found to weigh 400 gm., the left ventricle being 2 cm. thick; an old infarct was found on the endocardial surface of the anterior wall of the left ventricle near the base, involving the contiguous part of the interventricular septum; the corresponding branch of the left coronary artery was thrombosed, the remaining coronary arteries showing only slight atheroma. The brain showed only slight atheroma of the basal vessels and of the left and right middle cerebral arteries traced as far as the insula. A yellowish cyst 5 x 5 x 3 mm. was found in the left putamen in the same vertical plane as the mammillary bodies.

Of the 11 patients fully reported earlier (12) 3 died out of the hospital from apoplexy 3 years, 1 year, and 3 months respectively after their attacks. The brain was examined post mortem in only 3 cases. All 3 patients died of malignant hypertension with severe arteriolar lesions, particularly of the kidney. Cases 1 and 3, already described, each showed a cyst of the putamen clearly ischemic in origin, though no evidence on the nature of the arterial obstruction was obtained. In Case 1 an old myocardial infarct due to arterial thrombosis was also found. Case 2 presented a large number of small yellowish brown cysts about 2 mm. in diameter scattered through the basal ganglions of both hemispheres and two similar areas in the left pons. These findings in general agree with the more numerous and detailed observations of Rosenberg (13) in showing that focal ischemia has occurred in cases presenting transient paralytic attacks.

From what has been said already, it will not surprise you to hear that I am reluctant to accept the hypothesis of local vascular spasm as a basis of these attacks. If, in fact, without apparent cause a cerebral vessel suddenly contracts so strongly as to paralyze temporarily or permanently the function of the tissue it supplies while the other cerebral vessels remain widely open, this must occur as a result of a sudden release of the powerful vasoconstrictor substance to which the cerebral vessels are unusually susceptible. Such a conclusion could not fail to have important consequences for the general theory of the cause and mechanism of essential hypertension. But it is quite unnecessary to postulate vascular spasm as the cause of these attacks. The attacks are, in fact, quite like what one would expect if a small cerebral artery or arteriole were suddenly occluded. The speed of recovery would obviously depend (1) on the size of the area initially ischemic, (2) on its relation to the main motor and sensory tracts of the brain, and (3) on the speed and freedom with which the collateral supply was re-established. This latter would obviously depend very largely on the health of the other cerebral vessels. Support for the organic nature of such an attack comes from two sources. In the first place, as has been shown, there is no sharp dividing between attacks that are purely focal and briefly transient and those that are initially general and leave a permanent residuum. By general consent the latter are due to organic cerebral artery obstruction. It is my contention that the former are also. But the most important evidence for this view comes from the observation that precisely similar attacks occur in patients suffering from mitral stenosis and auricular fibrillation, where the cause of ischemia is almost certainly embolism of the cerebral arteries.

I have published the case histories of 10 patients with auricular fibrillation, with or without mitral stenosis, who experienced attacks that were in every way similar to those experienced by patients with hypertension (12). In 9 patients the disturbance was a hemiparesis, and in 1, loss of vision in one eye. The duration of the paresis was 1 hour or less in 4 patients, and in the remainder longer, the paralysis clearing slowly in periods up to a few months or persisting as an incomplete residuum. Consciousness was retained during the attacks, though the patient often felt apprehensive or confused at the time. As in the patients with hypertension, there was no sharp dividing line between attacks that were briefly transient, and those in which paralysis cleared slowly and incompletely. Examples are as follows:

Case 13. A. N., a schoolmaster aged 52, had noticed irregularity of the heart since 1941. In 1942, while returning from watching a boxing match, he noticed that he was walking badly and went into a public house to get a whisky. He could not get the money out of his pocket because his left hand was useless, and he could not talk. He was recognized, and some men in the public house carried him home in a hand chair; he was perfectly conscious and remembers clearly seeing the people pass by. When he reached home, he was laid on a couch, unable to move his left hand or left leg and unable to talk. He remained so for half an hour, and then quite abruptly and within a minute or two, he found he could talk normally and move his limbs. He had never had a similar attack before nor has had one since. Examination 2 years later showed mitral stenosis and auricular fibrillation which was paroxysmal, but no abnormal signs in the central nervous system and a normal blood pressure.

Case 14. J. F., with mitral stenosis, was known to have had auricular fibrillation since October 1942. In the evening of October 30, 1943, just after a routine visit to his physician, he felt dizzy on reaching home and lay down on a couch. He did not lose consciousness, but his wife noticed that he was confused and that the left side of his face and his left arm and leg were paralyzed. His nephew, a doctor who had just been my house physician, and his own physician were called and arrived 30 minutes later to find left hemiplegia and confusion of thought. The paralysis cleared gradually during the next 30 minutes, and after receiving "omnopon" (a proprietary mixture of opium alkaloids, papaveretum B.P.C.), he slept with periodic breathing. In the morning he was still confused, but was said to present no trace of paralysis. I examined him later in the day and found him still rather confused and with only the slightest weakness of the left upper limb and of movements of the left ankle. The tendon reflexes were brisk and equal and the plantar responses normal. By November 4 he had lost even these trivial signs. In May 1944, when I last heard from him, he had had no further attacks.

Case 16. C. S., a girl of 15 years suffering from mitral stenosis and auricular fibrillation, was treated with quinidine and her rhythm restored to normal in 1927. In 1928 she was readmitted to University College Hospital under Sir Thomas Lewis, with auricular fibrillation and congestive failure and was treated with digitalis. At 1:45 P.M. on November 12, 1928, she was noticed to be throwing herself about; the right corner of her mouth was down, and she was trying to make herself understood but could only repeat words such as "jing." She understood what was said to her and could answer *yes* or *no*. She exhibited facial weakness on the right side and a flaccid paralysis complete in the right arm and nearly complete in the right leg, the plantar responses were flexor on the left, extensor on the right. There was no loss of consciousness. At 5:30 P.M. she could talk well, and the weakness had passed off to a considerable extent. On November 13 she appeared a little drowsy but otherwise normal mentally. A slight weakness of the right side of the face and upper and lower limbs persisted, and the right plantar response was still extensor. On November 14 no weakness was found, but the plantar response was not tested. On November 15 the right plantar response was recorded as flexor. She was discharged on February 6, 1929, still fibrillating, but with no signs of failure or hemiplegia. She died in the hospital of terminal bronchopneumonia on January 6, 1932.

Her brain was examined post mortem by Dr. R. T. Grant, who provided me with all her case notes. The brain, sliced horizontally, was normal except for a yellowish cyst, 14 mm. long, 4 mm. wide, and 7 mm. deep, in the putamen of the left lenticular nucleus. To find the vascular lesion responsible for this cyst, the middle cerebral artery and its chief branches were opened up under the dissecting microscope; the arteries seemed normal. A block of tissue extending from the lesion to the base of the brain was cut in transverse serial section 10 microns thick. No lesion was found in any artery of the block.

Case 17. A married woman of 30 was walking across the hall to her office one day in the autumn of 1939, when she felt queer and had to sit down. Onlookers thought she looked ill and sent for a physician, who sent her to Charing Cross Hospital; there she was kept for the afternoon and then sent home to bed. Her memory of the attack is that she felt hot and giddy but never lost consciousness; her face became drawn to the right and she talked queerly; her left leg dragged, and her left arm was useless when she went to bed. On the first day she had difficulty in controlling her bladder. Her limbs recovered gradually, but she has since noticed that her left arm twitches and becomes useless for a few minutes when she is tired. She was admitted to the hospital in November 1941 with congestive cardiac failure, mitral stenosis with normal rhythm and normal arterial pressure (140 systolic and 100 diastolic). No abnormal signs were found in the central nervous system. She was treated with digitalis and discharged home. On July 21, 1942, her husband found her normal on leaving home in the morning but unconscious on his return at night. She was admitted to the hospital in coma with stertorous respiration. The right side of her face was flabby and her right arm motionless, and both plantar responses were extensor; she was incontinent. She had congestive cardiac failure, but her rhythm was still normal. She slowly emerged from her coma, regaining control of the sphincter on July 25, and showing some recognition of her husband. She was discharged on October 24, 1942, with a severe residual spastic paralysis of the right arm and leg and weakness of the right face. She recognized what was said to her and could reply by a nod of the head, but her articulation was so imperfect that few could understand her.

Since these patients do not die in the attack, it has up to now been impossible to identify the site of the embolus at post mortem. The only post mortem obtained was in Case 16 4 years after the attack, when the cyst in the left putamen was found. This obviously represented the area in which ischemia lasted long enough to kill the nervous tissue. The area in which ischemia paralyzed but did not kill was obviously larger and presumably involved the internal capsule. How long this lasted, and how long an interval elapsed between the return of the blood flow and the recovery of function must, in the present state of our knowledge, remain conjectural. In some of these cases the recovery of function was abrupt, as in Case 14. It is possible that in such cases the embolus moved from its initial site to become impacted in a smaller and more distal artery.

In the following case the embolus must have lodged in the left internal carotid artery proximal to the origin of the ophthalmic artery.

Case 15. W. M., an insurance clerk aged 28, had suffered from rheumatic heart disease with auricular fibrillation for many years, but still traveled 20 miles (32.2 kilometers) by train to London each day to his work. In 1935, while he was at his office desk, his right hand abruptly became weak and clumsy, and he found himself unable to hit the keys on his typewriter. At the same time he found himself unable to see out of his left eye. He was quite sure of this, for he covered first his left eye and then his right eye with his left hand. He felt confused and was unable to speak clearly, he believed. The attack lasted about an hour and then passed off completely, but my notes do not say whether the end was sudden or gradual. I saw him 3 months later and found signs of mitral stenosis and auricular fibrillation with aneurysmal dilatation of the left auricle. There were no signs in the central nervous system, but unfortunately the fundi were not examined. He died of cardiac failure a few years later without further attacks. There was no necropsy.

While, therefore, the comparison between the attacks of cerebral embolism and those occurring in hypertension lacks something in detail, they are like enough to suggest that in both the ischemia is due to organic arterial obstruction and that the site and duration of the ischemia will depend on the artery obstructed and the efficiency of the collateral circulation in restoring the blood flow. In hypertension the arteries obstructed are probably the smaller arteries or arterioles, which are usually diseased. A sudden occlusion would most probably be due to thrombosis or to a sudden swelling of the arterial wall. The former is known to occur. The latter may occur in hemorrhage into the wall or conceivably in fibrinoid necrosis, but of the time relations of this latter we are still completely ignorant.

Before leaving this subject, I should like to refer to 2 cases, one of auricular fibrillation and mitral stenosis, and one of mild hypertension in an elderly man. In both, attacks of transient paralysis were repeated several times, each preserving the same general character as the first, and then ceased, not to recur during the succeeding years. These cases are as follows:

Case 18. L. C., a married woman of 41, was seen in 1941, when she had had 10 normal pregnancies, the last six years previously. In 1936, she had had an attack in which she suddenly felt a buzzing in her head, the room seemed to go round, and she fell to the floor without losing consciousness. When she tried to get up, she found that she could not for weakness of the left arm and leg. The left side of her face felt queer, and she had difficulty in pronouncing her words properly. She recovered completely in an hour. During the next 6 years she had four further attacks similar to the first, in which weakness of the left side lasted about an hour, and three where it lasted 2 or 3 days; but she had not lost consciousness in any. On February 26, 1941, she had just come in from shopping when something "seemed to go click" in her head and she fell to the ground. Again there was no loss of consciousness and her left side was paralyzed. She could see normally, but her mouth felt pulled over. The left leg recovered its power to some extent in the next few days, but when she was brought to the hospital six days after the attack, she was found to have a spastic paralysis of the left arm, paresis of the left leg, and weakness of the left side of the face of the upper motor neuron type, mitral stenosis with auricular fibrillation, and a heart rate of 160 per minute. The plantar response was extensor on the left, flexor on the right. The arterial pressure was 144 systolic and 95 diastolic. Lumbar puncture on April 8 showed a clear colorless fluid not under pressure. By May 6 the left leg had recovered completely, but there was still slight weakness of the left side of the face and the left upper limb. In 1944 she had her eleventh confinement, before which she was admitted to the hospital with congestive cardiac failure, from which she made a good recovery. She was last seen in March 1946, when she had no signs of cardiac failure but was still fibrillating. She had had no further attacks, and the signs in the central nervous system had disappeared.

H. H. A business man of 62 had experienced in the past 6 months three attacks of right hemiparesis. The first began in February 1948; while he was watching a football game, he noticed the backs of the thighs getting numb. On getting up, he felt with the right foot as though he were walking on air. After he had walked 400 yards, his speech went. He got into a bus, where he read the paper and smoked a cigarette. He noticed numbness of his right arm and leg. His voice was spluttering; that is to say, he could not form the words properly.

He changed buses, and after he had traveled three fourths of a mile, everything went right again. A month later he had a left Bell's palsy lasting 8 days. Three weeks later he had his second attack while sitting in his office. His right leg began to feel funny; half an hour later his right arm went. His speech was then all right. After half an hour he was driven 13 miles home. On the journey his speech got bad. When he got out of the car, he could not use his right leg. His symptoms began to improve as he walked upstairs. He went to bed, and 5 minutes later the symptoms suddenly passed off. Three weeks later he wakened at 4:20 A.M. and noticed weakness and numbness of the right side again. At 5:50 A.M. the attack suddenly passed off. A twitching sensation was noticed in the right leg as it recovered. In all these three attacks his mind was clear and he knew exactly what was going on. In each the onset and end were sudden. I examined him 3 weeks after the last attack. He was a big man moderately obese, with a high color. His arterial pressure was 195/105. The heart was slightly enlarged radiologically, the enlargement being left ventricular. The rhythm was regular, and no signs of valvular disease were found. Renal function was good, and no signs were found in the central nervous system. The Wassermann reaction was negative. I saw him on three further occasions up to May 1950, when he had had no further attacks. There was no essential alteration in his condition. In particular, his mind remained alert and his memory good.

It is, of course, very tempting and very easy to explain these attacks as due to vascular spasm. But there is no hint concerning the stimulus to vascular contraction. Since these attacks were repeatedly of the same nature, I think we have to suppose that ischemia involved roughly the same area in each case. There may have been a permanent vascular obstruction, the attacks being produced either by renewed organic occlusion proximally or by a general fall of arterial pressure. The absence of observations during the attacks or of post-mortem examination makes further discussion purely speculative.

Before concluding this section, I should like to refer to the detailed investigations of Rosenberg (13), who examined the brains carefully in 17 cases of malignant hypertension and in 15 controls. In the cases of hypertension, massive cerebral hemorrhage was found in 4 cases, and small and spotty hemorrhages with numerous infarcts of similar size were found in 5 cases. Single large infarcts occurred in 3 cases. He was impressed with the frequency of multiple miliary infarcts, which he found in 12 cases in the basal ganglions, cortex, white matter, brain stem, and cerebellum; they varied in size from 5 to 6 mm.

across to minute softenings only seen with the aid of a microscope. These small lesions had been ascribed to vascular spasm by Westphal and Bär (14) and by Spielmayer (15) because no adjacent organic arterial lesion could be found. This was often Rosenberg's experience, but he found some infarcts adjoining thrombosed vessels. Rosenberg concluded that "in this study it was always possible to demonstrate regions of cerebral destruction where focal cerebral symptoms had been present during life, and in instances where the brain showed no destructive lesions the history revealed that episodic focal symptoms had not been present during life." He suggested from his anatomic studies that cerebral symptoms were of three kinds in malignant hypertension: (1) due to increased intracranial pressure (headache, vomiting, drowsiness), (2) due to multiple miliary cerebral lesions (a wide variety of transitory disturbances often without physical signs), and (3) due to large cerebral vascular accidents. Rosenberg's observations support the idea that attacks of transitory paralysis in hypertension are due to focal ischemia of the brain, but leave undecided the problem of whether the ischemia is due to spasmodic or organic arterial obstruction, though in some cases the latter was clearly the cause.

The reasons I have given you lead me to believe that the obstruction is organic and not spasmodic. The position as I see it may be summarized as follows. As in cerebral embolism, so in hypertension, local cerebral attacks are most probably and usually due to the sudden organic occlusion of a cerebral vessel. The nature and extent of the symptoms, whether there is aphasia, monoplegia, hemiplegia, blindness, or other sensory disturbances, will depend on the site and extent of the area rendered ischemic and thus on the site and size of the vessel occluded. The speed of recovery will depend on the size of the vessel, the location of the vessel, and the efficiency of the collateral circulation. A small area of permanent cerebral destruction situated in the internal capsule or other main conducting tract may be associated with a permanent residue of paralysis. A small area of permanent cerebral destruction situated, for example, in the putamen, as in the cases cited here, or other so-called silent areas of the brain, may leave no residual nervous signs, though the initial area of ischemia may have been large enough to involve conducting tracts such as those of the internal capsule and so to produce transient paralysis. Collateral vessels may be expected to be more capable of dilatation in young subjects than in old, and so we should expect transient paralysis to be more frequent in the young, as appears to be the case.

In hypertension the nature of the sudden vascular occlusion must remain speculative until post-mortem material is obtained sufficiently early after an attack. Three lesions are possible, a hemorrhage into the vessel wall, a thrombosis of the vessel probably developing on an intimal plaque, and an arteriolar necrosis. For as Dr. Goldblatt has pointed out, arteriolar necrosis which expands the vessel wall at the expense of its lumen may develop quickly and, if Byrom's work be confirmed, in a matter of minutes.

The third main variety of cerebral attacks occurring in hypertensive disease is very different from the foregoing, and has been termed acute pseudo-uremia (Volhard, 1) or hypertensive encephalopathy (Oppenheimer and Fishberg, 2). The best-known variety of these attacks is the eclamptic attack occurring in the toxemia of pregnancy; precisely similar attacks occur in other forms of hypertension of recent origin, such as acute nephritis, or in chronic hypertension with a recent exacerbation, such as certain cases of so-called malignant hypertension. The attack characteristically begins with severe headache, followed by vomiting, drowsiness, convulsions, and coma. These attacks may be preceded or followed by focal symptoms and signs, and clear up without residual nervous phenomena. Volhard pointed out the similarity of the clinical picture to that found in acutely raised intracranial pressure. For this reason and because of the frequent presence of papilledema, he suggested that the attacks were due to acute edema of the brain, an explanation previously suggested by Traube (16) and subsequently adopted by Zwangemeister and others. Gorke and Topplich (17), Blackfan and Hamilton (18), Volhard (19), and others have described cases in which death occurred after attacks of this kind and in which evidence of cerebral edema was found post mortem. Acute edema of the brain may therefore be provisionally accepted as the pathologic basis of such attacks. I say provisionally because there are some reservations. Edema of the brain is notoriously difficult to demonstrate post mortem, and some distinguished pathologists, notably Sheehan in Great Britain, are unsure if this is the anatomical basis of eclampsia. The water contents of the brain have not to my knowledge been correlated with hypertensive attacks. In 2 cases that I studied intensively I was not able to observe any correlation between the cerebrospinal fluid pressure and the attacks (20). Both cases had albuminuric retinitis; both had raised cerebrospinal fluid pressures, but in each the cerebrospinal fluid pressure was the same during coma following a fit as in the intervals when there were no symptoms. But I did observe 1 case of acute hypertension due to periarteritis nodosa, when fits were associated with signs of a block in the subarachnoid space at lumbar puncture and where necropsy revealed a pressure-cone apparently due to edema of the brain.

With this reservation we may proceed to discuss the cause of the edema. Traube regarded it as a passive consequence of a diminished blood protein and a raised arterial pressure. He supposed that both of these factors usually operated and that a sudden fall in the blood protein or a sudden rise in the arterial pressure might further increase the passage of fluid out of the cerebral vessels into the brain substance and precipitate a cerebral attack. At that time neither of Traube's two operative factors could be measured. No clear evidence has since been produced to show that plasma protein plays any part. Hypertension has been found invariable, and Volhard; Oppenheimer and Fishberg; and McAlpine (21) among others have shown that a further rise in the arterial pressure often immediately precedes the attacks. Traube's explanation implies that the cerebral arterioles are relatively feebly constricted by the agent raising the arterial pressure in hypertension, so that the cerebral capillary pressure is raised. The feeble contractility of the cerebral arterioles to constrictor agents supports the hypothesis, as does the relationship that exists between the pressure of the cerebrospinal fluid and the diastolic arterial pressure in hypertension.

The current view as to the origin of cerebral edema is, however, quite different, and was put forward by Volhard, who supposed the cerebral edema due to ischemia of the brain. He considered that the cerebral arterioles were not less but more constricted than those elsewhere, so that the cerebral blood flow became so small that the capillaries were damaged by anoxia, and so allowed abnormal amounts of fluid and protein to pass out into the cerebral substance. The chief evidence produced for this widely accepted hypothesis is that a rise in the arterial pressure precedes the attacks; this fact is of no great value as evidence, for it had been envisaged as a possibility by Traube when he was formulating a precisely opposite hypothesis. In 3 cases which I have observed myself and reported briefly elsewhere, the protein in the cerebrospinal fluid was not significantly different in and out of the attacks. But the strongest argument against the hypothesis is that the cerebral arterioles have never been found to constrict more strongly to a constrictor agent than arterioles elsewhere; in fact, the reverse is true.

And so I came to my final conclusion, which is this. On the evidence which has been made available in published writings, there is no proof that excessive constriction or spasm of the cerebral vessels is an important factor in the genesis of the cerebral attacks occurring in the course of hypertensive disease. I have put before you alternative explanations which, while they remain also unproved, at least violate no cardinal principle in vascular behavior.

• • • • • • • • • • • • • • • • • *by* GEORGE A. PERERA

The Natural History of Hypertensive
Vascular Disease

"THERE is something fascinating about science," said Mark Twain; "one gets such wholesale returns of conjecture out of such a trifling investment of fact." Today's student of medicine might even have trouble in obtaining sufficient facts on which to base the conjectures. Take, for example, the medical literature. A San Francisco newspaper reports that "scientists fight high blood pressure—the greatest killer of the middle-aged." A popular monthly digest states as follows: "High blood pressure? Don't be alarmed. . . . When the facts become known, a brooding and paralyzing fear should lift from the land."

Certainly all the facts are not evident. Indeed, it is surprising how little we know about so many serious and common problems in medicine. So today I shall not present the whole story and shall studiously avoid giving both sides. Instead, I plan to present my own unilateral, biased, and prejudiced opinion with what few bits of evidence can be mustered in my defense.

I should like to suggest that the diagnosis of hypertensive vascular disease is difficult and often made incorrectly, that the incidence of this disorder—although still an unpleasant and popular one—is less than generally supposed, and that we are dealing with a disease the first manifestations of which begin in youth and early adult life. And finally, I should like to present to you some of my data concerning the course and natural history of patients who develop this condition.

Diagnosis

The diagnosis of hypertensive vascular disease is not easy because it depends on a rough measurement modified by position, age, activity, obesity, and particularly by the emotional state of the subject. There is scarcely agreement on the definition of hypertension, and it is exceedingly difficult to draw a sharp distinction between normal and abnormal blood pressure readings.

A labile arterial tension is often an early finding in those subsequently shown to have vascular disease, but some persons—on constitutional or other grounds—persist in demonstrating extreme fluctuations extending well into the definitely abnormal range without ever developing the characteristic earmarks of a pathological process.

Anxiety may produce marked transitory hypertension, but permanent disease is not an essential sequel.

The label of essential hypertension is attached frequently to patients of more advanced years with blood pressures of from 160/80 to as high as 200/110. However, we have recently obtained pathological data indicating that the incidence and the degree of renal vascular damage in this group approximate those found among comparable age groups with normotensive backgrounds. Many of these people live a normal life span. The greater incidence and degree of renal arteriolosclerosis in young, documented hypertensives afford but two alternatives. Either there is a mild, benign form of the disease among the elderly, or—more likely—hypertension in many patients in this category results from degenerative arteriosclerotic changes completely independent of the disease under discussion.

To further confuse the issue, even hypertension of long duration can disappear under certain conditions. In our experience, the "resting" blood pressure of some 15 per cent of patients with uncomplicated hypertensive vascular disease will fall to normal after prolonged bed rest and relaxation. Others will have a drop in tension for days, weeks, or even months after a myocardial infarction or a cerebral vascular accident. Hence the absence of hypertension does not always exclude antecedent or concomitant disease.

I believe the label of hypertension is applied too readily and must be reserved until time, hindsight, and critical judgment have excluded such factors as lability, anxiety, and the degenerative changes of the more elderly. Hypertension should be suspected when diastolic values exceed 90; it becomes increasingly probable the more often this occurs; it becomes a certainty only after careful appraisal. As for hypertensive vascular disease, this diagnosis is one of exclusion reserved for those with definite hypertension after other causes—such as affections of the kidneys and adrenals, central nervous system disorders, or coarctation of the aorta—have been eliminated as best one can.

Incidence

It is traditional to say that about 25 per cent of the population will develop hypertension. The available statistics are generally derived from single sources—insurance, military, or industrial files or the records of hospitals or private practitioners. They are difficult for me to interpret because of varying criteria of diagnosis, the predominance of selected groups, casual or single blood pressure readings, and inadequate documentation. Many of the factors already discussed are not considered in some of these surveys.

We have made repeated analyses in different age groups, and, provided we have limited our material to those with established disease, which can only be done by adequate follow-up studies, we have never observed an incidence greater than 6 per cent in any series. Evidence will be presented that essential hypertension does not as a rule begin after the age of 50 or so; if this is true, the often quoted statement that there is more hypertension with each decade of life applies to blood pressure values but scarcely to the incidence of one disease. Six per cent does not belittle the issue; essential hypertension is still a common disorder affecting many millions in this country alone.

Age of Onset

Although it has been suggested by a few that careful examination would show the beginnings of hypertensive disease in childhood and youth, most investigators have regarded this disorder as associated more with old age. The menopausal period is mentioned frequently, but several studies have made it clear that this is a favorite time for the patient to consult the doctor or to have antecedent disease accentuated by vasomotor and autonomic factors.

We examined the records of more than 2,000 patients with hypertensive vascular disease, distributed in all age groups, and having a mean age of 40 years. It was possible to document the onset in 200 by virtue of records in which repeated previous normal observations had been made. Recurrent abnormal elevations of the blood pressure were evident in all before they reached the age of 48, and the peak age of incidence was in the thirties. As there were frequent gaps of several years before a definite normotensive was discovered to be a definite hypertensive, the true curve in this study can only be pushed back rather than ahead.

In my experience, whenever hypertension is proved beyond doubt to have developed for the first time after the age of 50, some other cause for an elevated blood pressure has almost always been disclosed. It is my conviction that hypertensive vascular disease can be detected in early adult life in the majority of instances.

Course

An accurate and complete picture of essential hypertension is not readily achieved. It is doubtful that the whole story has ever been written or will be for some time. In addition to the problems already enumerated, the need to avoid selection, to follow case material from the very incipience of the disease until its final outcome, and to obtain a large enough group to be statistically valid presents obvious difficulties. It is of interest that the natural history becomes longer with the literature of each decade; it seems fair to predict that the true picture will be better than it has appeared in the past.

I should like to report, with all of these reservations in mind, on a clinical survey of 300 closely followed patients, none of whom had received specific therapy. The basis of selection consisted only in the documentation of hypertensive vascular disease and a sufficient period of observation to permit complete routine studies and the elimination of subjects whose hypertension was transient. I should be the first to admit that all selective factors have not been eliminated in this group and that many of these people had their disease before a diagnosis was made. I can only state that this is as unselected a series as is possible in an urban area in one geographical location, and that the clinical material was obtained in large part from an outpatient clinic in continuous operation for 30 years with practically the same medical personnel (Table 1).

TABLE 1. Characteristics of a Group of 300 Hypertensive Patients
Observed for from 1 to 41 Years

Mean period of observation .... 14 years
Percentage still living 82
Average age at time of diagnosis .... 40 years
Average age at time of diagnosis in cases
    where date of onset was known .... 33 years
                                 (9–48)
Percentage of women 68
Percentage having a family history of hypertension 30

These 300 patients were observed for from 1 to 41 years. Eighty-two per cent are still alive after a mean period of observation of 14 years. Obviously the average duration of disease in this group will exceed 14 years. By subtracting the age of onset in cases where the date of onset was known from the average age at death as known from our experience and derived from multiple sources of pathological material, one is forced to conclude that essential hypertension begins earlier and lasts longer than is generally supposed; that although it is a disorder with serious consequences, causing death most frequently in the fifties, its average span encompasses close to a 20-year period. There is fairly general agreement that women are affected with somewhat greater frequency and that familial and genetic factors cannot be ignored.

An analysis of symptomatology and complications brings out many noteworthy features for discussion (Table 2). The average patient in

TABLE 2. Symptomatology and Complications among 300 Hypertensive Patients Observed for from 1 to 41 Years

Clinical or Laboratory Findings	Percentage of Patients	Reversibility	Relation to Prognosis
Headache			
None 31			
Mild 23	⅔	0	
Moderate 40	⅔	0	
Severe 6	⅔	0	
Retinopathy			
None 17			
Changes in vessels 60	0	0	
Exudate and/or hemorrhages 18	⅓	+	
Papilledema 5	Rare	+++	
Cardiac enlargement 68	0	0 unless condition was marked	
Congestive failure 27		+	
EKG "damage" 52	0	+	
Angina 10		+	
Myocardial infarction 9		+	
Cerebral vascular accident 10		+	
Albuminuria 14	0	+	
Nitrogen retention 6	0	+	

this group spent many more years than not in an uncomplicated stage of the disease and might have absolutely no complaints. Although essential hypertension can kill in relatively short order, it is surprising how many persons sustained decades of an elevated blood pressure without troubles or rapid progression. With reference to the blood pressure itself, persistently high or rapidly rising diastolic values were statistically less favorable prognostic signs, but not necessarily so in individual cases. In fact, I would emphasize that the blood pressure level, as it is recorded casually in office or clinic, bears remarkably little correlation with symptoms, rate of progression, or the subsequent development of complications.

Note that 31 per cent of this series never complained of a headache, and that, whether the headaches were mild, moderate, or severe in intensity (the last appearing in only 6 per cent of the entire group), the majority of patients were spontaneously relieved in time. Note that retinitis, as demonstrated by hemorrhages and exudate, improved or actually disappeared in approximately one third of these patients, but that papilledema—observed in 5 per cent of the series to date—almost never showed spontaneous remission. Note that 32 per cent, despite the length of the period of observation, had no demonstrable increase in the heart size. In some instances cardiac hypertrophy was conspicuously absent at autopsy even after years of marked hypertension. And finally, significant regressions in the heart size were not observed as a spontaneous occurrence.

It would be a great advantage if we could predict the future course of an individual patient from the data obtained from past history, physical examination, and laboratory studies. So we set about to analyze this group of 300 from the standpoint of prognosis. The following conclusions were drawn. In general, the initial height or even the maintained level of the blood pressure bore little relationship to the eventual outcome, although, as previously stated, very high diastolic values or progressive increases in arterial tension over relatively short periods were statistically, but not individually, less favorable. Headaches and other subjective symptoms were of no significance, and even mild to moderate degrees of cardiac hypertrophy did not appear to shorten the course. Retinal changes, limited to deviations in the caliber of the arteriolar lumen or to compression at the arteriovenous junctures, could exist for many years and were of no prognostic import. On the other hand, such definite and irreversible organic changes as congestive failure, coronary artery disease, cerebral vascular accidents, renal damage, or renal insufficiency were indicative of an unfavorable prognosis. Retinitis with exudates and hemorrhages fell into a similar category; and of all signs, papilledema, of other than a transitory variety, was very frequently associated with death within a year or two. It was found, however, that these were statistically valid considerations only, for there were innumerable individual exceptions. Thus we have observed patients who were alive 21 years after retinal hemorrhages were first recorded; we have seen survival for 18 years after a cerebral thrombosis, for 12 years after the onset of congestive failure, and for 10 years after the development of a persistent, low-grade nitrogen retention.

Comment

I do not ask you to believe these facts and figures or to draw the same conclusions that I have drawn from the evidence at hand. The story is obviously incomplete, and the facts are few and far between. But I hope you will agree with me that much of what has been said and written bears revision, that we must remain critical until the facts are known, and that only through accurate information concerning the natural history of hypertensive vascular disease can we learn to take care of our patients intelligently and evaluate the newer forms of therapy correctly. I read recently that a child almost died after taking her grandmother's hypertensive pills; let us keep in mind the possibility that the fears we invoke and the "cures" we prescribe may be worse than at least some forms of the disease.

Questions and Discussion

DR. GEORGE E. FAHR: I have seen a large number of physicians in the audience, and this is certainly a paper they can and, I suspect, would like to discuss. Naturally, this doesn't exclude the men who have done fundamental work in the laboratory, but I think the clinical men are somewhat startled by some of the data Dr. Perera has brought out.

I don't think any of us are startled when we hear about the occasional case that lasts for 30 years with a very high blood pressure. I mean cases where the blood pressure was taken frequently and followed very carefully. But I am somewhat startled by the apparently small number of cases of hypertension whose life expectancy and physical fitness have been very much affected by it!

I think that clinical men might want to discuss this. The paper is open for discussion now.

DR. IRVINE H. PAGE: Dr. Perera has brought up an interesting, and unfortunately seldom considered subject, namely, whether essential hypertension has a single origin. Is it not perfectly possible that the extraordinarily protean clinical manifestations of the disease are really due to different fundamental mechanisms?

At last it is generally being recognized that arteriosclerotic hypertension and essential hypertension differ basically and that their prognosis and management are quite different. Often the two are inextricably intertwined, and to dissociate their effects on the patient offers the greatest difficulty. The recognition of their difference is a start at least.

When attempts are made to compare large groups of patients before and after, say, sympathectomy, the lack of uniformity among the patients is abundantly clear. And, in my view, comparisons currently can only be of the roughest sort because of this inability to separate and measure the various mechanisms which express themselves in the single measurement of arterial pressure.

It is of the greatest clinical importance that we find signs and

370

symptoms which will more clearly delineate the various varieties of disease that are now lumped together as essential hypertension. The sphygmomanometer is no longer a sufficient instrument for the purposes of modern cardiovascular diagnosis.

There are today methods which give important insight into the varied mechanisms concerned in elevation of the blood pressure. Unfortunately, they have been too little understood and too little employed by physicians. For instance, despite the excellent modern methods of examination of the renal vascular bed, few clinicians use methods any more advanced than those employed by Mr. Bostock for Dr. Bright. There are many Mr. Bostocks around today who have been insufficiently employed.

Another point I think of great clinical importance is to determine the rate of progress of the vascular deterioration. This is why we have over the past 20 years insisted on graphing the progress so that we may follow simply with the eye the rate of change in the patient. We employ blood pressure measurements averaged over a period of a week rather than single measurements for these graphs. It is surprising when this form of recording is employed how stable the blood pressure becomes. The instability of the arterial pressure is largely confined to the minute and hourly changes, not to the average changes from week to week.

To me the decision of what sort of treatment to employ depends chiefly on what sort of fire we are trying to put out. If the disease is malignant and rapidly progressing, heroic measures are demanded. If no progress is demonstrable in any important vascular bed over a period of years, then why handicap the patients with drugs and diets, many of which are of questionable value?

We have a long way to go before we shall be able to measure participating mechanisms and the rate at which they are destroying the patient, but to me it is the major theme of modern diagnosis as it is the underlying theme of treatment.

DR. SIBLEY W. HOOBLER (ANN ARBOR): I want to congratulate Dr. Perera on a study which I think is fundamental in terms of understanding clinical hypertension.

And I should like to clarify too a point that has never been quite clear to me: namely, just how did he select these patients? Did the study include all the patients he was seeing in his clinic or just those patients who had a long history of hypertension in their clinical records and had survived up to the time of the study?

In other words, did he have a straightforward selection of hypertensives as they come, or did the conditions of selection exclude patients with the worst forms of the disease? I ask this question because obviously, to evaluate the over-all prognosis in a disease, one has to select a group of patients in whom the future course of it is unknown. We have tried to do that, and have just completed a study of 117 patients who were studied in the University of Michigan Hospital 10 years ago. We didn't know anything about their future records. We took them from the files of those patients who were not subsequently operated upon.

We found out what became of all of them 10 years later by personal return visit or letter. The figures were a little bit different, and I think we were able to get some valuable prognostic information from reviewing the records of the initial study. We selected only patients who on several visits to the clinic had diastolic pressures of 110 or greater, so that we might be certain not to get patients in the early labile and perhaps not fixed hypertensive stage. Secondly, of course, we excluded people who were moribund from cerebrovascular accidents or from coronary thrombosis or uremia. We also took people under the age of 52 so that we might not get into the older age groups. Otherwise we took consecutive cases and followed every one of them to see what had become of him.

We found 50 per cent of the cases living 10 years later, which is not a bad figure for comparison with Dr. Perera's, considering that our cases were relatively unselected. We did find, however, as he did, that the blood pressure initially made little difference in the outcome.

We had many women who had diastolic pressures as high as 140 who came back to see us 10 years later and apparently were quite well. So that I should quite confirm the fact that the blood pressure is not of major prognostic value.

We did find, however, that the signs of vascular damage that were present on the initial examination were of prognostic importance. These included cardiac enlargement as determined by X-ray measurements, electrocardiographic abnormalities, persistent albuminuria of 1 plus or more, or a history of cerebrovascular accident. These things, which might well be called vascular complications of hypertension, completely switched our survival statistics.

At similar blood pressures 80 per cent of patients without these complications were living 10 years later. If we selected only those patients with the vascular complications of hypertension, only 20 per cent were living 10 years later.

I make this point specifically because we tend to forget that high blood pressure doesn't kill people—it is the vascular damage that does. Perhaps, as Dr. Page indicates, if we can observe the early signs of vascular damage or its progression, we can predict that this patient has a serious prognosis unless some sort of radical therapy is instituted. Whereas, with another patient, regardless of his blood pressure level, who doesn't have vascular damage, one is tempted to "sit tight" and wait a little bit and see before advising radical treatment.

It was interesting, however, that while some did develop vascular damage, as defined above, 10 years later, a good many of them over the 10-year period didn't show any of the vascular complications, despite a sustained high blood pressure for a long period.

Just one other comment that is rather interesting—and I haven't got a good explanation for it. We followed the blood pressure of all of these people either through letters from their doctors or through their return visits, and in none of them had it changed significantly. Their blood pressure had stayed about where it had been, of those living; and of those who had died it was the same up to the time of death.

So we were forced to the conclusion that after the early labile stage of the disease is past (presumably the disease when we picked up the study was in a fairly stable form since we defined a diastolic blood pressure of 110 or greater as our initial level), there isn't much change. The scatter-graphs showed that over 10 years the subjects had just about the same blood pressures.

There was one blood pressure that had fallen to normal; one that we felt was significantly greater, over 20 mm. The others all came within the ±20 mm. diastolic range. A very few had risen. The subjects who died had not had a rise in the blood pressure before death. We develop a certain sense of false security if we keep following the hypertensive patient for years and his blood pressure doesn't go up. The mere fact of its remaining stable doesn't mean he won't die of his disease. Once the high blood pressure is established, it rarely, it seems to me, rises further unless malignant exacerbation supervenes.

And death, I should like to emphasize again, is probably related to the rate of progression of vascular complications, which can be identified to some extent even with our crude methods if one looks for a history of cerebrovascular damage, signs of renal damage, enlargement of the heart, or definite abnormalities on the electrocardiogram.

DR. HAROLD G. WOLFF: I enjoyed hearing, and I share, many of Dr. Perera's frankly biased opinions, especially as regards the evidence of and the natural history of symptoms in patients with hypertension.

In the studies I shall discuss more fully this afternoon, I have been able to show that among many patients with hypertension who had no evidence of renal or cardiac failure, the symptoms and the level of the blood pressure are not closely related.

I should like to comment at this moment especially upon the relation of headache to the level of the blood pressure among those patients with hypertension but without hypertensive encephalopathy. Dr. Perera's studies indicated that only a third of the patients ever had headache at all. Our own and the studies of Robey suggest that perhaps only half of the patients with hypertension have headache. The half that do, do not necessarily have higher blood pressures than the half that do not. Those that have headache with their hypertension do not necessarily have headache at the time when their own blood pressure level is highest. We have several patients who have their headaches predictably when their blood pressures are lowest. We have several patients who have lost headache as a symptom as the blood pressure became even more elevated with the mounting age of the patient.

It has seemed to me that these facts support rather strongly the idea that symptoms are not a manifestation (excepting always the group of patients with renal and circulatory failure) of the level of the blood pressure and therefore allow an entirely different orientation for their management.

DR. CECIL J. WATSON (MINNEAPOLIS): I should like to add just one comment on a point that may be obvious to many of you, namely, that what we really need in following patients with hypertension, with reference in particular to the progress of their disease and its prognosis, is a method of measuring the mean blood pressure during the 24-hour period.

Obviously, that is an ideal that we can't very well attain. But it does seem to me that we can get much better information as to progress and prognosis by determining the lability of the blood pressure. I used to be perplexed by patients such as you have just heard about—especially women in surprisingly good condition whose blood pressures for many years were found, in the office (and usually in the afternoon), to be from 200 to 250, with a high diastolic pressure—but I am not greatly surprised now because those that I have been able to study more carefully have usually been found to have a labile hypertension. Their blood pressures declined remarkably during sleep.

We are all acquainted with this phenomenon, but we don't take it into account often enough. You have just heard about the lack of correlation between the initial blood pressure reading and the subsequent course of hypertension or the prognosis. I am really not very much surprised at this because the initial blood pressure reading is often taken under adverse circumstances. If the patient is put at rest and the blood pressure taken during sleep, either induced or natural, one often finds that it drops to even normal levels.

I am convinced that if we study the lability of the blood pressure rather than just the blood pressure reading at 2 o'clock or 4 o'clock in the office, we shall get much farther with this question of prognosis.

DR. REGINALD H. SMITHWICK: I rather hesitate to say anything at this point because I have been allotted 20 minutes to talk about this general matter shortly. But I should like to echo the remarks that Dr. Watson just made and also to support those of the gentleman from Ann Arbor who spoke a moment ago.

As you will see shortly, Dr. Perera's results, if we call them results of no treatment, are vastly superior to the results in my surgically treated patients, and also to those in our nonsurgically treated control series. I think that the type of material that you are exposed to is very important and I can't overemphasize the importance of the overall amount of cardiovascular damage that exists at the time of the first observation of the patient. There is no question whatsoever that the prognosis varies according to the amount of cardiovascular disease which exists when you first see the patient.

I should also like to point out and emphasize that people who have transient forms of hypertension rarely have cardiovascular disease of consequence. It is only when the blood pressure has been persistently elevated for a considerable period of time, with exceptions in certain males, that cardiovascular disease begins to make its appearance.

If you were to review all the literature on this question of prognosis as I have tried to, I think you would find only one study in which the blood pressure levels of the patients were determined under resting conditions. Virtually all of the data have to do with ambulatory patients, and I am not at all surprised at the lack of correlation between prognosis and blood pressure levels on the basis of data of that sort.

We have seen patients, such as those I commented upon yesterday, with very high levels—blood pressures of 250/150—on an ambulatory basis. You put them in bed—and you don't have to put them in bed for a month, you put them in bed for a couple of days—and the blood pressure may be perfectly normal.

I think that a short period of observation at bed rest will differentiate patients in the transient phase from those who are beginning to have a persistently elevated blood pressure. Then you will find that if the blood pressures are elevated after 48 hours of bed rest, over 90 per cent of the patients will have cardiovascular changes.

If you start at that point and divide them according to the degree of cardiovascular disease in the various areas, you will find a very clear-cut relationship between prognosis and vascular disease. Also you will find a perfectly definite and clear-cut relationship between the severity of the hypertension, as judged by the resting diastolic level, and the mortality rate.

DR. PERERA: I should like to thank the discussors who have made so many helpful and critical remarks and comments. I certainly agree with Dr. Page's suggestion that we may be dealing with more than one disease.

It amuses me to think that hypertensive vascular disease may exist without hypertension, may be more than a vascular disorder, and as Dr. Page suggests, may represent more than one disease.

Dr. Hoobler asked about the way in which we selected our series. During the course of these years, we followed a group of consecutive patients, but we limited the selection to those in whom we were able to document the disease and about whom we were able to obtain sufficient data to determine their status in everything respecting the existence or absence of complications.

I quite agree that this still remains a selected group until the day when we finally characterize the disease from its beginning to its end. But Dr. Hoobler's series selects by virtue of an arbitrary blood pressure value.

My plea is not that one series is right or another wrong, but that we have yet a great deal to learn, because only when we can start with the beginning and go to the end can we evaluate the total story. As to the suggestion of what blood pressure means, I too feel strongly that the casually recorded blood pressure is of the least significance. There are those who say the "floor" is important and those who regard the "ceiling" as important, contending that the peaks of pressure may do the damage. I personally feel that the floor is much more important and that until we obtain further documentation we shall not be able to evaluate patients correctly.

I agree completely that those patients capable of lowering their blood pressure floor with rest or relaxation, no matter what their casual pressures may be, appear to have the best outlook. There is great need of a better index than blood pressure to gauge the development and course of hypertensive disease.

DR. FAHR: The fate of the patient with hypertension is determined by his blood vascular system. Approximately 30 per cent die from cerebral vascular disease. I think no one will deny that it is the state of the blood vessels that determines the outcome in cerebral vascular disease.

Approximately 10 per cent die from renal insufficiency and uremia. The state of the small arteries and the arterioles determines the renal insufficiency and the uremia.

Sixty per cent die of heart failure or coronary insufficiency with or without infarction.

It seems to me that more and more patients with hypertension are succumbing to coronary insufficiency. Here again it is the state of the coronary vessels that decides their fate. After many years of study of the heart in hypertension, I have come to the conclusion that the accompanying coronary arteriosclerosis is at least as potent a factor in producing congestive heart failure as the increased work of the left ventricle. The first case with a very high blood pressure that I studied for a long period, from 1912 to 1934, died without ever having a very active life throughout this period. Dr. Bell at autopsy found his coronary arteries like a young man's. He never developed any renal insufficiency as tested by the best methods of that period. He had no more renal small artery sclerosis and arteriolosclerosis than the amount that a man of his age without hypertension would have.

His death was caused by softening of the brain, and he died from a stroke. The vessels of the brain were severely arteriosclerotic.

We must get criteria as to the state of the blood vessels if we want to know how a case of hypertension is progressing, and what the prognosis is. Therefore I was delighted when Dr. Watson made the suggestion that we ask Dr. Gofman to come here and talk to us on his recent work on the study of atheromatosis and the size of the blood cholesterol molecules.

We know that diabetes accelerates the rate of progress of the arteriosclerosis to which we are all prone ultimately. We know that hypertension is also a factor which very definitely accelerates it. Many of us are convinced that plasma cholesterol is one of the factors that accelerate the development of arteriosclerosis. Dr. Gofman's work shows the correlation between the size of the cholesterol particle in the plasma and the tendency for diabetes and hypertension as well as high blood cholesterol values to speed up the process of arteriosclerosis.

I think the work that Dr. Gofman has done is epoch making in the field of atheromatosis, and I want everyone to hear from his own lips something about this work on the cholesterol particle in the blood plasma. I am going to allow him more than the 20 minutes allotted to each paper. It gives me personally a very great pleasure to introduce Dr. Gofman to this audience.

· · · · · · · · · · · · · · · · · by JOHN W. GOFMAN

Blood Lipid Transport in
Hypertensive Patients and Its Relation to
Atherosclerotic Complications

ATHEROSCLEROSIS, a common enough source of disabling vascular disease, is a proper subject for this symposium, in view of the reasonably well accepted evidence that it is an important complication in the course of hypertensive disease and is a disease process accelerated in general in the presence of hypertension.

Concepts concerning the pathogenesis of atherosclerosis are numerous and conflicting, even as to the sequence of steps in the natural evolution of the lesions. Although controversial, a body of evidence has accumulated over the past 30 years indicating that in some way certain of the blood lipids, especially cholesterol and its esters, are involved in the production of the disease in human beings as well as in rabbits, dogs, and chickens. Briefly, we know from the animal data that certain procedures which result in the production of a sustained hypercholesterolemia are effective in producing lesions of striking similarity to those in human atherosclerosis. In the human being there does exist a group of syndromes and disease states, associated with hypercholesterolemia, in which premature and excessive atherosclerosis is characteristic. Among these are essential familial hypercholesterolemia, myxedema, the nephrotic syndrome, xanthoma tuberosum, biliary cirrhosis, and diabetes mellitus (in some cases). However, all these states together account for a relatively small fraction of the large number of persons in whom clinical manifestations of atherosclerosis, such as occlusive coronary, peripheral, or cerebral artery disease, occur. Serum cholesterol studies on this large bulk of the atherosclerotic patients have been contradictory, with many workers refuting the

NOTE. This study is based upon the collaborative researches of John W. Gofman, Thomas P. Lyon, Frank T. Lindgren, Hardin Jones, and Beverly Strisower.

evidence that any significant elevation of serum cholesterol is present in this group. In no small measure this problem is complicated by the great difficulty of ascertaining what a normal serum cholesterol level is, when we consider that of the apparently well persons who may be chosen to make up a "normal" series, as many as 50 per cent or more have significant atherosclerosis already.

It was with the hope of escaping this apparently futile controversy that a group of us at Donner Laboratory initiated investigations (1–3) directed toward the possibility that perhaps the total concentration of such blood lipids as cholesterol might be of less importance with respect to atherosclerosis than the physico-chemical nature of the molecules actually involved in blood lipid transport. This general idea had been previously suggested by such workers as Hueper (4), Hirsch and Weinhouse (5), and Rosenthal.

Evidence accumulated by numerous workers over the past 15 years and by us has demonstrated that the largest part of the serum cholesterol (free or esterified) circulates in the blood *not* as individual molecules, but rather as building blocks of "giant" molecules that may contain as many as several thousand cholesterol or fatty acid units per single giant molecule. A basic need for the evaluation of the possible existence of a defect in the physical chemistry of the molecules transporting lipids has been a method of characterizing such molecules in the serum of an individual patient or animal. Under special conditions of use, we have found the ultracentrifuge to be particularly suited to this purpose.

The ultracentrifuge is useful because it allows us to characterize the individual giant molecular types and to determine their respective concentrations in a serum sample as a result of the different rates of migration of the individual species under an impressed gravitational force of from 200,000 to 300,000 times gravity. With such forces proteins, lipids, or lipoproteins can be made to sediment or float at observable rates in the ultracentrifuge cell, depending upon whether the density of the particular molecule of interest is greater or less than that of the medium in which it is dissolved. From the ultracentrifuge optical diagram (see Figure 1) two major types of data are obtained. First, a sedimentation or flotation rate *characteristic* of that molecule under specified conditions is calculated. This rate is a physical constant just as are such more familiar properties as melting points and boiling points. Second, the area under or over the "peaks" in the diagram is proportional to the concentration of the molecular species giving rise to the peak. In the study of atherosclerosis the lipoproteins of interest can be best studied by the expedient of raising the serum density with sodium chloride, floating these lipoproteins in the preparative ultracentrifuge (with simultaneous concentration and purification), and then studying the isolated group of lipoproteins in the analytical ultracentrifuge. In the analytical centrifuge flotation rates are described in terms of S_f units (Svedbergs of flotation), where 1 S_f unit means a rate of 10^{-13} cm/sec/dyne/gram.

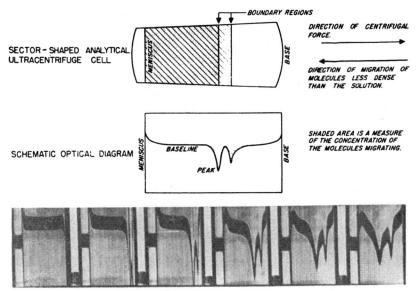

FIGURE 1. A diagram showing details of a sector-shaped analytical ultracentrifuge cell, a schematic optical diagram, and an actual series of photographs taken during an analytical run. The successive pictures are at 0, 6, 12, 22, 30, and 38 minutes after the full speed of 52,640 RPM has been reached. (This pattern was obtained from the serum of a patient with xanthomatous biliary cirrhosis.)

In Figure 2 are seen the various types of low-density components observed in the ultracentrifuge patterns of human subjects. These components may be categorized as follows:

1. The chylomicrons. Such aggregates, primarily neutral fat, are so large that they migrate across the field of view well before the centrifuge has reached full speed. The isolation of chylomicrons in our laboratory by Lindgren has revealed that they contain less than 1 per cent cholesterol. In view of this we feel it is dubious that they are directly involved in atheroma production.

2. Species which migrate with S_f rates greater than 40 units.

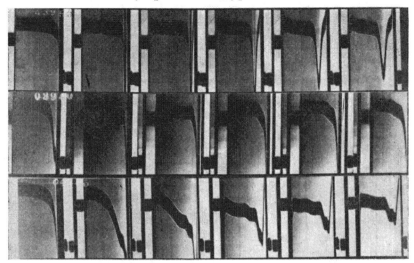

FIGURE 2. The ultracentrifugal patterns of the low density lipoproteins (density less than 1.063) from 3 different persons, demonstrating the major types of patterns obtained. Rotor speed 52,640 RPM. Temperature 26° C. Time intervals as in Figure 1. (The lowest picture is from a patient with the nephrotic syndrome.)

3. Species which migrate with S_f rates between 20 and 40 units. In this group there appear to exist a large number of components whose S_f values are so close to each other that they appear indistinguishable from a continuous series. The components of both the 20–40 and greater than 40 S_f classes are influenced acutely by meals.

4. Species which migrate with S_f rates between 10 and 20 units. These components are present in the blood only of certain human beings and are hardly affected acutely by meals. In this group several discrete molecular species are present.

5. Species which migrate with S_f rates between 3 and 10 units. One or more of the components of this class will be present at measurable concentrations in all human serum. In this group discrete molecular species are present. They are inappreciably influenced acutely by meals.

Before concerning ourselves with human atherosclerosis and a possible relationship of any of the above described components thereto, it is instructive to inspect the serum lipids and lipoproteins of the rabbit developing atherosclerosis as a result of cholesterol feeding.

Extensive studies of normal rabbit sera have shown only one prominent species in the low-density class of lipoproteins. This component, migrating with S_f rates between 5 and 10 units (variable within this range from rabbit to rabbit), is a lipoprotein containing approximately 30 per cent cholesterol and 25 per cent protein, as well as phospholipids and other constituents. The feeding of cholesterol to such rabbits results in a variable rate of increase in the concentration of the already existing lipoprotein of the S_f 5–10 class. Following this preliminary period, most rabbits show in addition new types of cholesterol-bearing lipoproteins in the serum, differentiable from the original lipoprotein by two major features:

1. The new lipoproteins migrate with rates greater than 10 S_f units in contrast to the normally occurring lipoprotein, which migrates with rates between 5 and 10 S_f units.

2. These new components of flotation rates greater than S_f 10 are of successively lower densities than the normally occurring lipoprotein.

The new components appearing in the course of cholesterol feeding have been found to be primarily in the S_f 10–30 class, although lower concentrations of components of S_f values greater than 30 are also seen. In general, the components appear in the order of increasing S_f

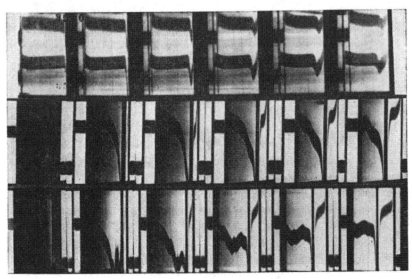

FIGURE 3. A diagram showing the appearance of lipoprotein molecules of successively higher flotation rates in rabbit serum during the progress of a cholesterol-feeding experiment. The upper and lower ultracentrifugal patterns of the top film are those taken respectively at the outset and after 2 weeks of cholesterol feeding. The center film shows the ultracentrifugal pattern 6 weeks later, and the bottom one 15 weeks later.

value, with appreciable concentrations of molecules in one particular range of flotation rates developing before those of even higher S_f rates appear in significant concentrations. Once the elevation of the normally occurring lipoprotein of the S_f 5–10 class has reached its peak, essentially all the increment in serum cholesterol in such rabbits is in the form of the components of S_f values greater than 10 units. (See Figure 3.)

Autopsy of some 35 rabbits at the end of a 15-week feeding period has revealed that the severity of gross atherosclerosis increases with the increase in the final concentration of molecules of the S_f 10–30 class, whereas the severity correlates poorly with the final concentration of molecules of the S_f 5–10 class. These observations indicate that the newly developed molecules of the S_f 10–30 class (and possibly those of even higher S_f rates) are in some way involved in the sequence of events leading to atheroma formation, if they are not indeed the etiologic agents. Contrariwise, the molecules of the S_f 5–10 class appear to represent a transport mechanism in the rabbit which is less noxious and which fails to handle the cholesterol (and possibly other lipid) excess beyond a certain limit. It is to be emphasized that individual rabbits differ in their tolerance to cholesterol feeding, some developing neither appreciable levels of molecules of the S_f 10–30 class nor atherosclerosis in spite of the ingestion of a full ration of cholesterol-containing food.

A study of the ultracentrifugal diagrams from human beings in various categories of age and state of health reveals that two major types of patterns occur:

1. Persons who shown only lipoprotein components with S_f values between 3 and 10 S_f units, in variable concentration. This picture bears a resemblance to the normal rabbit picture or to that of the rabbit in the early stage of cholesterol feeding.

2. Persons who show, in addition to the components of the S_f 3–10 class, variable concentrations of molecules of S_f 10–20, and in some cases S_f 20–40 molecules. Those showing such additional lipoproteins (of lower density than the S_f 3–10 class) show thus a striking similarity in their serum lipid transport to rabbits developing atherosclerosis.

It is an obvious step, therefore, to raise the question whether the additional lipoproteins in the human being, i.e., the S_f 10–20 class (and possibly the S_f 20–40 class), may be related to the development of human atherosclerosis in a manner analogous to the situation in the rabbit. The evidence presented below indicates that this question can be answered in the affirmative, at least for the S_f 10–20 class of molecules in man. It may be that the S_f 20–40 molecules in man are also involved, but since these components are more acutely influenced by meals than those of the S_f 10–20 class, it was felt that they represented less well the steady state of a person's lipid metabolism; hence consideration of the role of the S_f 20–40 class was deferred. Considerations of this class of molecules will be published elsewhere.

Unfortunately there exists no way clinically of appraising the extent or even the existence of atherosclerosis in the living human being. At best we may take a disease entity, e.g., myocardial infarction, and state that in well over 90 per cent of cases coronary atherosclerosis will be present in significant degree in at least one branch of one coronary artery. Even this allows one to say little or nothing about the extent of atherosclerosis in other regions of the vascular bed of such persons. However, significant incriminatory evidence can be marshalled by a study of the occurrence of the S_f 10–20 class of molecules associated with clinical entities occurring superimposed upon atherosclerosis of certain vascular beds, other entities known to predispose to excessive atherosclerosis, and in various classes of presumably normal people. One must decidedly qualify "normal" by the word *presumably,* since moderate or extensive atherosclerosis may be present in the absence of a clinical vascular manifestation.

The pertinent data concerning the occurrence of appreciable concentrations of molecules of the S_f 10–20 class are presented graphically in Figure 4. From these data certain observations and conclusions pertinent to the possible relationship of their presence may be made:

1. "Normal" females in the age group 20–40 show a much lower average concentration of S_f 10–20 molecules than do corresponding males.

2. Both sexes show an increasing average concentration of these molecules with increasing age, at least up to 60 years, the effect being particularly striking in the female. Further, the difference between the male and female blood picture is progressively obliterated with increasing age, at least up to 60 years.

These data are consistent with the more frequent occurrence of atherosclerosis and its complications in young males than in young females and with the clinical observation that females lose this relative protection, especially above the age of 40 years. The data are further consistent with the over-all increase in atherosclerosis with age in both sexes. The observation that presumably normal persons often show appreciable levels of these molecules is highly consistent

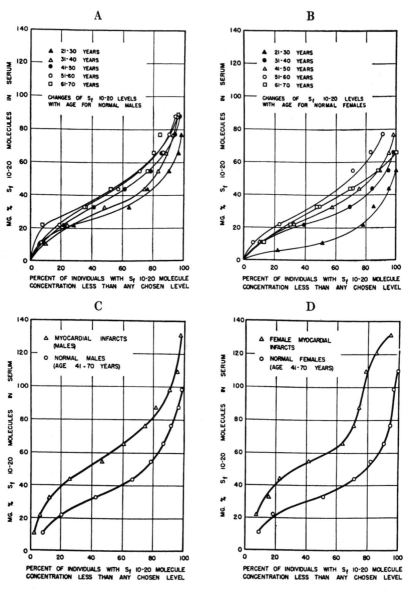

FIGURE 4. Seven diagrams illustrating certain trends in the blood level of S_f 10–20 lipoproteins in various circumstances. As a result of calibration changes, the lipoprotein levels reported throughout this figure have been revised upward as compared with previous data reported in reference 2. The revision in no way alters the interpretations given in that reference. A and B of this figure show the blood levels of S_f 10–20 lipoproteins in normal males (data based

E

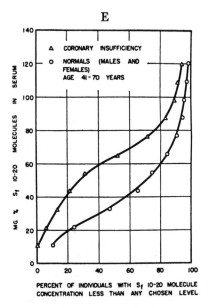

F

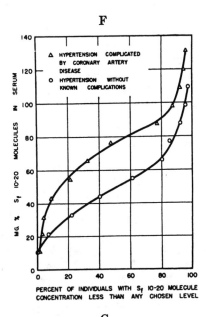

on 291 cases) and normal females (data based on 309 cases) 20–70 years of age, showing the trend with age. C and D show, for males and females respectively, the higher blood levels of S_f 10–20 lipoproteins in patients with myocardial infarction than in normal persons of corresponding age. All patients with infarction were at least 6 weeks beyond the infarction date. (Data for males based on 203 cases of myocardial infarction and 241 normals, and for females on 27 cases of infarction and 139 normals.) E, F, and G show the comparative blood levels of S_f 10–20 lipoproteins for various other groups. As no significant differences were found between the sexes, the plots are composite for males and females. E compares results based on 63 patients with coronary insufficiency (as manifested by angina pectoris) and 380 normal subjects. F compares results based on 95 patients with hypertension complicated by coronary artery disease and on 139 hypertensives without such known complications. G compares results based on 15 patients with diabetes complicated by hypertension and/or coronary artery disease and on 58 diabetics without known vascular complications.

G

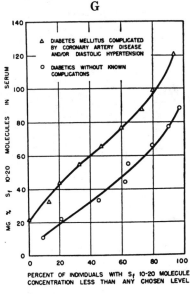

387

with the thesis that a relationship exists between the S_f 10–20 class of lipoproteins and human atherosclerosis, since so many of the presumably normal persons do have appreciable atherosclerosis. In fact, one would be highly suspicious of any supposed index of atherosclerosis that was negative in the large majority of human beings beyond the age of 40.

3. Patients with myocardial infarction or angina pectoris show much higher average levels of S_f 10–20 molecules than do corrèsponding normals. This is fully anticipated for molecules that may be related to atherosclerosis, since myocardial infarction and angina are nearly always sequelae of atherosclerosis, at least of the coronary arteries.

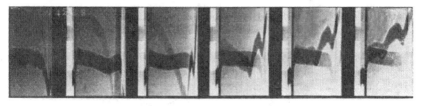

FIGURE 5. The ultracentrifugal pattern of the low-density lipoproteins in a patient with myxedema. The upper of the two patterns in this figure is the one from the myxedema case. (Note the similarity to the pattern in xanthoma tuberosum, Figure 6.)

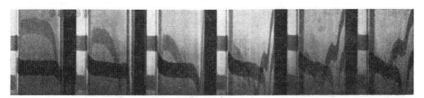

FIGURE 6. The ultracentrifugal pattern of the low-density lipoproteins in a patient with xanthoma tuberosum. (Note the exceedingly high levels of molecules of the S_f 10–20 class and of higher S_f rates, without a corresponding elevation of molecules of the S_f 3–8 class.) The pattern involved is the upper of the two on this figure, the lower pattern being from a different person, but run at the same time.

4. Patients with diabetes mellitus and hypothyroidism, both diseases which predispose to atherosclerosis, show higher concentrations of S_f 10–20 molecules than do corresponding normals. Figure 5 shows the lipoprotein pattern in a case of myxedema. Worthy of note is the fact that the S_f 3–10 class of molecules is not appreciably elevated over the normal, whereas the S_f 10–20 class is fantastically high. This would suggest that, as in the rabbit, the group of components of S_f 10 or less

may not be related to atherosclerosis, whereas the S_f 10–20 class is so related.

5. Observations not shown in the summary diagram (Figure 4) have been made which show that in the nephrotic syndrome (see Figure 2, e), in xanthoma tuberosum, being studied in collaboration with Dr. James McGinley (see Figure 6), and in biliary cirrhosis (see Figure 1), there are exceedingly high levels of molecules of the S_f 10–20 class, without corresponding elevations of the S_f 3–10 class. Inasmuch as these states also predispose to atherosclerosis, the presence of high levels of S_f 10–20 molecules in the serum of patients with these diseases supports the hypothesis of the relationship of such molecules to atherosclerosis.

Returning to the central subject of this symposium, hypertension, we may re-emphasize the excessive atherosclerosis which frequently accompanies the hypertensive state. A study of 75 patients with essential hypertension, including those already manifesting angina or having had a myocardial infarction, shows that the average level of molecules of the S_f 10–20 class is considerably higher in these patients than in corresponding normals. This is consistent with the clinical observations of excessive atherosclerosis in hypertensives. However, it should be noted that a small percentage of the hypertensive group show very low levels of the S_f 10–20 class of molecules, which is in agreement with the autopsy data indicating that some hypertensives do *not* develop appreciable atherosclerosis. Also worthy of note are the observations that the level of S_f 10–20 molecules does not correlate well with either the known duration of the hypertensive state or with the actual level of the pressure. The data as a whole would suggest that the elevated average levels of S_f 10–20 molecules in hypertensives could account for excessive atherosclerosis as a complication of hypertension *without* invoking the pressure elevation as the responsible factor. It will, of course, now be imperative to observe a group of hypertensives over an adequate period to determine directly whether those hypertensives with the most elevated S_f 10–20 levels do in fact develop more atherosclerosis than do the hypertensives with low levels of these molecules. Only in this way can an ultimate evaluation of the relative importance of pressure per se versus blood lipids in the development of atherosclerosis in hypertensives be made.

A consideration of the relation between the blood level of S_f 10–20 molecules and analytical serum cholesterol levels provides a possible answer to the question of the discrepancies reported between serum cholesterol elevations and atherosclerosis. In normal persons and in patients in various disease categories the routine analytical blood cholesterol determination is of *no* predictive value as to the level of S_f 10–20 molecules that will be found ultracentrifugally. The S_f 10–20 molecule level may be high when the serum cholesterol is low, and vice versa. It is true, however, that, considering average levels and without concerning ourselves about the individual patient, there is a general trend toward increasing levels of S_f 10–20 molecules with increasing serum cholesterol levels. The observations thus indicate that there is at least a semi-independent mechanism for the control of one group of lipoproteins, no matter what the level of certain others may be.

If our thesis of the relationship of molecules of the S_f 10–20 class to atherosclerosis should be correct, it would be readily understandable that certain patients, for example, diabetics, with low total serum cholesterol levels but with high S_f 10–20 levels, could develop extensive atherosclerosis. This might remove some of the paradoxes of the relation between serum cholesterol and atherosclerosis.

Any ultimate understanding of the significance of the S_f 10–20 molecules and others of the lipoproteins of serum will require an understanding of the factors responsible for the maintenance of any particular level of these molecules in a steady state. One approach to this which has already provided some clues has been via dietary alterations in human subjects.

In human beings, normal or with vascular disease, the restriction of the total fat intake to from 25 to 50 gm. per day (vegetable and animal fats) and of cholesterol to 100–200 mg. per day results in a decrease in the blood level of S_f 10–20 molecules in the majority of cases within 1–8 weeks, the response being variable in rate and extent from individual to individual. Accompanying the depression in the level of the S_f 10–20 class of molecules, there may be less striking, but definite, depression of the level of the S_f 3–10 class of molecules. These changes may be accompanied by appreciable, moderate, or negligible reductions in the serum cholesterol level as measured by the usual chemical techniques. That significant changes in the S_f 10–20 class may occur without appreciable alteration in the total serum cholesterol in some cases would be anticipated, since in many such cases only a very small percentage of the total serum cholesterol is in the form of S_f 10–20 molecules. The addition of fat back to the restricted diet, whether fat of animal or vegetable origin, results in a rise again in the level of S_f 10–20 molecules. Thus the dietary depression in the level of such molecules persists only if the dietary restriction is maintained.

Studies of hypothyroid patients receiving thyroid extract has already indicated that in such patients this drug does depress the level of S_f 10–20 molecules. Whether thyroid extract influences apparently euthyroid persons who show these molecules is now under investigation.

The possible prophylactic and therapeutic value of depressing the level of the S_f 10–20 class of lipoproteins with respect to atherosclerosis will necessarily require a longer-term evaluation than has been possible to date.

Questions and Discussion

DR. ANCEL KEYS (MINNEAPOLIS) : I am sure all of us here are in full agreement that we could spend the rest of the symposium discussing Dr. Gofman's paper and could find reason for relating that to the problem of essential hypertension which is the occasion of the meeting.

Perhaps we may hope at some future date that a symposium will be devoted to the general question of atherosclerosis and perhaps the other varieties of arteriolosclerosis over which the pathologists debate.

The questions, however, that are brought out by Dr. Gofman's paper are so important and so numerous that we must touch on a few of them.

In the first place, Dr. Gofman was exceedingly modest in his explanation of the physical system that he is working with. It is true, it is not difficult to comprehend the principles; but I must emphasize the tremendous amount of ingenuity and labor involved in getting the astonishing number of data, some of which he has only alluded to here. I think there is a great deal more material under analysis, according to what I understand from Dr. Calvin, who visited here a few days ago.

The problem that we begin with, to take up one of the early points raised by Dr. Gofman, is the question of "normality" and "normal" standards. These points have interested us at the laboratory of physiological hygiene for some time, not merely in connection with cholesterol in the blood, but in other connections as well.

I think it should be realized that when we are using, as we do in popular medical parlance, the term "normal," we merely refer to people who at that moment do not exhibit developed disease discoverable by our present techniques. In general, we gather together a group of people who, let us say, are acceptable insurance "risks" at the present moment, make our measurements on them, and take the average of whatever we have measured to be the center of normality.

This method merely gives us the popular "vote" of that group of people in regard to the item of measurement. We record as "normal" merely the most frequent or the most common characteristic. That does not *necessarily* have anything to do whatsoever with the *prognosis* for those persons, their future with regard to disease versus health. We have heard repeatedly throughout this symposium the plea for a long-time study of persons, for it is only by relating present findings on people to their future developments that we can begin to understand the meaning of a particular present finding.

Now, in connection with atherosclerosis, I think there is no doubt in the minds of most students of the problem that somehow or other cholesterol is, if not primary to, at least intimately associated with the development and progress of the atherotic condition in the vessel wall. It has also been obvious for some time that it is not a simple and straightforward connection, for many patients are seen who obviously have atherosclerosis, but who do not show major elevations in the total blood cholesterol, the free cholesterol, or any other fraction that has been studied hitherto.

The significance, it seems to me, of Dr. Gofman's work is that he is obviously bringing us much closer to the measurements of something which is more directly related to the atherosclerotic process. But perhaps, and I think that Dr. Gofman will agree, there are several other points which have not been mentioned at all in his discussion.

In the first place, you cannot have S_{13} molecules in the blood without having cholesterolosis in some form. Secondly, there is the question of why the cholesterol, so to speak, sets up housekeeping in the vessel wall. He has mentioned 8 per cent of his patients with unquestioned coronary disease who show no elevation in the S_{13} fraction in the blood. It is true he need not apologize for that 8 per cent, but they do represent people who apparently do not have abnormally high levels of this particular form of cholesterol and yet have all the signs of the lesions.

Where does that leave us? To me it means that possibly some of these patients have their lesions because of, let us say, past history. At one time they may have had a high level of S_{13} molecules in the blood, and the atherosclerotic lesions persist, but it is equally reasonable to suggest that these persons reflect the fact that the vessel wall itself has a major role to play. There is much other evidence to indicate the importance of the vessel wall. For example, we know the predilection of different persons for laying down cholesterol in different parts of the body. Cholesterol deposition is not all vascular; the dermatologist picks up the more external manifestations in patients who have no vascular symptoms. We ourselves have studied several of these people with xanthoma tuberosum. Such people usually have total cholesterol levels in the blood which are very high. They also have high levels of these large molecules which Dr. Gofman is studying. Nevertheless, although the majority of such persons may have a tendency toward vascular disease as well, many of them do not exhibit this tendency so that it can be recognized clinically. Many of us have seen patients of this kind who have enormous deposits of cholesterol in the skin but who get along very well indeed without the slightest sign of vascular disease and who continue that way, for some years, at least. For these and other reasons I must insist that there is some factor involved in the blood vessel wall which influences the deposition of cholesterol there.

Another question that has to be thought about very carefully here is one arising from the fact that among persons on the same diet, living the same kind of life, some have high concentrations of cholesterol in the blood, and some have low. Now this may be "explained" by talking about "constitutional differences," but that is really evading the issue of individual differences. The important point is that we conclude there is obviously some regulating machinery which affects the blood concentration and, very likely, the atherosclerotic process as well. There is some regulating machinery which determines the level at which the S_{13} molecules exist in the blood. So far, I have seen no clue whatsoever as to what that regulating machinery may be or how it operates. The individual level of cholesterol in the blood, and I believe of S_{13} molecules also, is largely independent of the diet; although we can produce modifications by drastic changes in the diet of the individual, he tends to maintain a particular individual level. Here is an enormous problem for future investigation.

One last word. I should like to ask Dr. Gofman if he would comment on his use of the term "molecule" for his particles. Many years ago when I studied physical chemistry, we had a simpler concept of molecules and atoms than has emerged in recent years. Nevertheless, I think we should still cling to some fairly rigorous terminology if we possibly can, and I wonder whether it is proper to speak of Dr. Gofman's particles as molecules. What is the criterion for calling them molecules? They have a particular density and size characteristic, and, as far as I know, that is all. I should inquire as to the forces which hold these cholesterol particles together. I should ask whether they are held together by covalence bonds, partial valences; whether protein factors are involved and, if so, how; and whether there is anything more than the loosest kind of physical force holding them together in *aggregation*. This is not academic quibbling; whatever factors and forces produce these aggregates or molecules, these are factors which obviously enter into the etiology of atherosclerosis if these particles are involved as such in the etiology of atherosclerosis.

DR. IRVINE H. PAGE: Mr. Chairman, I should like to tell you why I think this work bears all the earmarks of genial thinking. I can tell you because I can compare it with our own arteriosclerotic thinking.

Two years ago, the U.S. Public Health Service bought an ultracentrifuge for us, and we were so busy watching things go down that we forgot that they could go up. The genial thought—and I suspect it means that a man must be young, bright, and possibly from California—was that lipids usually float rather than settle. Now that looks like a very simple step, but it is a step that nobody but Jack Gofman took. It is a step of major importance!

Now I am also pleased to say that we have been able to confirm in essence almost everything that Dr. Gofman has said. That naturally gives us great pleasure, and while it doesn't add anything, I think, to Dr. Gofman's work, at least it comes from an entirely independent source.

You might ask what we had in mind in the first place in buying an ultracentrifuge. Dr. Lena A. Lewis and I were interested in comparing the changes we had found in the Tiselius electrophoretic pattern in patients with vascular disease with what might be found using another physical method of measuring changes in the macromolecules of the blood. It had become clear that the beta-lipoproteins in the Tiselius pattern were grossly disturbed, even in experimental renal hypertension. The ultracentrifuge seemed to offer a method which might aid us in further analyzing this problem. But we missed the boat, and it took Dr. Gofman to show us not only that we had made, but how to rectify, the mistake.

I think that none of us at present would want to jeopardize our thinking as to the final outcome of the work on the S_f 10–20 molecules. It will come out in the not distant future what they really mean in terms of the mechanism of atherosclerosis and in usefulness in clinical medicine. That they are present in the blood under some very interesting circumstances, as Dr. Gofman has shown, there can no longer be any doubt. That they occur in the blood of men more commonly than women is also unfortunately true. Which is just another way of bringing out the confounded superiority and durability of the female.

DR. EPHRAIM SHORR: I should like to refer very briefly to the question raised by Dr. Keys concerning a regulating machinery within the body itself that determines blood concentrations such as those described by Dr. Gofman. In this connection I should like to cite what may be relevant studies being carried out by Dr. Henry Simms, of the College of Physicians and Surgeons. Dr. Simms is using a tissue culture technique. Taking chicken fibroblasts which he washes free of the lipid granules which they are prone to deposit in the normal state of growth, he has been able to determine the presence of two families of substances. There are lipids which deposit lipfanogens within the fibroblast in the tissue culture. There are factors which appear to be in the albumin fraction which inhibit this deposition. Apparently in these fibroblasts he has demonstrated the existence of varying ratios of these lipfanogens to antilipfanogens. The antilipfanogens, for example, are heat labile and can be removed from a particular specimen, allowing the lipfanogens to exert their action unopposed. His initial studies have established a ratio of lipfanogens to antilipfanogens in the so-called normals, and he has begun a study of patients with coronary disease and of patients with diabetes.

In the patients with coronary disease, the ratio of antilipfanogens to lipfanogens has been profoundly reduced.

Dr. Gofman, I believe, is about to carry out studies correlative to those of Dr. Simms, so that it may be possible to relate these findings on the species of substances to a ratio of inhibitors which set the pattern for each individual—another example of homeostasis.

DR. L. L. WATERS (NEW HAVEN): Arteriosclerosis is a focal process. It develops in a characteristic pattern in the aorta at the mouth of the intercostal arteries and at the origins of the great thoracic and abdominal branches. If the blood pressure is raised acutely in experimental animals, damage to the vessel wall occurs at precisely these sites. This damage is essentially an inflammatory process. Particulate matter including India ink, dyes, and lipids may localize in these areas. I should like to ask Dr. Gofman if his molecules would be likely, because of their physical properties, to localize in such areas of inflammation? Further, would not local factors be important in determining the localization of any lipid particles derived from the blood?

DR. GOFMAN: I might start with Dr. Keys. I will start with Dr. Keys' comments about the 8 per cent who don't show these molecules in the blood itself. I think that as far back as Virchow, and possibly before that, it has been recognized that atherosclerosis is a focal process.

Whatever the reasons for this are, I don't know them. I think we must take that into account.

There is the fact that there are many, many cases that come to autopsy with the left coronary artery involved with atheroma and with the aorta completely clear. There are cases with the aorta involved and the coronary arteries clear. There are cases with other muscular or muscular-elastic arteries involved and others clear.

We don't understand what the factors are which determine why a certain vessel is involved. Certainly this is one of the major problems to settle. But if, in any event, it may be that having a certain set of molecules or a certain lipid metabolism is the sine qua non of the developing of the disease, the actual site of the disease may well depend upon the local factors.

There has been considerable discussion with respect to Dr. Waters' question about the possible injuries at a particular local site which might determine that this site itself is the site of atheroma formation.

I don't think we know what those injuries are. There has been discussion of injury to the elastic tissue, its fraying, and so on, but I believe it is wholly reasonable to think that given certain substances that do form atheroma, specific local factors in the vessel will be highly important in determining where these molecules will appear.

Again, about this 8 per cent, I should like to say that among many of these people we know very definitely that after their coronary episodes they have been eating far less than before of the foods that we know will raise these molecules in concentration. If anyone takes a series of coronary thrombosis patients and weighs them a year after they have had their coronary episodes, he will find their weights lower than before the coronary episodes. The patients, we know, have been eating less, probably because their doctors advised them to lose weight, if they were at all overweight, even though making no suggestions with regard to specific items of diet.

Whether it is this advice alone or not, it is unquestionably true that the patients who have had a myocardial infarction are in general lighter afterward than before. Possibly Dr. Clawson might also want to make some statement, but there is no question that a certain percentage—possibly 5 per cent, maybe 10 or more—of patients who have a myocardial infarction have it on some basis other than atherosclerosis. We should therefore not be greatly surprised to find some of these people negative.

Now about the patients with xanthoma tuberosum that Dr. Keys spoke of, of whom we say they don't have vascular disease—I think this is very dangerous. Even though we say they don't have vascular disease, they may have extensive vascular disease. For that matter, we know there are many, many people who come to autopsy at the age of 80, who have never had a symptom of coronary disease or peripheral vascular disease, yet have vessels that are loaded with atheroma far in excess of what patients have who have died at 40 of a myocardial infarction. That is the perplexing part about atherosclerosis and its great difficulty.

Patients can have a good deal of atherosclerosis if they just don't happen to have it in a critical area or to have superimposed upon it the accident that we don't understand at all—namely, a hemorrhage into a plaque or a thrombosis. To us they look normal. To my knowledge there is no clinical way of looking at these people and saying they are or they aren't in trouble. Certainly the vast amount of evidence on patients who have xanthoma tuberosum and have it for a while is that they do have a fair amount of atherosclerosis in their vessels.

There again one might find a patient with xanthoma tuberosum whose coronary arteries are free but whose aorta is loaded. But the mere fact that a patient appears clinically well indicates nothing at all about how much atherosclerosis he may have, for the amount can be terrific without any clinical manifestations.

About the regulating machinery, I am in full agreement that we haven't even touched on the regulating machinery which determines why some people who eat a high fat, a high cholesterol diet—eat it day in and day out and eat more of it than other people—don't show these molecules. They are among, let us say, the superior persons.

The great future problem of this sort of research, I think, is to determine just what the nature of the regulating mechanism is. But it is absolutely true that one can make no blanket statement to the effect that if one eats these foods he will have these molecules. I tried it myself, tried eating an exceedingly high fat, high cholesterol diet for a period of time to see whether I could produce the molecules; what I succeeded in doing primarily was to raise the level of my own molecules of the 4 S_f class. This is very similar to the rabbit situation early. Possibly if I could have tolerated this diet for a period of longer than the three weeks during which I tried it, I might have developed an appreciable level of S_f 10–20 molecules. At the rate I was gaining weight, the diet was a little bit difficult to continue.

With respect to the third problem, whether or not we should use the term molecules or aggregates. I have a very, very strong opinion on this point. These are molecules. I think that the progress of science, especially the science of large molecules, has been held up more by the concept that we should distinguish between a so-called aggregate and a so-called molecule than by any other thing that the colloid chemists have done, and I think that the weight of high-powered thinking in the chemical field is that one should not establish a difference between a loose force and a strong one.

There are many, many important chemical forces—the so-called Vander Waals forces—which are in existence between any two atoms that are close enough together. These forces play the most important of roles in the structure of molecules, and hence to make a differentiation between a covalent link, an ionic link, and a Vander Waals link (or a weak link, so-called) is really to lose sight of the fact that all chemistry is based upon the combination of such linkages rather than upon the existence of only covalent links. If there were only one type of linkage existing in chemistry, it would have long since been a simple problem, but in the vast field of immunology and antibody reactions the conditioning factors are undoubtedly primarily these so-called weaker links.

The fact that these substances have a repeatable composition and a perfectly distinct classification with respect to sedimentation rates, density, and other properties would indicate they are a distinct species. Whatever the forces involved in holding them together, they absolutely and unequivocally deserve the term molecules rather than aggregates.

As to Dr. Page's comments, well, I am certainly grateful for his generosity, but particularly grateful to him for the statement that we aren't imagining all these things. Concerning what Dr. Shorr had to say, it will be very interesting to see whether and how our work correlates with the work of Dr. Simms and others. I think I have covered Dr. Waters' point.

DR. GEORGE FAHR: I think you all have had enough in what Dr. Gofman and some of the others have brought forward today to realize that atherosclerosis is the central point in the prognosis and the etiology of factors that bring about a decrease in physical fitness in hypertension. The atherosclerotic is by far and away the great problem for discussion.

• • • • • • • • • • • • • • • *by* ROBERT W. WILKINS

The Hemodynamic Effects of Various Types of Therapy in Hypertensive Patients

STUDIES of the hemodynamic effects of procedures designed to lower the blood pressure in hypertensive patients are of interest not only in connection with the specific cases studied, but also in relation to the general problems of the nature of the disease and the proper aims of therapy. First of all, such an approach will quickly demonstrate to any investigator who cares to try it that under controlled laboratory conditions the blood pressure of hypertensive patients can be lowered. This is of some importance, particularly now when there seems to be increasing adherence to the view that the pressure in hypertensive patients is naturally so variable as to cast doubt on the significance of any lowering that may occur after a therapeutic procedure. Secondly, such studies will demonstrate that the blood pressure of hypertensive patients may be lowered in a variety of ways, and with a number of different hemodynamic adjustments, some of which may be, at least theoretically, more desirable than others. In this laboratory attention has been devoted chiefly to the effects of lumbodorsal sympathectomy and of certain hypotensive drugs. Other laboratories have studied, in addition, adrenalectomy, spinal anesthesia, pyrogens, and diet. It seems possible that from all these studies will stem, if not an effective form of treatment, at least a better understanding of the disease.

Lumbodorsal Sympathectomy

Lumbodorsal sympathectomy (Smithwick, 1) has now been in use for 12 years for the relief of essential hypertension. One of the hemodynamic effects most commonly observed, particularly early after this operation, is postural hypotension presumably due to the reduction in sympathetic vasopressor responses to the upright position. Indeed, some observers have ascribed the clinical improvement that they have observed in patients after operation chiefly to this effect (2). While in time postural hypotension appears to lessen or at least to become less bothersome to patients, who usually cease to complain of it from 6 to 12 months after the operation, it is our impression that the autonomic vasopressor responses to the upright position are impaired for an indefinite period. We have found them to be markedly reduced as long as 9 years following lumbodorsal splanchnicectomy. We believe that patients learn to accommodate for their loss of autonomic control through a conscious or unconscious activity of the voluntary muscles in the lower parts of the body.

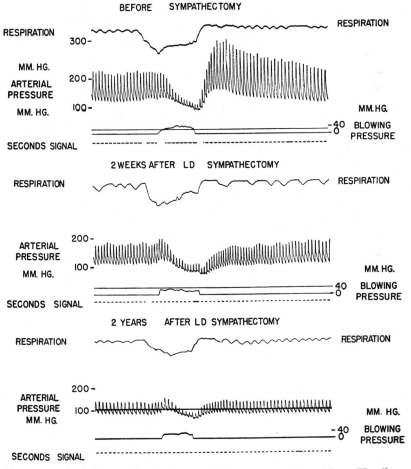

FIGURE 1. Optical records of the arterial pressure taken with a Hamilton manometer showing responses to the Valsalva maneuver in a hypertensive patient before, 2 weeks after, and 2 years after a lumbodorsal sympathectomy.

There are other sympathetic nervous vasopressor responses that are somewhat easier to relate to the extent of surgical sympathectomy and to the presumed reactivity of the sympathetic nervous system. These are brief overshoots of arterial pressure that occur as pressor responses to even a few seconds of arterial hypotension produced by any maneuver that does not itself impair vasomotor reactivity (3). The Valsalva test is one of the easiest and simplest of such maneuvers to perform. After an extensive sympathectomy a patient fails to have an overshoot after this test in contrast to the marked responses usually present before operation (Fig. 1). Since during such overshoots the arterial pressure may rise to dangerously high levels, it is reassuring to speculate on the possibility that their abolition may be clinically valuable to the patient. The impairment of these responses also has been observed 9 years after operation.

A peculiarity of the pulse rate in hypertensive patients was noted during recent studies of the effects of epinephrine and norepinephrine in a group of hypertensive, as compared with a group of normotensive,

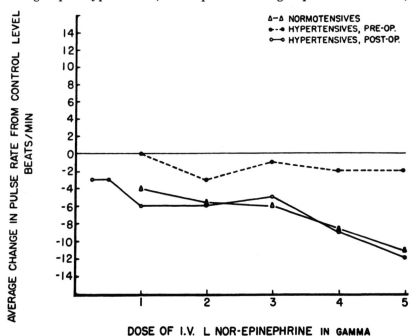

FIGURE 2. A chart showing the average change in the pulse rate during pressor responses to various intravenous doses of norepinephrine in 5 normotensive subjects, and in 6 hypertensive patients before and after lumbodorsal sympathectomy.

subjects (4, 5). Although the blood pressure responses of the two groups to both these pressor drugs was the same, the pulse rate responses were different. The normotensive subjects slowed their pulse rates during pressor responses to these agents, but the hypertensive patients failed to slow their pulse rates normally. Lumbodorsal sympathectomy, however, restored the normal slowing of the pulse rate in hypertensive patients during pressor responses to epinephrine or norepinephrine (Fig. 2). It was further interesting that on re-examination of the pulse rates during the overshoot responses to the Valsalva test, the hypertensive patients were again found not to slow their pulse rates as much as normotensive subjects (6). However, one could not assess the effect of sympathectomy on this type of pulse retardation since the operation abolished the overshoot itself which presumably was responsible for the slowing.

Measurements of the cardiac output, renal blood flow, and peripheral blood flow have not revealed them to be consistently changed after sympathectomy, at least with the patient resting under laboratory conditions (7). Similar results have been obtained for the cere-

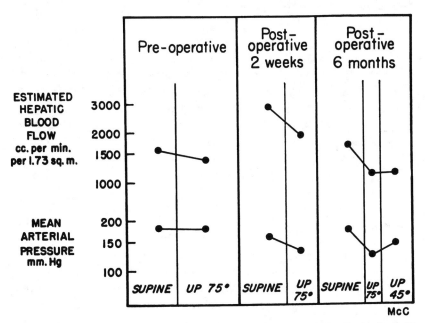

FIGURE 3. A chart of the estimated hepatic blood flow and the "mean" (half systolic plus diastolic) arterial pressure measured in the horizontal and upright positions on a hypertensive patient before, 2 weeks after, and 6 months after lumbodorsal sympathectomy.

bral blood flow (8). The resting hepatic blood flow, on the other hand, was usually increased early after the operation but then slowly subsided so that by from 6 to 8 months it had resumed its preoperative resting level. The hepatic blood flow in the upright position before operation in hypertensive patients, as in normotensive subjects, was usually less than in the resting horizontal position, although the mean arterial pressure was essentially the same, denoting splanchnic vasoconstriction in the erect posture (Fig. 3). After splanchnicectomy, however, there was no evidence of splanchnic vasoconstriction in hypertensive patients in the upright position, the hepatic blood flow decreasing only in proportion to the postural hypotension (9). Thus the resting blood flow through the body was essentially unchanged after sympathectomy, whether or not the resting blood pressure was greatly reduced. These results indicate that after sympathectomy the circulation remains adequate in the major vascular areas under resting conditions, although under conditions of stress, as, for example, during exercise and/or the assumption of the upright position, it may be diminished in certain regions, particularly when there is a major reduction in the arterial pressure.

Drugs

To be suitable for therapy in essential hypertension, a drug should lower the blood pressure without undue side effects and should be active, when taken by mouth, over long periods of time. There are as yet no drugs available which satisfy these requirements. However, those that have at least some of the desired properties have been studied to determine what types of drugs would be desirable (10). The agents that have been used may be divided into the sympatholytic and the non-sympatholytic drugs.

SYMPATHOLYTIC DRUGS

Dihydroergocornine. The rationale for the use of sympatholytic drugs is, of course, the same as that for surgical sympathectomy. The prototype of the group that has been studied most in this laboratory is Dihydroergocornine (DHO-180) (11). Active by mouth, this drug might have been suitable for long-term clinical trial had it not been found to lose its hypotensive effect after continuous oral administration for several weeks (12).

Like surgical splanchnicectomy, DHO was found to cause postural hypotension and the abolition of vasopressor overshoots to blood-

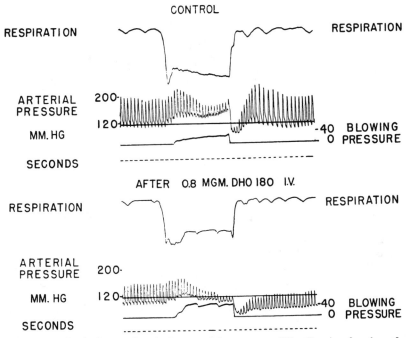

FIGURE 4. Optical records of the arterial pressure (Hamilton), showing the responses to the Valsalva maneuver in a hypertensive patient before and after the intravenous administration of 0.8 mgm. of Dihydroergocornine.

pressure-lowering procedures (Fig. 4). Also, like a sympathectomy which includes the heart, DHO usually produced bradycardia. However, on acute administration its effects upon the blood flow in different vascular areas were much less consistent than those of surgical sympathectomy. Characteristically, although the cardiac output did not fall, the blood flow in the kidneys and liver decreased with the drop in the arterial pressure, although in some instances it later returned to control levels while the pressure continued to be reduced. The cerebral blood flow has been reported to remain at control levels during falls in the arterial pressure due to DHO (13). The peripheral blood flow in the arms and legs increased or remained unchanged.

NON-SYMPATHOLYTIC DRUGS

Veratrum viride. Veratrum viride is a hypotensive but not a sympatholytic agent (14). Consequently, in therapeutic doses it was found not to cause postural hypotension or to reduce the vasopressor overshoot reactions (Fig. 5). In this respect it was interesting since

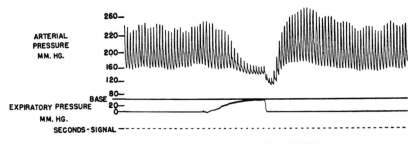

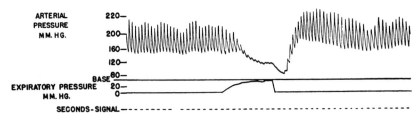

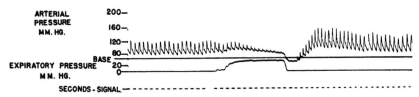

FIGURE 5. Optical records of the arterial pressure (Hamilton), showing the responses to the Valsalva maneuver in a hypertensive patient before, 5 minutes after, and 28 minutes after the intramuscular administration of Veratrum viride (Veratrone).

it apparently changed the pressure level to which the vasomotor system was set. Thus, after Veratrum the blood pressure responded to hypotensive stimuli similarly, but at a lower level, than before the administration of the drug.

Preparations of Veratrum viride suitable for parenteral use have conclusively demonstrated the powerful hypotensive effects of the drug in hypertensive patients on acute administration (15). The persistence of its action on chronic oral administration is more difficult to assess accurately, but in some patients appears to be real. On intravenous infusion of the drug (Fig. 6) hypotensive effects appeared within 10 minutes and were related directly to the dose, which was

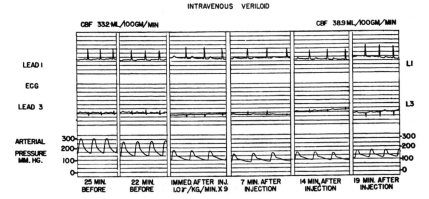

FIGURE 6. Electrocardiogram (leads 1 and 3) and arterial pressure (Sanborn electromanometer) tracings in a hypertensive patient before and at various intervals (as noted below) after the intravenous administration of Veriloid. Cerebral blood flow (Kety) measurements, as noted above, were made during the time of the first two (control) and the last two (postdrug) tracings.

less per kilogram of body weight in hypertensive patients than in normotensive patients for a given hypotensive response. The retardation of the pulse rate through vagal action was a usual and contributory, although not a necessary, component of the hypotensive effect of Veratrum viride. Physiologic evidences of myocardial strain, such as a decreased cardiac output, pulsus alternans, or negative T waves in the first lead of the electrocardiogram, were often improved (Fig. 6). The total cardiac output and blood flow through the kidneys, liver, and extremities apparently remained adequate, at least after adjustment to the initial sharp drop in the blood pressure on acute administration of the drug (14). Preliminary measurements of the cerebral blood flow made by us (16) and also by the Philadelphia group (17) have shown no consistent change during the hypotension produced by Veratrum (Fig. 6).

Comment

Hemodynamic studies during the effects of certain procedures designed to lower the blood pressure of hypertensive patients have revealed that the blood pressure can be lowered and that the circulation may remain adequate in a number of different organs in spite of quite sizable lowerings of the pressure. These observations are reassuring in the face of the argument that hypertension is merely an adjustment to organic vascular disease and that to disturb this adjustment will cause circulatory embarrassment. The studies do not, of course, indicate that hypertension does not occur in association with vascular disease or that too great a lowering of the pressure will not cause ischemia. However, they do emphasize that essential hypertension in many cases is a disease primarily of disturbed physiology, with perhaps some, but by no means universal, organic vascular pathology.

It is still important today to make the distinction between pathologic physiology and pathologic anatomy in disease first emphasized by Sir James MacKenzie years ago. It is important because when both types of disturbance occur together in a patient, the organic changes may in part be due to, or at least aggravated by, the physiologic changes. To insist that therapy should be directed at and judged by the improvement of only organic and not physiologic disturbances may mean abandoning all therapy, for in some cases it may be presumed to be too early, while in other cases it may be presumed to be too late. The prevention of organic lesions by the amelioration of physiologic disturbances is the cardinal aim in the use of hypotensive therapy in hypertensive patients. It must be emphasized again that only long-term studies are capable of establishing the efficacy of such therapeutic attempts.

The most objectionable feature of long-term therapeutic studies is that they take such a long time. There are many lesser objections that hinge on this one. There is great difficulty in keeping patients continuously on a given therapy over long periods of time. Here surgeons have a great advantage over internists. Indeed, there seems to be something satisfyingly final about removing portions of the human anatomy. In cases where the sympathetic nerves are removed for the treatment of hypertensive disease, patients simply have to continue undergoing the effects of such therapy whether they like it or not! Speaking seriously, this may constitute one of the chief favorable characteristics of surgical treatment, namely, the continuity of its effects. By now, as you will hear from others, enough surgical cases have been followed for sufficient periods of time for the results to be statistically significant when compared with non-surgically treated cases. The evidence of the prolongation of life and the reduction of vascular disease seems clear. It is disconcerting, however, to hear some critics of therapy accept the evidences of organic improvement after surgery but object to certain associated physiologic disturbances, such as "symptomatic debilitation" of the patient, and on the other hand accept evidences of physiologic or symptomatic improvement after medical treatment but object to the lack of evidence of organic improvement.

In time, of course, both organic and physiologic evidence for the efficacy of all the various forms of therapy now in use in hypertension will be forthcoming. Even at this point, however, it is obvious that none of these forms of therapy is ideal or, for that reason, likely to be the ultimate. Nevertheless, by carefully studying the available procedures that lower the blood pressure in hypertensive patients, enough evidence has been obtained to indicate that the ideal therapy—namely, one that decreases the peripheral resistance, lowers the blood pressure (in early cases to normal), and maintains the cardiac output and blood flow in the various organs of the body at adequate levels without undue side effects—is not beyond the realm of possibility.

· · · · · · · · · · · · · · · · · *by* MARK NICKERSON

Sympathetic Blockade in the Therapy of Hypertension

IN THE absence of clear-cut evidence regarding the extent and manner in which the sympatho-adrenal system is involved in the development and maintenance of most cases of human hypertension, there is little theoretical basis for the treatment of this condition by sympathetic blockade. However, continued reports of partial, although highly variable, relief obtained from surgical sympathectomy have kept alive the hope that chemical adrenergic blockade might provide similar benefits.

In the treatment of neurogenic factors in hypertension the desired action is the peripheral inhibition of excitatory, vasoconstrictor responses to sympatho-adrenal activity. Blockade of the inhibitory effects of the sympatho-adrenal system and of the activity of other divisions of the nervous system is not only unnecessary but also frequently undesirable. Chemical blockade may occur at many points along the reflex arcs controlling sympatho-adrenal activity. However, in order to achieve a desirable degree of specificity, it is necessary to produce the blockade at the efferent neuro-effector junctions. Blockade within the central nervous system alters many vital regulatory reflexes, respiratory activity, and particularly vagal activity, even when consciousness is not impaired. Blockade by most agents acting on the autonomic ganglia indiscriminately interrupts all efferent impulses passing over both the sympathetic and parasympathetic pathways.

Agents which block the responses of the effector cells to sympatho-adrenal stimuli may be appropriately termed *adrenergic blocking agents* because it is only at this point that adrenergic mediators are involved in the transmission of the nerve impulse. This term is preferable to the frequently employed term "sympatholytic," for it is now clear that such blockade does not involve "lysis" of the nerve ending, the mediator, or the effector cell. Much confusion has resulted from the indiscriminate inclusion under the term sympatholytic of all agents which in any way reduce the activity of the sympathetic nervous system. Such a grouping would of necessity include the barbiturates, local and general anesthetics, certain antimalarials, tetraethylammonium, Dibenamine, and many other agents which obviously have little in common.

Preliminary efforts to employ adrenergic blocking agents in hypertension fall into two categories, diagnostic and therapeutic. In the former, outstanding success has been achieved in the differentiation of hypertension due to pheochromocytoma from other types of hypertension. The benzodioxanes were first employed for this purpose (1) because certain members of the series (particularly 933F [Benzodioxan] and 1164F) block the responses to circulating epinephrine much more readily than those to sympathetic nerve activity (2). In contrast to their depressor effect in cases of pheochromocytoma, these agents induce an increase in the blood pressure, sometimes alarming, in patients with essential hypertension (1, 3), probably as a result of hypothalamic stimulation (2). The duration of the blockade which they produce is much too short to allow them to be used for preoperative maintenance therapy, and unpleasant side effects are not uncommon.

Although Dibenamine and its congeners block excitatory responses to both circulating epinephrine and sympathetic nerve activity (2, 4, 5), their effective use in differentiating pheochromocytoma from other causes of hypertension (6, 7, 8) derives from the fact that the responses to circulating epinephrine are inhibited more readily and by lower doses of the blocking agent. In addition, sympatho-adrenal factors are probably of limited significance in most other types of hypertension. Dibenamine has been employed both in the diagnosis of pheochromocytoma and for relatively prolonged preoperative maintenance of patients with this type of tumor. The results recorded have been excellent. Injections at about 72-hour intervals provide complete symptomatic relief prior to operation. During the period of Dibenamine administration, the Roth-Kvale histamine test is consistently negative, although it is strongly positive in these patients prior to adrenergic blockade.

Because of the multiplicity of their pharmacological actions, Priscoline, Regitine (7337), and the dihydro ergot alkaloids would not be expected to be of great value in the diagnosis of pheochromocytoma. Regitine has been employed in the preoperative preparation of one patient (9).

On theoretical grounds, an agent such as Dibenamine which produces a highly specific and effective blockade of peripheral sympathetic vasoconstriction (2, 4, 5) would be expected to be an ideal diagnostic agent for predicting the blood pressure response to subsequent sympathectomy. Indeed, single injections of this agent have been reported to produce a significant depressor response lasting from 24 to 72 hours in patients with early or moderately advanced benign hypertension, but not in those with more advanced organic changes in the cardiovascular system (10). However, this observation has not been confirmed, and much more study will be required before a clear evaluation of the presympathectomy prognostic value of members of the Dibenamine series is possible. The results obtained with Priscoline, Regitine, the ergot alkaloids, tetraethylammonium, the barbiturates, and spinal anesthesia would seem to have even less diagnostic specificity because important effects in addition to sympatho-adrenal blockade are involved.

In practice, none of the many pharmacological tests proposed for the selection of patients for sympathectomy has proved to be a reliable index of the response to that operation. In some reported series it would appear even that the persons with the greatest apparent "neurogenic" component in their hypertension responded the least favorably to sympathectomy (11). Because of this poor correlation between the results of pharmacological tests and of subsequent sympathectomy, a majority of surgeons working in this field are now placing their reliance almost entirely on clinical criteria of operability.

The failure of any of the proposed chemical tests accurately to measure the contribution of the sympatho-adrenal system to a given case of essential hypertension is probably related to the multiplicity of the factors involved in the maintenance of the blood pressure. The paravertebral sympatho-adrenal system is clearly not essential to the maintenance of a normal (12, 13, 14, 15) or even an elevated (14, 15, 16, 17, 18, 19) systemic arterial pressure in animals or men. The factors involved in the regulation of the blood pressure (largely a matter of adjusting the peripheral resistance) in normal or hypertensive laboratory animals and in men after the complete removal of the paravertebral sympathetic nervous system have not been clearly defined. However, aberrant sympathetic fibers which have their ganglia in the ventral primary rami of spinal nerves and do not enter the paravertebral chains may play a significant role. These have been demonstrated functionally and anatomically in men (15, 20, 21), cats (13), and dogs (22, 23), although some workers consider them to be of limited functional significance in dogs (13).

However, additional factors must be involved because the blood pressure may still be maintained at normal or elevated levels after procedures which would be expected to eliminate the vasoconstrictor effects of all sympathetic pathways. These include anterior rhizotomy (24) or complete spinal cord destruction (25, 26, 27, 28) in animals, and blockade with large doses of Dibenamine in laboratory animals (4, 29, 30) and men (31).

In the absence of all sympathetic control of the peripheral vascular system, one or more poorly understood factors must come into play to maintain the systemic pressure. In cases of renal hypertension, nephrogenic factors are undoubtedly involved, and it is quite possible that these may also be activated by the initial hypotension and the hemodynamic changes incidental to the loss of sympathetic control of the renal circulation. The participation of humoral pressor factors from other areas has been suggested (32, 33, 34), but is less well established.

Local vascular tone is probably a major factor in the maintenance of a relatively normal peripheral resistance after the loss of sympathetic control. Tonus in the absence of nervous stimulation is one of the fundamental properties of most smooth muscle, and marked muscularis hypertrophy has been noted in small vessels after prolonged denervation (35). The blood flow through the hand is very high immediately after denervation, but returns to essentially normal levels within one week (36), long before regeneration could account for the change. The vessels of completely denervated limbs have also been noted to regulate the blood flow in response to cold and irritants applied locally, although reflex vascular changes are completely absent (37, 38). Perhaps the most direct evidence for the development of autonomous tone in denervated vessels is derived from observations on the arterioles and small arterio-venous shunts in transparent chambers in the rabbit ear (39). These vessels have been noted to relax after denervation, but to regain a high degree of tone from 10 to 14 days later, although the rhythmic fluctuations in tone characteristic of innervated vessels are still absent.

We still know very little regarding the extent to which inherent vascular tone, antagonized by locally produced metabolites and perhaps by the activity of dorsal-root vasodilator fibers (40), may maintain vascular homeostasis in various organs and in the body as a whole.

The depressor response to sympathectomy or to sympathetic blocking agents may depend more upon the rapidity and the magnitude of compensatory changes than upon the extent to which the sympatho-adrenal system was involved in the maintenance of the initial pressure. It would be difficult to attribute the hypertension of advanced senile arteriosclerosis to excessive activity of the sympatho-adrenal system. Yet patients with this condition frequently respond to spinal anesthesia with a precipitous fall in pressure. Here the explanation for the extent of the response must lie in the inability of the rigid vessels to compensate for the loss of vasoconstrictor tone. It is of interest that these same patients tend to be hyperresponsive to depressor agents which act through a variety of mechanisms.

Although the requisite clinical studies have not yet been carried out, prolonged blockade of sympatho-adrenal activity might provide a more reliable indication of the results of subsequent sympathectomy than does short-term administration. Prolonged blockade would allow compensatory mechanisms, with the exception of the activity of extra-paravertebral sympathetic fibers, to operate in much the same way as after the surgical procedure.

Figure 1 illustrates a possible sequence of adjustments during the development of neurogenic hypertension and its subsequent "cure" by sympathectomy or sympathetic blockade. Column A represents the normal condition, B the situation after the development of hypertension, and C, D, and E stages in the postblockade or postsympathectomy adjustment. Stabilization may occur under the conditions depicted in either D or E. Few quantitative data are available regarding most of the factors illustrated. However, it is clear that some such over-all adjustment does occur.

None of the specific adrenergic blocking agents inhibits vascular responses to angiotonin (2, 41), and the mechanism by which adrenergic blockade or sympathectomy brings about even a partial reduction of the blood pressure in renal or human essential hypertension has not been clearly established. However, it has been definitely demonstrated that vasomotor reflexes are fully active in the presence of nephrogenic hypertension in animals (19, 42, 43, 44, 45) and men (46) and in human essential hypertension (46, 47, 48). Consequently, it may be assumed that all or a major part of the observed decrease in pressure is due to the elimination of relatively normal sympatho-adrenal factors. Observations indicating augmented pressor responses to reflex activation of the sympatho-adrenal system cannot be loosely interpreted as indicating hyperactivity of the sympatho-adrenal system. In accordance with Poiseuille's law, a given amount of neurogenic

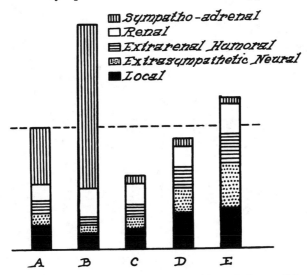

FIGURE 1. A diagrammatic representation of the possible contributions of various factors to the maintenance of the systemic arterial pressure during neurogenic hypertension and its subsequent "cure" by sympathectomy or adrenergic blockade. A, normal; B, neurogenic hypertension; C to E, sequential stages in the recovery of the blood pressure after sympathectomy. The pressure may stabilize at either D or E. (Reproduced, by permission of the copyright owner, from Nickerson: Am. J. Med. 8:344, 1949.)

vasoconstriction may produce a greater increase in the peripheral resistance when exerted upon vessels which are already of a smaller caliber than normal.

If a significant element of neurogenic renal vasoconstriction is involved in human essential hypertension, a second factor in the hypotensive effect of adrenergic blockade may be the increase in the renal blood flow which could be induced. Both high spinal anesthesia and inflammatory processes have been reported to reduce renal vascular resistance in human essential hypertension and experimental nephrogenic hypertension in dogs (49, 50), but the relationship of this alteration to the associated fall in the blood pressure is far from clear. Sympathectomy fails to alter the renal blood flow or glomerular filtration in many cases of essential hypertension (51).

Possible interrelationships among various factors supporting the blood pressure in renal and perhaps essential hypertension are dia-

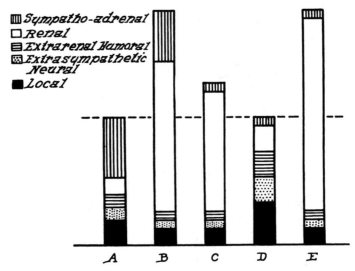

FIGURE 2. A diagrammatic representation of the possible contributions of various factors to the maintenance of the systemic arterial pressure during renal (and perhaps essential) hypertension. A, normal; B, renal (and perhaps essential) hypertension; C, immediately after extensive sympathectomy or effective adrenergic blockade; D, a case of essential hypertension in which the pressure continued to drop for some time after treatment, presumably because neurogenic alteration of the renal blood flow was a significant factor in the original hypertension; E, a common end result of sympathectomy, which may or may not be preceded by an initial fall in pressure such as that depicted in C. (Reproduced, by permission of the copyright owner, from Nickerson: Am. J. Med. 8:347, 1929.)

grammed in Figure 2. However, the highly variable response of renal and essential hypertension to sympathectomy or sympathetic blockade makes it impossible to present any diagram which adequately covers all cases. Column A represents the normal and B the hypertensive condition; C depicts a case in which sympathetically mediated renal vascular tone is assumed to be a significant factor in maintaining the elevated pressure; and D illustrates possible changes in the few cases of human essential hypertension in which a gradual fall in pressure is noted for some time after sympathectomy, perhaps also on the basis of changes in the renal blood flow. Column E represents a common result of sympathectomy or adrenergic blockade in renal and essential hypertension; this result may or may not be preceded by some early fall in pressure as in C.

The application of adrenergic blocking agents to the practical management of hypertension has been very limited, largely because of the present lack of any really effective oral preparation. However, some preliminary observations in this field deserve comment.

The parenteral administration of Dihydroergocornine and other hydrogenated ergot alkaloids may produce a significant reduction in the recumbent blood pressure of patients with essential hypertension, and orthostatic hypotension is .usually a prominent result of their administration (52, 53, 54, 55). However, the response of different patients varies widely and as yet unpredictably. The known pharmacology of the hydrogenated ergot alkaloids indicates that the observed fall in the blood pressure is due to two major factors—central stimulation of the vagal nuclei, with a resultant decrease in the heart rate, and central depression of the postural cardiovascular reflexes. Because of the latter action, the prominent orthostatic hypotension observed after the administration of these agents cannot be considered evidence of the production of an adrenergic blockade, i.e., of a so-called sympatholytic action. The reduction in the blood pressure by the hydrogenated ergot alkaloids does not parallel the suppression of vasomotor reflexes (e.g., digital vasoconstriction in response to body cooling) (53), and an increase in the dose usually causes an increase rather than a further decrease in pressure. Single injections of these agents usually reduce the heart rate and blood pressure; the blood flow in the extremities may be unaltered or increased, while the cardiac output is unchanged or decreased (53, 54, 56, 57, 58). The effective renal blood flow is considerably reduced, and the glomerular filtration may also be depressed (59).

It is interesting to note that the pulse pressure is markedly decreased during the hypotension induced by the dihydro ergot alkaloids in hypertensive patients (Fig. 3); an unaltered or increased pulse pressure would be expected if the fall were primarily due to adrenergic blockade with a resultant peripheral arteriolar dilatation. The ergot alkaloids are less than 10 per cent as potent when administered orally as when injected, and the response is even more variable (52, 57, 60). Tolerance to the blood-pressure-lowering effects of Dihydroergocornine develops rapidly (55).

Although the dihydro ergot alkaloids are the most potent (i.e., mg/kg) adrenergic blocking agents known at the present time, they all stimulate the emetic center in doses smaller than those required to produce blockade in man (2). Even with the very small doses usually administered to human beings (0.5 mg. or less) nausea and vomit-

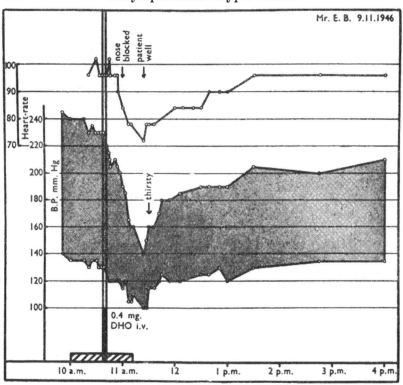

FIGURE 3. Changes in the blood pressure and heart rate following the intravenous injection of 0.4 mg. of Dihydroergocornine (DHO) in a patient with malignant hypertension (52). (Reproduced, by permission of the copyright owner, from Bluntschli and Goetz: South African M. J. 21:390, 1947.)

ing are frequently observed (52, 53, 56). As a result, it has never been possible to administer an amount adequate to block effectively the peripheral responses to sympathetic nerve activity in man. Unfortunately, hypertensives appear to be even more sensitive than normotensive persons to the emetic action of the ergot alkaloids (52, 54). The respiration may be depressed by even very small doses (54).

Priscoline has been tested in a few cases of human hypertension, but the results have been disappointing (61, 62). Although this agent is capable of producing significant adrenergic blockade and considerable direct peripheral vasodilatation in doses tolerated by human beings, little reduction in the blood pressure occurs in most cases. The failure to obtain a depressor response is probably due to the fact that Priscoline is a strong direct cardiac stimulant, and the increase in the cardiac output balances or even overshadows the vasodilatation. Even a massive dose of Priscoline taken with suicidal intent caused no lowering of the blood pressure (63). Indeed, this agent (64), as well as the benzodioxanes (3), may actually cause an alarming increase in the blood pressure. Regitine (7337) has pharmacological properties qualitatively the same as those of Priscoline, and a recent report of a greater depressor response to the former (65) is difficult to evaluate as the doses employed produced a very limited blockade of pressor reflexes.

Dibenamine has been employed with encouraging results in the treatment of rapidly progressive, malignant hypertension in which other therapeutic measures had failed to give relief (66). In most individuals in the series reported, the blood pressure was lowered significantly, but it usually remained considerably above the normal range. The relief of sequelae such as oliguria and hypertensive encephalopathy and retinopathy was marked in almost all cases and appeared to be greater than could be accounted for simply on the basis of the decreased blood pressure. Whether the release of sympa-

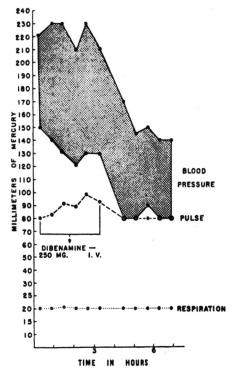

FIGURE 4. Changes in the blood pressure and pulse rate after the slow intravenous infusion of 250 mg. of Dibenamine in a patient with severe hypertension (67; courtesy of Dr. F. Simeone). (This figure is reproduced, by permission of the copyright owner, from Bridges and White: M. Clin. North America 31:1110, 1947.)

thetically mediated local vasospasm is involved in this therapeutic response can be only a matter of conjecture at the present time. Dibenamine may significantly reduce the pressure in some cases of benign essential hypertension (Fig. 4) (10, 67). However, consistent reductions are not obtained, and no adequate basis has yet been proposed for predicting the response in a given case.

As discussed earlier in this symposium, the role of the sympatho-adrenal system in human essential hypertension may be predominantly one of initiating repeated bouts of increased pressure which induce hemodynamic or metabolic changes capable of sustaining a largely non-neurogenic hypertension. On the basis of this concept it might be assumed that the most effective employment of adrenergic blockade would be as a prophylactic measure or as a buffer to temporary rises in the blood pressure in the very early stages of clinical hypertension or in persons with hyperactive vasomotor reflexes whose blood pressure is usually still within normal limits. Obviously none of the agents currently available for clinical use possesses the requisite effectiveness, prolonged action, and activity after oral administration for the studies required to establish this point. However, members of the beta-haloalkylamine (Dibenamine) series of blocking agents meet the first two of these requirements, and it is quite probable that more complete enteric absorption of certain more potent congeners of Dibenamine will allow them also to satisfy the third. Studies involving the prolonged administration of such agents to patients with very early hypertension will be awaited with interest.

In established hypertension prolonged sympatho-adrenal blockade with an effective adrenergic blocking agent may be expected to produce results much the same as those of surgical sympathectomy. A "chemical sympathectomy" would be capable of inhibiting the effects of all sympathetic vasoconstrictor fibers, including those which do not pass through the paravertebral ganglia—a result not feasible surgically. In addition, it would have the advantages of reversibility, ease of administration, and day-to-day control of the extent of the "sympathectomy," i.e., the completeness of the blockade.

Summary

Adrenergic blocking agents have received only limited trial in human hypertension. Although at least the more specific agents, such as Dibenamine, might be expected to be ideal agents for preoperative tests to predict the depressor effects of surgical sympathectomy, the multiplicity of the factors involved in the maintenance of the systemic blood pressure has made it impossible for pharmacological tests to define with any precision the magnitude of the sympatho-adrenal "neurogenic" component in a given case. The extent of the fall in the blood pressure in a given case may be determined as much by the extent and rapidity of compensation for the absence of sympatho-adrenal activity as by the magnitude of the sympatho-adrenal component. Cases of pheochromocytoma represent a special problem in which sympatho-adrenal factors are so predominant that adrenergic blockade provides an excellent method of diagnosis and of preoperative maintenance therapy.

None of the presently available adrenergic blocking agents is pharmacologically suitable for the maintenance therapy of patients with hypertension. However, current pharmacological investigations suggest that fully effective oral preparations may soon be available. Such preparations may be anticipated to produce essentially the same therapeutic effect as surgical sympathectomy. In addition, the results of prolonged prophylactic administration of such preparations to patients in the very early stages of hypertension will be of great theoretical and practical importance.

Questions and Discussion

DR. REGINALD H. SMITHWICK: At the risk of talking too much, I should like to make one or two very brief comments, particularly with regard to the selection of patients for surgical treatment.

That has been a very difficult problem. Naturally, in the beginning we had no conception which patients might be benefited and which might not. The problem has always arisen as to what is the best yardstick for measuring the value of a form of therapy. Should the yardstick be changes in the blood pressure levels? Should it be symptomatic improvement? Should it be the reversal of cardiovascular disease? Should it be an increased life expectancy?

The last is the only real measure we can use today which is strictly accurate. The difficulty of measuring the blood pressure levels, which you are all aware of, and the impossibility, from any preliminary tests of a pharmacological nature such as have been described today, of drawing conclusions concerning what will happen to the blood pressure, have made it unsatisfactory to select patients on that basis.

So we have had to rely on mortality rates, and our feeling is that at the present time that is really the only sound basis for selection. If you can demonstrate conclusively that patients in certain categories have their life expectancy prolonged to a statistically significant degree, that seems to me the most accurate method of selecting patients for splanchnicectomy at the present time.

It is of interest that the physiological changes which Dr. Wilkins has shown to occur following splanchnicectomy, as well as some of those that have been shown by others in other areas such as the renal area, may be very important. It is not necessarily the effect on the blood pressure levels alone that is important.

It may be that these intermittent variations in pressure, which can be very striking and which can be significantly modified by splanch-

422

nicectomy so as favorably to modify the hepatic and the renal blood flow, are important physiological effects.

The fact remains that regardless of whether or not the blood pressure levels are lowered after sympathectomy, our figures indicate that mortality rates have been significantly reduced in both groups, although the patients with the most marked lowering of the blood pressure have done the best. Nevertheless, those who show no significant change in the blood pressure levels still live longer than non-operated control patients and may have their cardiovascular disease reversed.

DR. ARTHUR GROLLMAN: Despite the desirability of lowering the abnormal elevation in the blood pressure seen in hypertension, it is now generally recognized that this alone, assuming that it could be done, would not constitute an adequate or satisfactory therapy for the disorder. The normal level to which the pressure of the hypertensive patient sometimes declines following a coronary occlusion or cerebrovascular accident certainly does not constitute a satisfactory therapeutic response. This fact accounts for the general failure of depressor drugs to be of value in the treatment of hypertension. Except insofar as they may exert incidentally a sedative effect, these drugs when used in doses sufficiently large actually to lower the blood pressure appreciably, usually worsen the condition of the patient and may even induce alarming symptoms.

The available evidence suffices to permit one to conclude that hypertension as it is observed clinically or experimentally is not a result of abnormalities of the autonomic nervous system. Hence, as Dr. Smithwick has already emphasized, sympathectomy cannot be considered a fundamental solution of the therapeutic problem of hypertension. At best, it is only a method of protecting the patient against the ravages due to an uninhibited and excessive rise in the blood pressure, with its detrimental consequences.

The use of sympatholytic drugs is open to the same objections as have been raised against other depressor drugs or sympathectomy. An effective sympatholytic drug reduces the patient to the status observed during the days immediately following sympathectomy. The removal of the sympathetic chain has the advantage over drug therapy of being followed by compensatory changes which overcome to some extent the undesirable features which follow operation. Drug therapy has the advantage of being reversible by cessation of the therapy, but at best can only be looked upon as a temporary measure for use in such emergencies as in the acute crises of hypertensive encephalopathy.

On the basis of our present knowledge, it must be concluded that current methods of therapy are at best only symptomatic, and at worst, in some cases at least, actually harmful and irrational. In view of the difficulty of evaluating therapeutic measures in this disorder in the human being, one must insist that any advocated procedure be proved effective not only in consistently lowering the blood pressure but also in prolonging the life and ameliorating the clinical state of the experimental hypertensive animal. Only by the use of such objective experimental methods is it possible to avoid deluding ourselves by observations based on the subjective responses or the spontaneous and unpredictable fluctuations encountered in the human patient.

DR. NICKERSON: I should like to say a few words here about the adjustments which occur in the human body as well as in the animal after the administration of drugs which block responses to the sympathetic nervous system.

Our observation has been that adjustments occur in almost exactly the same manner as they do after surgical sympathectomy. In a number of patients in the age group of from 40 to 50 years, not hypertensive, but probably with some rigidity of the vascular tree, we found that extensive blockade of the sympathetics by Dibenamine produced an orthostatic hypotension which prevented the patient from sitting up for periods of from 24 to 36 hours. However, within 3 days, the patients were again able to stand, and at the end of a week the adjustment was to a very large extent complete, although repeated administrations maintained the blockade as complete as it was in the beginning.

Another case which we studied very recently was that of a little girl 9 years of age with erythromelalgia, who was apparently capable of very normal cardiovascular adjustments. A high degree of orthostatic hypotension was produced by the Dibenamine injection. However, within an hour she could stand, and within from 3 to 4 hours she was running around the ward playing with the other children. I believe that the difference between drug blockade and sympathectomy is only one of degree and that the non-neurogenic vascular adjustments which I mentioned earlier this morning can occur to the extent that the subject may carry on his usual activities in the presence of a complete chemical blockade of the sympathetic system.

DR. WILKINS: Since Dr. Nickerson, and very properly, has been accorded two rebuttals, I think I will take the privilege of one, even though the time is short.

The main thesis we were trying to develop in the paper that I read was to emphasize the point that Dr. Nickerson just made—namely, that arterial hypertension itself may do harm. We do not believe that it is always a "good" response to a "bad" disease, in the sense that it compensates for a fundamental fault and allows normal profusion to take place through diseased vessels. We believe it may be a "bad" response, establishing a vicious circle that may aggravate the underlying disease.

It appears that the fear we all once had that ischemia, particularly of the kidneys, would result if the blood pressure of a hypertensive patient were lowered by any means, is an unnecessary fear. The kidney appears to have remarkable ability, through intrinsic or other adjustments, to return to the same level of blood flow at lower blood pressures (within limits) as it had at higher levels. Now as we extend these observations in the kidney (which I believe have been well substantiated not only in our own but in many other laboratories) to the liver, to the brain, and to the peripheral areas, it looks as if the whole body were able to adjust itself to significantly lower levels of the blood pressure without tissue ischemia, even though marked hypertension has existed previously.

This was the first hurdle to get over in our therapeutic approach. There are, of course, many other criteria for judging whether a therapeutic procedure is worth while. The papers this morning have stressed one point, namely, that we can continue to try to lower the blood pressure in hypertensive patients on the assumption that we shall not necessarily cause severe ischemia of the tissues if we succeed.

· · · · · · · · · · · · · *by* REGINALD H. SMITHWICK

The Effect of Sympathectomy upon the Mortality and Survival Rates of Patients with Hypertensive Cardiovascular Disease

THE complications of hypertensive cardiovascular disease involving the cardiac, cerebral, and renal areas are responsible for many deaths and for much premature disability among young and middle-aged people. Together, these complications are generally thought to cause more deaths each year than cancer. It is clear that an attempt to lower the mortality rate for hypertensive cardiovascular disease is desirable.

In evaluating a therapeutic measure for this disorder, consideration must therefore be given to its effect upon mortality and survival rates. This is true whether one is discussing dietary, pharmacologic, or surgical therapy. Much has been written in recent years about the effect of various forms of treatment upon the blood pressure and symptoms. Less attention has been given to the effect of therapy upon the rate of progress of cardiovascular disease, and few facts have been recorded concerning the effect of these various forms of treatment upon mortality rates. In evaluating therapy, one should also have in mind the fact that the cause of hypertension and hypertensive cardiovascular disease is unknown. Consequently, all existing forms of therapy must be regarded as more or less empirical in nature.

To demonstrate that a particular therapeutic measure influences prognosis significantly requires that a large number of cases be followed for a long period of time. It is also necessary that data on comparable cases treated otherwise or untreated be available for comparison. In spite of the fact that over 14,000 articles dealing with hypertensive cardiovascular disease have been published since 1920, the available control data are not wholly satisfactory at the present time.

During the past 10 years over 2000 hypertensive patients have been referred to me by physicians from various parts of the world for study and for consideration of surgical therapy. About 75 per cent of the cases elected to be operated upon and 25 per cent did not. These two groups of patients have been followed very carefully for up to 10 years. Consequently, sufficient data are now available to begin to evaluate the effect of this particular therapeutic measure upon mortality and survival rates. This discussion may be regarded as a preliminary report upon this matter, to be followed from time to time by further reports, since the data will become increasingly significant each year.

This series of patients is, of course, a selected one and not representative of hypertensive cases as a whole. They were referred because they had unusually severe forms of the disorder, because they were not doing well upon current therapy, or because the status of the patients indicated an extremely poor prognosis. Data concerning the total material are presented in Table 1. It seems best to summarize

TABLE 1. Surgically and Non-Surgically Treated Patients with Hypertensive Cardiovascular Disease, Followed 1–10 Years

	Surgical Series	Non-Surgical Series	Total
Females	845	242	1087
Males	748	330	1078
Total 1593		572	2165

representative reports from the literature dealing with the prognosis for patients not treated surgically before considering this material in greater detail.

The Mortality among Hypertensive Patients Not Treated Surgically

From time to time since the introduction of the sphygmomanometer at the turn of the century, physicians have recorded mortality rates for groups of hypertensive patients. The first of these reports was by Janeway in 1913 (1). Other representative papers have followed: Blackford, Bowers, and Baker, 1930 (2); Keith, Wagener, and Barker, 1939 (3); Rasmussen and Boe, 1945 (4); Bechgaard, 1946 (5); Palmer, Loofbourow, and Doering, 1948 (6); Perera, 1948 (7); and Hammarström and Bechgaard, 1950 (8). The mortality rates which these authors have noted for groups of patients followed for varying periods of time are given in Table 2. The mortality rates vary tremendously, from 17 per cent to 91 per cent. Although there is also a considerable variation in the duration of the follow-ups, this does not appear to be an adequate explanation for the marked differences between the various series. It seems much more likely that the patient material making up the different series also varies a great deal. Most of the authors referred to in Table 2 have also given the mortality rates for females and males separately. These figures are given in Table 3. It will be noted that the mortality for males is

TABLE 2. The Mortality among Hypertensive Patients Not Treated Surgically

Author	No. of Cases	Years Followed	Per Cent Mortality
Janeway (1913)	244	5–10	81
Blackford, Bowers, and Baker (1930)	202	5–11	50
Keith, Wagener, and Barker (1939)	219	5–9	91
Rasmussen and Boe (1945)	100	6	52
Bechgaard (1946)	1038	4–11	28
Palmer, Loofbourow, and Doering (1948)	430	8 (average)	61
Perera (1948)	250	12 (average)	17
Hammarström and Bechgaard (1950)	435	2–10	51

TABLE 3. The Mortality among Hypertensive Female and Male Patients Not Treated Surgically

Author	Percentage of Females	Percentage of Males
Janeway (1913)	69	86
Blackford, Bowers, and Baker (1930)	39	70
Keith, Wagener, and Barker (1939)	88	93
Rasmussen and Boe (1945)	43	71
Bechgaard (1946)	22	41
Palmer, Loofbourow, and Doering (1948)	52	72
Hammarström and Bechgaard (1950)	37	69

higher in every series, the difference being sufficiently great in five of the seven series to indicate the advisability of discussing the prognosis for the two sexes separately. It is also apparent from a study of the material in certain of the series that the subdivision of patients into groups on the basis of the changes in the cardiovascular system at the time of the original observation is also highly desirable.

The Prognosis for Hypertensive Patients Grouped according to the Criteria of Keith, Wagener, and Barker

Keith, Wagener, and Barker were the first to recognize the need of subdividing hypertensive patients into groups in order to judge the prognosis for a particular patient with greater accuracy. They divided their patients into four groups on the basis of the vascular changes

432   A Symposium on Hypertension

noted in the eyegrounds and found that the prognosis varied for each group. The patients in Group 1 had mild narrowing or sclerosis of the retinal arteries. Those in Group 2 had moderate to marked sclerosis of the retinal arteries characterized especially by exaggeration of the arterial reflex and arteriovenous compression. Group 3 contained patients with angiospastic retinitis characterized especially by edema, cotton-wool exudate, and hemorrhages in the retina, superimposed upon a combination of sclerotic and spastic lesions in the arteries. If measurable edema of the optic discs was added to this picture, the case was placed in Group 4.

Keith, Wagener, and Barker divided their 219 patients into four groups on this basis and calculated the mortality rate for each for a period of observation of from 5 to 9 years. They also published survival curves for each group. They felt that their data could serve as control material by which the merits of a particular form of treatment might be judged, since treatment consisted of general measures,

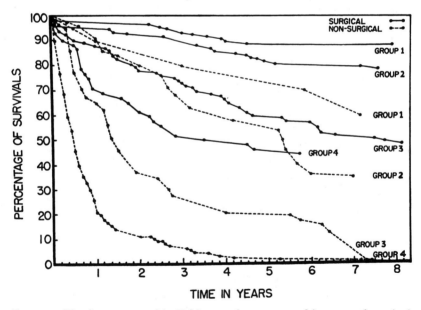

FIGURE 1. The data presented in Table 4 are here expressed in terms of survival curves. The survival rates are higher in all groups in the surgical series. The differences observed are statistically significant for Groups 2, 3, and 4.

TABLE 4. The Mortality Rates for 219 Non-Surgically and 376 Surgically Treated Patients with Hypertensive Cardiovascular Disease, Grouped according to the Criteria of Keith, Wagener, and Barker

| | | Non-Surgical Series (K., W., B.) | | | | | Surgical Series (Smithwick) | | | |
| | No. of Cases | No. of Deaths | | Per Cent Mortality | | No. of Cases | No. of Deaths | | Per Cent Mortality | |
Group		At 5 Years	From 5–9 Years	At 5 Years	From 5–9 Years		At 5 Years	From 5–9 Years	At 5 Years	From 5–9 Years
1	10	3	4	30	40	122	13	14	11	12
2	26	12	17	46	65	109	20	23	18	21
3	37	30	34	80	92	93	37	48	40	52
4	146	145	145	99	99	52	28	29	54	56
All groups	219	190	200	75	91	376	98	114	26	30

433

especially with regard to diet and rest and the regular use of certain sedatives. I have compared the mortality and survival rates of comparable numbers of consecutively treated surgical patients with their control data. The mortality rates for both their cases and mine are given in Table 4, and the survival rates are compared in Figure 1. It is apparent that the mortality rates are lower in all groups treated surgically. There are too few cases in the Group 1 control series to make statistical study possible, but the difference for Group 2, 3, and 4 cases appears to be significant. This difference is clearly indicated by the survival curves. It would therefore seem that splanchnicectomy has lowered the mortality rate significantly for Group 2, 3, and 4 patients.

This was demonstrated several years ago for Group 4 patients by the late Dr. Peet, whose pioneering interest in this problem is well known and whose sudden death is a great loss to the medical profession. On reference to Table 2, it will be noted that the mortality among the Keith, Wagener, and Barker cases is the highest of all. The reason for this becomes clear on reference to Table 4, since the vast majority of their patients were in Groups 3 and 4. This clearly indicates the need of subdividing hypertensive patients into more comparable groups and the impossibility of comparing mortality statistics for undivided groups of patients. One can safely presume that few cases in the series having the lowest mortality rates had Grade 3 or 4 eyeground changes.

The Prognosis for Hypertensive Patients Grouped according to the Criteria of Palmer, Loofbourow, and Doering

In 1948 Palmer, Loofbourow, and Doering published data bearing upon the prognosis for hypertensive patients upon conventional medical management. They divided their cases into four grades, which differ slightly from those of Keith, Wagener, and Barker in that the most important change in any vascular area determines the grade. Their criteria for grading follows:

Grade 1. These patients have no changes or have minimal changes in the fundi as represented by narrowing of the arterioles; have normal hearts or no more than prominence of the left ventricle by X-ray study; exhibit no impairment of renal function by the tests used; and in the urine examination either are normal or occasionally show slight albuminuria and slight changes on microscopical examination of the sediment.

Grade 2. These cases include those with moderate organic changes in the fundi as represented by widening of the arteriolar light reflex, narrowing, caliber changes, and arteriovenous compression. The heart rarely is normal by X-ray study; it is usually prominent in the region of the left ventricle and sometimes more definitely enlarged, but without functional impairment. The kidney is normal; slight degrees of albumin and minimal numbers of formed elements are found in the urinary sediment; or there may be slightly impaired function.

Grade 3. The fundi are rarely normal, usually showing arteriolar narrowing, caliber changes, wide light reflex, and arteriovenous compression. Often there are exudates and hemorrhages; the heart is often moderately to markedly enlarged, commonly with symptoms and signs of actual or impending congestive failure or symptoms of anginal failure. The urine frequently shows albuminuria and casts, and renal function is often impaired, though actual failure (uremia) is not common; cerebral accidents occur in about 20 per cent of cases.

Grade 4. The cardinal—indeed, the obligatory—sign is edema of the optic discs, with or without exudates and hemorrhages, and always with marked narrowing of the arterioles. Cardiac enlargement and congestive failure may be present; renal impairment and failure are common.

The mortality rate for each grade was noticeably different. The mortality statistics were based upon 316 patients followed for an average period of 4 years and upon 430 patients followed for an average period of 8 years. The use of an average follow-up period makes it difficult to utilize their material as control data because some of their patients were followed for as short a period as 1 year and others for as long as 30 years. It is impossible for another observer to duplicate the time factor exactly. One should therefore have reservations concerning the validity of a comparison of other data with theirs. The mortality rates for my surgically treated patients for each year of observation are given in Table 8. It will be noted that 948 cases were followed for 4 years and 154 cases for 8 years. Thus all patients were observed for exactly the same period of time, which averages 4 and 8 years for each group respectively. I have used these cases to compare with those of Palmer, Loofbourow, and Doering. The 4-year comparison is given in Table 5 and the 8-year comparison in Table 6. In the latter the patients are subdivided not only into the four grades but also by sex. It is apparent from a study of these data that the mortality rates for surgically treated patients are much lower for all grades.

TABLE 5. The Mortality Rates for 316 Non-Surgically and 948 Surgically Treated Patients with Hypertensive Cardiovascular Disease Grouped according to the Criteria of Palmer, Loofbourow, and Doering

Grade	Non-Surgical Series (P., L., D.) (1–30 Years, Average 4 Years)			Surgical Series (Smithwick) (At 4 Years, Average 4 Years)		
	No. of Cases	No. of Deaths	Per Cent Mortality	No. of Cases	No. of Deaths	Per Cent Mortality
1 100	6	6		120	6	5
2 58	10	17		262	24	9
3 111	40	36		457	86	19
4 47	38	80		109	44	40
All grades 316	94	30		948	160	17

TABLE 6. The Mortality Rates for 430 Non-Surgically and 154 Surgically Treated Patients with Hypertensive Cardiovascular Disease, Grouped according to Sex and the Criteria of Palmer, Loofbourow, and Doering

Grade	Non-Surgical Series (P., L., D.) (Average 8 Years)			Surgical Series (Smithwick) (At 8 Years, Average 8 Years)		
	No. of Cases	No. of Deaths	Per Cent Mortality	No. of Cases	No. of Deaths	Per Cent Mortality
1 104	23	22		25	1	4
Male 38	13	34		12	1	8
Female 66	10	18		13	0	0
2 80	38	47		31	5	16
Male 26	15	48		10	2	20
Female 54	23	43		21	3	14
3 192	150	78		74	32	43
Male 96	80	83		33	12	36
Female 96	70	73		41	20	49
4 54	51	94		34	15	44
Male 32	31	97		15	6	40
Female 22	20	91		19	9	47

The impression one gathers from this is that surgery has significantly lowered the mortality rate for most hypertensive patients. One must, however, have certain reservations about this comparison because of the use of an average follow-up period in the control series. It would seem preferable to compare mortality rates on a year-to-year basis, every case being followed for exactly the same period of time. One would not, for instance, estimate the 5-year mortality rate for a group of cancer patients on the basis of an average 5-year follow-up period of cases observed for from 1 to 30 years. Since Palmer, Loofbourow, and Doering presented their data feeling that it offered a satisfactory control by which the value of a particular form of treatment might be judged, it seems wise to comment upon the difficulty which has been encountered, and at the same time to enter a plea for the presentation of data in a manner which will permit other observers to use it to best advantage.

The Prognosis for Hypertensive Patients Grouped according to the Criteria of Hammarström and Bechgaard

Hammarström (9) has published a detailed report on the surgical treatment of hypertensive cardiovascular disease, and Bechgaard has discussed the prognosis for patients not treated surgically. More recently these authors have compared the prognosis for operated and non-operated patients in a combined report. They found that they could not use the series of Bechgaard as a control for the operated cases because so few of the patients had changes in the cardiovascular system which were comparable in severity to those in the operated series. Consequently they selected a control series for the comparison. In order to obtain an adequate number of patients, they reviewed the records of over 130,000 patients who had been studied in various hospitals in Denmark and Sweden and selected 435 cases, which comprised the control group.

These authors appreciate the fallacy of comparing undivided groups of hypertensive patients and have laid down certain criteria for subdividing cases into four groups. Group 1 contains patients with uncomplicated hypertensive disease without marked subjective symptoms. The prognosis for patients of this sort is indicated by the report of Bechgaard (Table 2). No cases of this sort were operated upon, and none were selected for the control series. Group 2 includes those with marked subjective symptoms but without signs of myocardial damage. They may have a left-axis deviation and/or a relative enlargement of the left ventricle if the heart volume is within normal limits according to the teleradiography. The retinal changes are classified as Group 1 or 2 according to Keith, Wagener, and Barker. Group 3 includes those with the same eyeground changes or in addition retinal hemorrhages with or without signs of thrombosis of the retinal vessels. Patients in Group 3 further show one or more of the following signs of cardiovascular damage: negative T_1, heart volume above the predicted normal (500 ml/m^2 body surface in men and 450 ml/m^2 in women, or the transverse diameter of the heart greater than half the inner thoracic diameter), residues after cerebral insult, and constant albuminuria. In Group 4 they include all hypertensives with definite retinal exudates and/or papillary protrusion, since they found the life expectancy to be about the same whether the patients in this group had papillary protrusion or not. Their operated and non-operated patients were divided according to these criteria and into the two sexes as well. The mortality rates for a 2 to 10-year period of

TABLE 7. The Mortality Rates for 435 Unoperated Hypertensives Followed 2–10 Years and for 251 Hypertensives Followed 2–8 Years after Sympathectomy (Hammarström and Bechgaard, 1950)

	Unoperated			Operated		
Group	No. of Cases	No. of Deaths	Per Cent Mortality	No. of Cases	No. of Deaths	Per Cent Mortality
2 ....*164*	*30*	*18.3*		*87*	*4*	*4.6*
Male 42	9	21.4		29	4	13.8
Female 122	21	17.2		58	0	0.0
3 ....*177*	*101*	*57.1*		*85*	*17*	*20.0*
Male 83	57	68.7		35	9	25.7
Female 94	44	46.8		50	8	16.0
4 .... *94*	*92*	*97.8*		*79*	*34*	*43.0*
Male 69	68	98.7		38	18	47.3
Female 25	*24*	96.2		41	16	38.9

observation are given in Table 7. It is apparent in this comparison as in the others which have been made that the mortality rates for the surgical patients are much lower than for the non-operated cases.

The Prognosis for Hypertensive Patients Grouped according to the Criteria of Smithwick

With the preceding discussion as a background, the material referred to in Table 1 may be considered in greater detail. The mortality rates for 1593 surgically and 572 non-surgically treated patients are given in Table 8. The rates have been calculated by dividing the total number of deaths which occurred from any cause during each year of observation by the total number of cases which had been followed for each of the 10 years. In this first comparison the patients are not divided according to any criteria. It will be noted that the mortality rates are considerably lower in the surgical series. It also should be noted that the cases followed for more than 8 years in the surgical series and for more than 5 years in the non-surgical series are too few to be of statistical significance. Each year however, these data will become increasingly significant for longer periods of time.

The importance of subdividing patients according to sex has already been commented upon. The material presented in Table 8 is divided into two groups, the mortality rates for female patients being

TABLE 8. The Mortality Rates for 1593 Surgically and 572 Non-Surgically Treated Patients with Hypertensive Cardiovascular Disease

Years Followed	Surgical Series			Non-Surgical Series		
	No. of Cases	No. of Deaths	Per Cent Mortality	No. of Cases	No. of Deaths	Per Cent Mortality
1 1593	74	4.6		572	103	18.0
2 1420	105	7.4		418	120	28.7
3 1173	142	12.1		301	110	36.5
4 948	160	16.9		230	94	40.8
5 705	154	21.9		121	52	43.0
6 428	113	26.4		43	27	62.8
7 268	81	30.2		10	5	50.0
8 154	53	34.4		5	4	80.0
9 70	28	39.9		2	2	100.0
10 28	12	42.8		...	...	...

TABLE 9. The Mortality Rates for 845 Surgically and 242 Non-Surgically Treated Female Patients with Hypertensive Cardiovascular Disease

Years Followed	Surgical Series			Non-Surgical Series		
	No. of Cases	No. of Deaths	Per Cent Mortality	No. of Cases	No. of Deaths	Per Cent Mortality
1 845	28	3.3		242	28	11.5
2 740	36	4.9		172	32	18.6
3 619	46	7.4		121	27	22.3
4 516	61	11.8		96	24	25.0
5 363	52	14.3		42	12	28.6
6 231	47	20.3		15	5	33.4
7 144	37	25.7		5	1	20.0
8 93	29	31.2		1	0	0.0
9 40	15	37.5		1	1	100.0
10 19	6	31.6		...	...	...

TABLE 10. The Mortality Rates for 748 Surgically and 330 Non-Surgically Treated Male Patients with Hypertensive Cardiovascular Disease

Years Followed	Surgical Series			Non-Surgical Series		
	No. of Cases	No. of Deaths	Per Cent Mortality	No. of Cases	No. of Deaths	Per Cent Mortality
1 748	46	6.2		330	75	22.8
2 680	69	10.1		256	88	34.4
3 554	96	17.3		180	83	46.0
4 432	101	23.4		134	70	52.0
5 342	102	29.9		77	40	52.0
6 197	66	33.5		28	22	78.6
7 124	44	35.5		6	6	100.0
8 61	24	39.4		3	3	100.0
9 30	13	43.3		1	1	100.0
10 9	6	66.7		...	...	...

given in Table 9 and for male patients in Table 10. It will be noted that the mortality rate for male patients is somewhat higher than for females, but that for both sexes the mortality rates for the surgical cases are considerably lower than for the non-operated patients. This is in keeping with the data already presented.

The subdivision of hypertensive patients into groups according to the changes in the cardiovascular system is very important, as has already been pointed out. The criteria of several authors have been outlined. I have used a slightly different method of dividing patients into four groups in order to make the patient material in each group as similar as possible. For this purpose a numerical value has been assigned to each of numerous cardiovascular changes, and an attempt

TABLE 11. The Numerical Value of Various Factors Which Influence Prognosis

Factor	Numerical Value
Cerebrovascular accident without or with minor residual Abnormal EKG Enlarged heart Impending failure P.S.P. less than 25% in 15 minutes or less than 60% in 2 hours Age 50 or over Mild angina	1
Cerebrovascular accident with residual* Frank congestive failure, moderate angina P.S.P. less than 20% in 15 minutes Unsatisfactory response to sedation	2
P.S.P. less than 15% in 15 minutes	3
Nitrogen retention	4

* Cerebral deterioration or hemiparesis.

TABLE 12. Two Examples of a Method of Determining the Numerical Grade of a Hypertensive Patient

Factor Considered	Numerical Value
Example 1	
Abnormal EKG	1
Cerebrovascular accident without residual	1
P.S.P. 20% in 15 minutes	1
Numerical grade	3
Example 2	
Abnormal EKG	1
Enlarged heart	1
P.S.P. 10% in 15 minutes	3
Numerical grade	5

has also been made to take the response to sedation, the resting diastolic blood pressure level, and the age of the patient into consideration as well.

The resting diastolic level is the average of the readings in the horizontal position during the postural and cold blood-pressure test performed after 48 hours of hospitalization and physical inactivity, most of the time being spent in bed. This test has been described on numerous occasions. A sedative test was performed on all cases, 3 sodium amytal grains being given at 7:00, 8:00, and 9:00 P.M. and the blood pressure level being recorded at hourly intervals from 7:00 P.M. to 7:00 A.M. For patients with resting diastolic levels between 100 mm. and 119 mm., a fall in the diastolic level to 90 mm. or less was regarded as satisfactory. For those with diastolic levels between 120 mm. and 139 mm., a fall to 100 mm. or less was classified as satisfactory. For patients with resting diastolic levels of 140 mm. or more, a fall to 110 mm. or less was regarded as satisfactory. With regard to age, approximately 90 per cent of the series under consideration are below 50.

The numerical values which are assigned to the various factors which have been taken into consideration are given in Table 11. The numerical values for each case are totaled, and the resulting figure is called the numerical grade for the particular case. Patients with a numerical grade of less than 4 will fall into Group 1 or 2. Those with

TABLE 13. A Classification of Hypertensive Patients according to the Criteria of Smithwick

Group	Numerical Grade	Other Factors
1	Less than 4	Males and females eyegrounds Grade 0 or 1 Females eyegrounds Grade 2 or 4
2	Less than 4	Males eyegrounds Grade 2, 3, or 4 Females eyegrounds Grade 3
3	4 or more	Resting diastolic level below 140 mm. Changes are present in cerebral, cardiac, and/or renal areas, but they do not include the following: (a) C.V.A. with marked residual (b) Frank congestive failure (c) P.S.P. below 15% in 15 minutes associated with a poor response to sedation
4	4 or more	Resting diastolic blood pressure below 140 mm., combined with one or more of the following: (a) C.V.A. with marked residual (b) Frank congestive failure (c) P.S.P. below 15% in 15 minutes combined with a poor response to sedation Resting diastolic level of 140 mm. or more

TABLE 14. The Mortality Rates for 752 Surgically and 201 Non-Surgically Treated Patients with Hypertensive Cardiovascular Disease, Group 1 (Smithwick Classification)

Years Followed	Surgical Series			Non-Surgical Series		
	No. of Cases	No. of Deaths	Per Cent Mortality	No. of Cases	No. of Deaths	Per Cent Mortality
1	752	12	1.6	201	9	4.5
2	660	17	2.6	156	13	8.3
3	543	20	3.7	120	17	14.2
4	449	19	4.2	97	13	13.4
5	307	22	7.2	55	8	14.5
6	191	23	12.0	16	4	25.0
7	127	16	12.6	4	0	0.0
8	69	13	18.8	...	...	...
9	30	7	22.4	...	...	...
10	15	3	20.0	...	...	...

TABLE 15. The Mortality Rates for 390 Surgically and 114 Non-Surgically Treated Patients with Hypertensive Cardiovascular Disease, Group 2 (Smithwick Classification)

Years Followed	Surgical Series			Non-Surgical Series		
	No. of Cases	No. of Deaths	Per Cent Mortality	No. of Cases	No. of Deaths	Per Cent Mortality
1	390	13	3.3	114	11	9.6
2	352	18	5.1	91	17	18.7
3	263	35	13.5	55	20	36.4
4	212	38	18.0	36	16	44.5
5	165	36	21.8	16	7	43.8
6	92	22	24.0	6	5	83.0
7	64	18	28.0	1	1	100.0
8	34	15	44.0	1	1	100.0
9	13	4	31.0	...	...	...
10	7	5	71.0	...	...	...

TABLE 16. The Mortality Rates for 303 Surgically and 140 Non-Surgically Treated Patients with Hypertensive Cardiovascular Disease, Group 3 (Smithwick Classification)

Years Followed	Surgical Series			Non-Surgical Series		
	No. of Cases	No. of Deaths	Per Cent Mortality	No. of Cases	No. of Deaths	Per Cent Mortality
1	303	14	4.6	140	24	17.2
2	270	24	8.9	98	33	33.7
3	236	31	13.7	67	29	43.3
4	163	32	19.6	47	24	51.0
5	126	33	26.2	23	14	60.0
6	74	19	25.7	12	9	75.0
7	35	14	40.0	3	2	66.7
8	18	6	33.4	3	2	66.7
9	7	4	57.0	2	2	100.0
10	...	...	...	...	...	...

TABLE 17. The Mortality Rates for 148 Surgically and 117 Non-Surgically Treated Patients with Hypertensive Cardiovascular Disease, Group 4 (Smithwick Classification)

Years Followed	Surgical Series			Non-Surgical Series		
	No. of Cases	No. of Deaths	Per Cent Mortality	No. of Cases	No. of Deaths	Per Cent Mortality
1 148		35	23.6	117	59	50.5
2 138		46	33.3	73	57	78.0
3 131		56	42.7	59	44	74.6
4 130		65	50.0	50	41	82.2
5 103		63	61.2	27	23	85.0
6 71		49	69.1	9	9	100.0
7 42		33	78.5	2	2	100.0
8 21		19	90.4	1	1	100.0
9 14		13	92.7	...	...	...
10 4		4	100.0	...	...	...

a numerical grade of 4 or more will fall into Group 3 or 4. Two examples of determining the numerical grade are given in Table 12. The decision to divide patients according to a numerical grade of less than

SURVIVAL RATES FOR 572 NON-SURGICALLY AND 1593 SURGICALLY TREATED HYPERTENSIVE PATIENTS DIVIDED INTO 4 GROUPS ACCORDING TO SMITHWICK CRITERIA

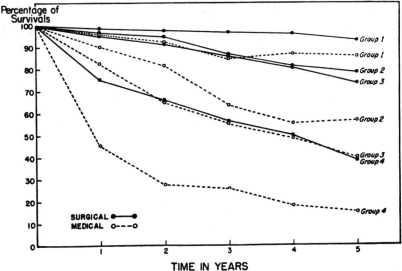

TIME IN YEARS

FIGURE 2. The data presented in Tables 14–17 are here expressed in terms of survival curves. The survival rates are higher in all groups treated surgically. The differences observed are statistically significant for Groups 2, 3, and 4.

4 or more than 4 was based upon the finding that the difference between the mortality rates for the two groups was most marked for this particular numerical grade.

Having determined the numerical grade of a particular case, one then proceeds to place the patient into one of four groups according to the criteria outlined in Table 13. My operated and non-operated patients have been divided into four groups on this basis, and the mortality rates are compared in Tables 14–17. A study of these tables indicates that the mortality rates for the surgical patients are con-

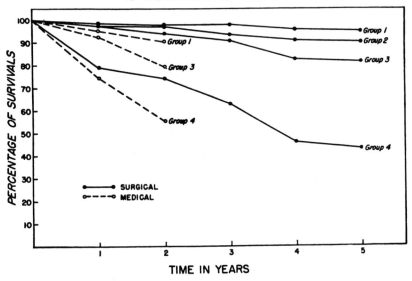

HYPERTENSIVE CARDIOVASCULAR DISEASE

SURVIVAL RATES FOR 845 SURGICALLY AND 242 NON-SURGICALLY TREATED FEMALE PATIENTS SUBDIVIDED INTO 4 GROUPS ACCORDING TO THE CRITERIA OF SMITHWICK

FIGURE 3. The data contained in Table 18 are here presented in the form of survival curves for surgically treated female patients followed up to 5 years. The curves cannot be carried out to this extent for non-surgically treated patients since the numbers do not permit it. It is possible to begin to construct the curves for Groups 1, 3, and 4 of the control series. These have been drawn in for the first 2 years of observation. The number of patients in Group 2 is so small that they have not been included. It can safely be presumed, however, that the curve for this group will fall between that for Groups 1 and 3 and will approximate 3 more closely than 1. A comparison of the survival curves for the surgically treated female patients with the curves for the surgically treated male patients (Fig. 4) indicates that the survival rates for females are higher group for group. The survival rate for Group 1 females probably approximates the survival rate for normotensive females very closely.

Table 18. The Mortality Rates for 845 Surgically Treated Female Patients with Hypertensive Cardiovascular Disease, Divided into 4 Groups
(Smithwick Classification)

Years Followed	Group 1			Group 2			Group 3			Group 4		
	No. of Cases	No. of Deaths	Per Cent Mortality	No. of Cases	No. of Deaths	Per Cent Mortality	No. of Cases	No. of Deaths	Per Cent Mortality	No. of Cases	No. of Deaths	Per Cent Mortality
1	530	8	1.5	110	3	2.7	143	4	2.8	62	13	21.0
2	450	10	2.2	101	3	3.0	132	8	6.1	57	15	26.4
3	363	8	2.2	77	5	6.5	122	12	9.2	57	21	37.0
4	311	14	4.5	65	6	9.2	80	14	17.5	50	27	54.0
5	211	11	5.2	49	5	10.2	59	11	18.6	44	25	57.0
6	138	16	11.6	27	4	14.8	34	7	20.3	32	20	62.5
7	96	15	15.6	20	7	35.0	12	4	33.3	16	11	68.6
8	63	12	19.0	14	7	50.0	7	2	28.6	9	8	89.0
9	27	6	22.0	6	3	50.0	1	0	0.0	6	6	100.0
10	13	2	15.4	4	2	50.0	...	...	...	2	2	100.0

Table 19. The Mortality Rates for 748 Surgically Treated Male Patients with Hypertensive Cardiovascular Disease, Divided into 4 Groups
(Smithwick Classification)

Years Followed	Group 1			Group 2			Group 3			Group 4		
	No. of Cases	No. of Deaths	Per Cent Mortality	No. of Cases	No. of Deaths	Per Cent Mortality	No. of Cases	No. of Deaths	Per Cent Mortality	No. of Cases	No. of Deaths	Per Cent Mortality
1	222	4	1.8	280	10	3.6	160	10	6.2	86	22	25.3
2	210	7	3.3	251	15	6.0	138	16	11.6	81	31	38.4
3	180	12	6.7	186	30	15.5	114	19	16.7	74	35	47.0
4	132	11	8.3	147	32	21.8	83	18	21.8	70	38	54.5
5	96	11	11.5	116	31	26.6	67	22	32.8	59	38	64.5
6	53	7	13.2	65	18	27.7	40	12	30.0	39	29	74.5
7	31	1	3.2	44	11	25.0	23	10	43.5	26	22	85.0
8	6	1	16.7	20	8	40.0	11	4	36.3	12	11	91.5
9	3	1	33.3	7	1	14.3	6	4	67.0	8	7	87.5
10	2	1	50.0	3	3	100.0	...	...	...	2	2	100.0

HYPERTENSIVE CARDIOVASCULAR DISEASE
SURVIVAL RATES FOR 748 SURGICALLY AND 330 NON-SURGICALLY TREATED MALE PATIENTS SUBDIVIDED INTO 4 GROUPS ACCORDING TO THE CRITERIA OF SMITHWICK

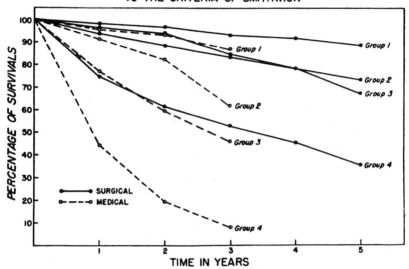

FIGURE 4. The data contained in Table 19 are here presented in the form of survival curves for surgically treated male patients followed up to 5 years. As in the previous figure, it is possible to include comparable data for our non-surgical control series for the first 3 years only. After that, the numbers of cases become too small to be of significance. It is apparent, however, that the mortality rates for the surgical patients are much lower than for the non-surgical cases, group for group. It also is apparent that this difference between surgical and non-surgical cases in mortality is greater for males than for females (Figure 3). On the other hand, the actual survival rates for surgically treated female patients are higher than for comparable male patients.

siderably lower than for the controls in each group, being more markedly so in Groups 2, 3, and 4 than in Group 1. This is best illustrated by the survival curves which are shown in Figure 2.

An examination of Tables 14–17 reveals that the number of cases followed for up to 5 years is adequate in the surgical series to subdivide the patients not only by groups but also by sex. This has been done in Tables 18 and 19. It is apparent that the mortality rates increase for both sexes as the amount of cardiovascular damage increases. It is also apparent that the mortality rates for male patients are higher in each group than for females.

Group 1 patients have the lowest mortality rates, the rate of the females more nearly approaching the normal than does the rate of any other category of patients. These findings are more obvious when expressed in the form of survival curves. Those for the female patients are presented in Figure 3 and for the male in Figure 4. It is not possible to subdivide our control material in this fashion because the number of patients followed for 5 years or more is not large enough. The survival rates for the first 2 or 3 years for non-operated females and males have been included in Figures 3 and 4 since there are 30 cases or more to use in calculating the rates. It is expected that the mortality rates for our control females will be considerably higher than for the surgically treated cases, group for group. The difference between the two series will be statistically of greatest significance for Group 2, 3, and 4 cases. On the other hand, the mortality rate of Group 1 females treated surgically will in all probability closely approximate that of normotensive persons. The difference between male patients treated surgically and those treated non-surgically will be more marked than for female patients. Of the most favorable cases in the surgical series, Group 1 patients, the males will have a higher mortality rate than the females. The survival rate for these male patients will not approximate the calculated mortality rate quite so closely as will that for Group 1 females.

Summary and Conclusions

1. The mortality rates for groups of hypertensive patients who have not been treated surgically and who have been followed for a varying number of years differ widely, from 17 per cent to 91 per cent.

2. The mortality rates for male patients are higher than for females. This indicates that it is advisable to discuss the prognosis for the two sexes separately.

3. If hypertensive patients are subdivided into groups according to the cardiovascular changes noted at the onset of observation or treatment, the prognosis varies according to the extent of the cardiovascular damage. Such a subdivision is essential to any discussion of prognosis. In this way, the patient material is made more comparable. The estimation of the mortality rates is rendered more accurate, and the effect of a particular therapeutic measure upon the course of the disorder can be better evaluated.

4. A comparison between the mortality rates for surgically and for non-surgically treated patients subdivided into groups according to the criteria of various authors reveals that the prognosis for surgically treated hypertensive patients has been significantly improved.

5. The greatest reduction in the mortality rates is noted in patients

with from early to moderately advanced cardiovascular disease, the comparison of such cases with those not treated surgically being statistically significant for all suggested methods of subgrouping.

6. The favorable effect of surgical treatment appears to be greater in males than in females. The explanation for this is not known.

7. While surgery has a more striking effect upon the mortality and survival rates of patients with the more advanced cardiovascular changes, the lowest mortality rates are noted in those patients operated upon before the onset of vascular damage of consequence. The mortality rates for surgically treated females are distinctly lower than for males. The mortality rate of Group 1 females (Smithwick classification) more closely approximates the expected mortality rate of normotensive persons than does that of any other group of patients.

Questions and Discussion

DR. ALFRED W. ADSON (ROCHESTER) : I shall confine my remarks to the surgical treatment of essential hypertension, since I was a participant in the studies and the development of the surgical procedures (extensive splanchnic sympathectomies) designed to ablate the control of the arterial system below the diaphragm by the sympathetic nerves. The purpose of ablating the sympathetic nerve control of a large vascular bed was to interrupt central stimuli and reduce vascular spasm, in the hope of creating a vascular reservoir below the diaphragm even though the non-sympathetized arteries above the diaphragm went into spasm. If this could be accomplished, it was hoped that the blood pressure after operation would not rise to a dangerous level.

This purpose has been achieved in a goodly number of patients who have had extensive operations on the splanchnic sympathetic nervous system for essential and malignant hypertension. I am fully in accord with Dr. Smithwick in that extensive resection of the splanchnic nerve at present represents a type of treatment for a selected group of patients suffering from malignant hypertension. Symptoms have been ameliorated, and life has been prolonged for patients that were unable to obtain relief from medical regimens. Surgical intervention (extensive resection of the splanchnic nerve) is not a cure-all. Our problem still is one of selecting the patient who will respond favorably to this type of surgery and to decide on the time in the course of the disease when the operation should be performed.

My interest in the treatment of patients with malignant hypertension was initiated by two observations: (1) Medical regimens frequently failed to control the disease or relieve the symptoms. (2) Spinal anesthesia during the 1920's not infrequently resulted in a fall in the blood pressure.

Since the spinal anesthetic anesthetized the spinal nerves, it was reasonable to assume that the vasomotor nerves also were anesthetized.

449

Since they were anesthetized, the arteries lost their central control and were unable to maintain their tonus; hence the fall in the blood pressure.

After studies were made of the effects of spinal anesthesia on patients with malignant hypertension, I proposed and performed an extensive rhizotomy, sectioning the anterior roots which gave off the vasomotor fibers bilaterally from the fifth dorsal caudally to and including the second lumbar motor roots.

The blood pressure often fell during the operation to such a degree that it could not be read. This prompted us to perform laminectomy and rhizotomy of the ventral roots in two stages. Even though this was done, the procedure was still a formidable affair.

In order to reduce the morbidity, other approaches were developed to interrupt the vasomotor sympathetic fibers to the arterial system below the diaphragm. Craig and I resected the splanchnic nerves, a portion of the celiac ganglia, and the upper lumbar sympathetic trunks on both sides after a subdiaphragmatic extraperitoneal approach. Peet, Poppin, and others sectioned the splanchnic nerves above the diaphragm. Smithwick combined the infradiaphragmatic with the supradiaphragmatic procedures and devised an operation known as the thoracolumbar splanchnic resection.

Grimson has performed the most extensive sympathectomy of us all, including all of the thoracic sympathetic trunks and upper lumbar ganglia. George Crile at one time advocated the manual removal of the celiac ganglion for the treatment of essential hypertension. Bronson Ray has performed an extensive resection of the splanchnic nerves and a rhizotomy of the ventral roots of the twelfth thoracic and first and second lumbar nerves. Kuntz, by anatomic studies, showed that a number of the vasomotor fibers by-passed the sympathetic ganglion and passed directly to arterioles along with nerve fibers in the peripheral nerves from the twelfth thoracic and first and second lumbar nerves. Apparently, these are so few in number that if left undisturbed they do not change the blood pressure when an extensive splanchnic resection has been performed.

In view of my 20 years of experience with operations on the sympathetic nervous system for the control of essential or malignant hypertension, I now am employing a procedure that is as effective as the extensive rhizotomy that I once employed. It is also as effective as the thoracolumbar approach without the necessity of opening the thorax. Thoracic approaches carry a considerable morbidity in surgical shock, pneumothorax, pleural effusions, and intercostal pain.

The procedure I now employ consists of a subdiaphragmatic extraperitoneal approach to the splanchnic nerves and the celiac and upper lumbar ganglia. The exposure is effected by a hockey-stick type of incision in the kidney region with the stock of the stick along the lateral borders of the rectus and spinous muscles. The latissimus dorsi muscle is divided, and the twelfth rib is resected. The fascia covering Petit's triangle is divided, which permits elevation of the kidney and liver. With the patient placed on his side, the kidney and liver are retracted ventrally with an illuminated retractor which exposes the splanchnic nerves and the celiac and lumbar ganglia.

In order to include sympathetic nerves that follow the aorta to enter the celiac ganglion, the entire ganglion mass is resected. The splanchnic trunks are divided as they penetrate the diaphragm to enter the abdominal cavity. Silver clips are attached to the proximal ends of the trunks to control bleeding and prevent regeneration, if that is possible. Following section of the splanchnic trunks, lateral traction is applied to the celiac ganglion in order to section all communicating rami. The celiac ganglion is then divided; half of the ganglion is removed during the first operation. The aorticorenal ganglion is removed with the celiac ganglion in order to interrupt the rami to the adrenal gland and kidney. The first and second lumbar sympathetic ganglia and the intervening trunk are removed also. A similar operative procedure is employed on the opposite side in a week or 10 days.

The operations are performed in two stages in order to minimize the sudden and severe falls in the blood pressure. Occasionally after surgery it becomes necessary to apply an abdominal support and even wrap the legs with ACE bandages for several months to maintain adequate blood pressure and prevent syncope.

The adjustment of the blood pressure to a normal or above normal level takes place spontaneously within from three to six months. Dyspnea on exertion may continue for years. The surgical mortality is less than 1 per cent.

The postoperative results following any one of the major operations on the splanchnic nerves and celiac and lumbar ganglia for malignant hypertension are very similar. Approximately a third of the patients will obtain good results, with a relief of clinical symptoms and the maintenance of a normal blood pressure. The second third will receive good clinical results, with a relief of symptoms but with a gradual return of the blood pressure to levels near those prevailing before surgery. The last third of the group of patients obtain very little from surgery. There is only a temporary relief of clinical symptoms. Blood pressures soon return to, or exceed, preoperative levels. Davis stated that although surgery has not been effective in relieving the symptoms in this last group, they have responded better to treatment with potassium sulfocyanate following surgery than they did before it.

The real problem that confronts those of us who are attempting to relieve the symptoms and prolong the lives of patients suffering from malignant hypertension is this: When should surgery be instituted?

It is obvious that medical management is an adequate and sufficient treatment for the major group of patients suffering from essential hypertension. However, it is rather disheartening to be asked to consider surgical treatment for a patient whose disease has progressed while he was on a medical regimen until changes have become irreversible.

If surgical treatment is to be considered, it should be employed for that group of patients who have "early malignant hypertension." This group usually does not respond well to medical management. The symptoms progress in severity rather rapidly, and they soon interfere with the patient's comfort and efficiency.

Before extensive sympathectomy is advised or performed, a careful evaluation of the vascular system should be made. One should make sure that the blood pressure is of the labile type, that it can be lowered by rest in bed or by the administration of a vasodilating drug. One should make careful studies of the kidney to determine whether a lesion is present that has resulted in ischemia and the development of a pressor substance, since such a lesion is a contraindication to surgery. However, if the renal lesion is unilateral, a combined operation of nephrectomy and sympathectomy may be indicated. Cardiac decompensation or a history of cerebrovascular accidents lessens the prospects of a satisfactory surgical result.

DR. WILLIAM T. PEYTON (MINNEAPOLIS): Hypertension is a variable disease and the sympathetic nervous system is a variable structure. It is not surprising that the results of sympathectomy have been somewhat variable. I think that the results Dr. Smithwick has reported are about what we should have got in our group if we had followed them for a longer period of time and had mortality rates.

For this discussion I tried to check up on our results following sympathectomy for hypertension. We have had a very small group compared to that on which data have been presented. Up to one year ago we had operated upon 154 patients. Perhaps because of a certain amount of luck, we had no mortality in the group.

It is quite a difficult problem to find these people and to get them back to the clinic for examination, so that our data on them are not at all complete. Seventy-six we did get back for re-examination, but in a clinic that is busy with many other things they didn't all get the routine tests planned. We did, of course, always get the blood pressure reading, but a funduscopic examination, P.S.P. excretion test, and an electrocardiogram were not made on all of them.

I will give you in detail only the results of the blood pressure readings and just mention in general what the other results were. We are perhaps a little out of date in reporting these patients, in reporting, that is, the effect of the operation on the blood pressure. This morning Dr. Smithwick said that reporting results according to the effect on the blood pressure is out of date and that he was now reporting results by giving the mortality or survival rates. We are still back in the stage of reporting the effect on the blood pressure.

Of course, our groups are so small that perhaps our data are not significant, but I think they do show the results an average clinic gets. The blood pressure reading we used in compiling results was the mean of all the pressures taken in the sitting posture when the patient returned to the outpatient clinic after operation. We divided patients into five groups according to the drop in the diastolic blood pressure.

The first group had a drop in the diastolic pressure of more than 30 mm. The next group had a drop of from 20 to 29 mm. The third group had a drop of from 10 to 19 mm. The fourth group had a drop of from 1 to 10 mm. or no drop at all, and the fifth group were those in which there was a rise in the diastolic pressure.

I will not go into detail concerning all of these groups. Twenty-nine per cent of our cases fell within the first two groups, those, that is, in which there was a rather significant drop in the blood pressure. That figure is not so good as the results Dr. Smithwick reported some years ago.

I thought that perhaps our selection of cases was not good, but Dr. Smithwick, as I understand from his discussion of this morning, has not used any definite criteria of selection. I understood him to say that the selection of cases for operation was by consideration of the survival rates for the various groups.

I should be very much interested to hear Dr. Smithwick tell us what he does use at the present time to determine whether or not the individual patient he is evaluating for operation is going to respond favorably to it. That is one of the things that bothers us. It is very unsatisfactory for a surgeon when discussing the advisability of operation to have to say to the patient that he does not know whether or not in this case the operation will be beneficial, that is, that the patient must gamble on the result. We can say to the patient that for the group as a whole the results are good and that, as Dr. Smithwick has shown, the survival period in general is lengthened. But unfortunately we can't pick out the individual patient and promise him that he is going to be one of those who get good results. We thought at one time that with the sedation test we were getting some selection that was worth while. But in the follow-up made for this report there does not appear to be a correlation between the response to sedation and to sympathectomy.

We thought at one time also that changes seen in the retina might be a lead to the proper selection of cases, but according to the follow-up, that is not reliable either. The renal function and even the kidney biopsy do not indicate what the response will be to operation. So we really have no way by which we can select a patient for sympathectomy with the certainty that he will get a good result. We have only a few cases where the patient was followed for many years by a physician who over this long period made a record of blood pressure readings. From such a record we can possibly best judge the lability of the pressure, and certainly that discloses the progress of the disease. This way may be the one by which cases should be selected for operation. I should like to hear Dr. Smithwick comment on it.

The relief of symptoms, of course, is a very satisfactory result, but it is not correlated with any drop in the blood pressure or improvement in the renal function, cardiac function, or changes in the retina.

I should be most interested in having Dr. Smithwick tell us just how at the present time he can predict to a certain patient that he is going to be the one that will be improved by the operation. Granting that he cannot always do this, what are his criteria for the selection of patients for sympathectomy?

DR. SMITHWICK: I should like to thank you, Dr. Peyton and Dr. Adson, for your discussions.

As I have already indicated, there are various yardsticks by which one might measure the result of any form of therapy in this disease. Naturally we are talking about hypertensive cardiovascular disease, and I think that it is the natural reaction of everybody to feel that what one should measure is the blood pressure. What we are really aiming at is to restore the blood pressure to normal. Nevertheless, we know that so far as the surgical treatment of hypertension goes, that can only be accomplished in a certain percentage of patients, a percentage that varies according to the material one has. Nobody as yet has been able to predict which patients will have a significant decrease in the blood pressure to normal or to near normal levels.

With regard to the question of symptoms, I think we can disregard this yardstick because it is not an accurate objective measurement of improvement and because almost any form of treatment, if judiciously followed, will relieve symptoms except in some of the very severe and terminal cases.

The third method is the evaluation of the progress of cardiovascular disease. I think that is very important. It is a very strange thing, but there is almost nothing in the literature as yet about that for non-surgically treated patients. When people write about the long-range prognosis for hypertensive patients who have not been treated surgically, there is little mention of the blood pressure, and nothing of any consequence is said about what has happened to the cardiovascular system.

That is a defect which ought to be corrected. We recognize that, and why has the job not been done? Well, the reason is that it is a perfectly stupendous task to keep track of a large group of patients, particularly such a group as mine, who have come from all over the world, and to get them to come back year after year after year for a follow-up study. Therefore, at the present time, there are no data that I can use for comparison except what I get from my own control medical series; there just isn't in the literature anything on cardiovascular disease except on electrocardiograms. Dr. Paul White has been interested in the problem, and he is about the only one who has made any effort to follow a series of non-surgically treated patients to see what happens to them in that particular regard. So for the cardiovascular system, there just aren't sufficient data for comparison at present.

I have been able to get back over a thousand operated patients in the 1 to 5-year period for a complete cardiovascular check-up and so far over 500 operated patients in the 5 to 10-year period. So I have a good many data on the surgically treated group and what happened to their cardiovascular systems. Sixty per cent of the surgically treated patients who have been followed for 5 years or more have cardiovascular systems which are better than they were originally. In 20 per cent there is no evidence of progress in the cardiovascular disease of consequence, and in 20 per cent there is a definite progression of the disease. So in addition to the improvement in survival rates, 80 per cent of the patients that I have been able to follow for 5 years or more after operation have cardiovascular systems that are either as good as they were originally or better in 60 per cent of the cases.

But when it comes to the non-surgical series, we have a great deal more difficulty. We can't follow them in so high a percentage of cases, even to the extent of checking the mortality rates. We use every device known to mankind to follow these patients, including the assistance of J. Edgar Hoover, who has been very cooperative in trying to find them, but we have a lot more trouble with these patients who have not been operated upon. They are scattered around. They are being treated by various doctors, in various ways. We don't have the contact with them that we have with the patients that we have operated on. The latter are a most cooperative group of patients, and we have very little difficulty following them. In the control group, however, so far as the rate of progress of the cardiovascular disease goes, we have a great deal of difficulty getting more than a very small percentage of them to come back for periodic observations.

As far as the selection of patients for surgery is concerned, I think that at the present time the only really practical basis is the survival rate. It's the only thing that we have accurate statistics on. One thing you can't argue about is whether a patient is alive or dead. You can argue about the blood pressure, and you can argue about symptoms. You can argue about the cardiovascular system, but if a patient is dead, he is dead, and that settles that.

Most of these patients who are beginning to show vascular changes or have fairly marked changes want to know whether you can do anything to prolong their lives. They want to live; they don't want to die. If you can assure the patients that on the basis of statistics you can promise them a significantly increased life expectancy, that is what they want to know. It is possible to offer this to cases falling into my Groups 2 and 3. Surgery should be advised for these patients.

· · · · · · · · · · · · · · · · *by* HAROLD G. WOLFF
and STEWART WOLF

The Management of Hypertensive Patients

Observations on the Pertinence of Life Situations, Attitudes, and Emotions to Variations in the Course of Essential Hypertension and to the Occurrence of Associated Symptoms

Every physician who attempts to manage a patient with essential hypertension exerts some effect merely because he is a physician. Moreover, the impression is widespread that by a skillful development of the patient-physician relationship a significant alleviation of hypertension and its accompanying symptoms may often be effected. Accordingly an attempt has been made to define some of the factors that may operate in these circumstances and if possible to sharpen them by emphasis.

To ascertain whether or not any appreciable modification in the course of essential hypertension can be effected, it is essential that its natural history be clearly evaluated. Although there are a number of reports (1–5) concerning the prognosis of malignant hypertensive disease in various phases ultimately ending in death, there are no equally complete considerations of that group of patients who at one time presented evidence of hypertension and who for one reason or another ceased subsequently to give evidence of the disorder.

Levy *et al.* (6) found that a significant proportion of men who exhibited a transient pressor response during examination for military service later developed sustained arterial hypertension. They found that "the rate of the later development of sustained hypertension is 3.6 times as high in the group with transient hypertension as in the group without it." These observations would seem to indicate that the

NOTE. This paper is based on studies carried out with the collaboration of Drs. Beatrice B. Berle, Herbert S. Ripley, William H. Dunn, and Edward M. Shepard.

The study was aided by grants from the National Institutes of Health, U.S. Public Health Service.

proclivity toward arterial hypertension is present in certain persons early in life, but that all persons who under stress show that they are such "blood pressure reactors" do not develop hypertensive disease in later life. Such a notion is further supported by the interesting studies of Hines (7) at the Mayo Clinic, who was able to relate initial blood pressure readings with the subsequent development of hypertension 10 (and 20) years later. It will be noted from reviewing his tables that those with the higher initial blood pressure readings were the most likely to develop subsequent hypertension. When both the systolic and diastolic readings were elevated, the incidence of subsequent hypertension was high. On the other hand, in those whose diastolic pressure was higher than 85 mm. Hg, even when the systolic blood pressure was less than 140 mm., the incidence of subsequent hypertension was high. It is of particular interest that none of those whose diastolic readings were less than 85 mm. later developed hypertension even though their systolic readings had been higher than 140 mm. The comparatively low diastolic pressures observed among these subjects suggests that the peripheral resistance too was relatively low and that their early elevation of the blood pressure was the result of an increased cardiac output. As pointed out elsewhere in this volume, it appears that high levels of arterial pressure due to an increased peripheral resistance are far more pertinent to the mechanism of essential hypertension than are those attributable predominantly to an increase in the cardiac output.

If Hines' observations are examined not so much in relation to the persons who do subsequently develop hypertension as in relation to those who do not, the interesting fact becomes apparent that approximately 20 per cent of those with a high initial blood pressure reading do not develop hypertension and approximately 14 per cent of those with initial diastolic pressures of even 100 mm. are normotensive 20 years later. In other words, in spite of a hypertensive proclivity, 10 to 20 per cent of persons so constituted remain normotensives.

Equally suggestive is Hines' observation that a similar proportion of persons who present evidence of vascular overreactivity to stress or pain do not ultimately develop essential hypertension. Unfortunately these studies also allow of but limited inferences since the initial readings may not have been representative of a state lasting more than a few minutes. There is no precise information as to how many persons who at one period were known to have more or less sustained hypertension may be normotensives 10 or more years later.

Hence in the following report of 90 patients known to be hypertensive for various periods with the indication that a certain portion have become normotensive during a period of management, it may be that certain "naturally occurring" remissions have been made easier or more possible. An attempt has been made to ascertain what in the life of a hypertensive who has become normotensive has been modified during the transition. Since the patient's reason for seeking help from a physician is chiefly related to the presence or absence of symptoms, it is necessary to consider the symptoms associated with hypertension before elaborating the results of the experience in the management of these patients.

The Relation of Symptoms to Hypertension

As indicated elsewhere in this volume,* it appears that certain persons, either by nature or experience, are so constituted as to invoke under stress protective adaptive reactions which appear to have been designed primarily for desperate struggle or mortal combat. Arterial hypertension may be part of such a reaction. There is no evidence, however, that an elevation of the blood pressure per se gives rise to symptoms. The only symptoms directly attributable to the hypertensive process are those due to the local vascular lesions in the brain, heart, and kidneys in advanced cases. Associated with the hemodynamic changes which underlie hypertension, however, there may often be observed evidences of other more or less unrelated adaptive patterns, especially those designed to meet the needs of violent effort or flight. Many of these give rise to sensations and evident impairment in function, so that troublesome symptoms occur. Others do not give rise to unusual sensations or conspicuous changes, but may none the less persist for long periods and make their existence known to the subject only after secondary and perhaps irreversible changes in body structures have ensued.

STIFFNESS, DISCOMFORT, BACKACHE, AND GENERALIZED ACHES AND PAINS

Although the mechanism of these complaints has not been clearly established, it appears that sustained contraction of the skeletal muscles can play an important role in their genesis. Holmes, therefore, undertook a study of the participation of the skeletal muscula-

*Stewart Wolf and Harold G. Wolff, "A Summary of Experimental Evidence Relating Life Stress to the Pathogenesis of Essential Hypertension in Man," p. 288.

ture in patterns of behavior in a variety of settings; the subjects were patients with backache and other muscle pain and control subjects without such complaints (8). Although these studies were not made primarily on hypertensive persons, from the similar nature of the symptoms and manifestations among hypertensive subjects there is reason to believe that the mechanisms are identical in both normo- and hypertensive persons.

It was possible to assess the contractible state of the muscles by re- cording action potentials on an eight-channel ink-writing oscillograph of the Grass type by means of bipolar needle electrodes (not con- centric) applied bilaterally to the skeletal muscles of the torso and extremities. These data were correlated with the presence of pain, the intensity of which was estimated by the subjects on the basis of an arbitrary scale 0 through 10+, 10+ representing maximal or "un- bearable" pain. A correlation was also made with the subject's life situation, emotional reactions, attitudes, and mood.

When these patients complaining of backache were given a simple test of motor function which might easily have been performed by the skeletal muscles of one right arm and shoulder girdle, distant muscle groups were called into play which neither take part in nor facilitate the action. Such generalized participation of distant muscle groups was a striking feature in all the backache patients observed.

In contrast, the reaction of non-backache subjects in similar ex- periments was, in general, characterized by conservation of muscular activity. Not only were distant muscle groups usually not involved, but there was even less intensity of the muscle contraction in the extremity performing the purposive act.

This "action" pattern involving generalized and sustained hyper- function of the skeletal musculature was characteristic of other as- pects of the behavior of the patients with backache and was especially apparent in the intensity and vigor with which they participated in social and athletic activities and discharged their responsibilities. In their efforts, then, to maintain their sense of security by "giving a good account of themselves" and "turning in a good performance," the entire skeletal musculature was mobilized for participation in the test.

A similar pattern accompanied discussions of threatening life situa- tions engendering conflict and feelings of resentment, frustration, humiliation, and hostility. In contrast, although a discussion of sensi- tive topics with non-backache subjects also provoked states of con- flict with strong emotions, hyperfunction of the bodily musculature was not a striking feature of the reaction, and when it did occur, it was often confined to the muscles of facial expression. The time interval between the onset of sustained muscle contraction and the appearance of pain was considerably longer after prolonged relaxation than after brief relaxation. Also, with the blood flow to the forearm intact and then occluded by a sphygmomanometer cuff, the time interval between the onset of sustained muscle contraction and the occurrence of pain was measured daily under a variety of life situations. In a setting of prolonged conflict and anxiety, the time interval required for the occurrence of pain in the muscles with the blood flow intact and in ischemic muscles was relatively short and approximately the same. In contrast, in a setting of relaxation and tranquillity, the time interval required for the appearance of pain in the muscles with the blood flow intact was considerably longer than (more than twofold) that from ischemic muscles. This relationship between muscle activity and deep pain suggests that the mechanisms involved in the production of pain in these experiments and in the backache syndrome are similar in nature to those described by Lewis in ischemic muscles, and depend on the accumulation in the tissue spaces of a metabolite designated by Lewis as "Factor P" (9).

HEADACHES

There are two types of headaches frequently associated with hypertension. Neither bears a direct relationship to the level of the blood pressure. One type, due to a sustained contraction of the skeletal muscles, referred to above, was studied in detail by Simons et al. (10). The other is a vascular headache, dull, diffuse, deep aching, usually intermittent but occasionally continuous. Such headaches characteristically throb, especially at the onset. They may be generalized, unilateral, or occipital, and are commonly worse in the early hours of the morning, beginning at some time between midnight and 4 A.M. and reaching their peak intensity about daybreak or shortly before rising time. They usually awaken the patient in the early hours of the morning and commonly diminish in intensity after he gets up, takes a cup of hot coffee, and assumes the duties of the day. Patients often discover after the onset of the headache that they are more comfortable in the sitting position, and a few have the notion that sleeping in the "head up" position minimizes the headache, and perhaps even prevents it. The headache is increased in intensity by bodily effort, stooping over, and coughing, and, as will be demonstrated, closely resembles migraine headache in other ways.

Among 448 patients with hypertension, Robey found 218 who had never had headaches; in short, one half the patients with hypertension had no headache whatever (11). In a group of 303 outpatients with hypertension, 50 had headaches as a chief or major symptom, but these persons had practically the same levels of systolic and diastolic blood pressures and of pulse pressure as did 150 patients who never had headaches. Furthermore, those with headaches did not necessarily have them when their blood pressures were at their highest.

The fact that the high level of the blood pressure among hypertensive subjects is not a sufficient condition for headache does not justify the assumption, however, that these phenomena are unrelated. Indeed, this too would be contradicted by the facts of common experience, since some persons with hypertension had never had headaches until the hypertension became established. It seems reasonable to postulate that a cranial artery only slightly relaxed for whatever reason would not distend so much, and possibly not to the point of producing pain, if the blood pressure was low. If, however, the sustained level were raised, distention would be created and therefore pain might readily follow. In other words, a degree of change in the contractile state of the arterial wall, compatible with comfort when the blood pressure was average, would be associated with pain when the blood pressure was elevated. An improvement in the contractile state of the cranial arteries, with a reduction or loss of headache, often occurs in the absence of any change in the systemic arterial pressure and, indeed, sometimes in the face of an actual rise in the arterial pressure (12).

PALPITATION, DYSPNEA, AND PRECORDIAL PAIN

Troublesome symptoms, including palpitation, dyspnea, and precordial pain, are often noted in hypertensive subjects in whom there is no evidence of structural cardiovascular disorder. In an earlier study of cardiovascular dynamics by G. A. Wolf, Jr., it was shown that such symptoms, occurring at times in healthy as well as hypertensive subjects, are actually associated with inefficient and overfunctioning of the cardiovascular apparatus, marked chiefly by the persistence of elevations in the cardiac output following minor exertion (13).

Some patients with precordial symptoms in situations of stress are morbidly interested in their hearts, which they feel are functioning in a peculiar way. Actually, as has been demonstrated, the hearts of many persons during periods of duress may function differently, in that there are an increase in the cardiac output and the force of the contractions and an increase as well in arrhythmias, all of which may give rise to unusual chest sensations, regardless of whether the person is normotensive or hypertensive.

Dyspnea is also often an accompaniment of stress (14). The X-ray studies of Stewart Wolf (14) demonstrated a difference in the action of the diaphragm during a period of emotional turmoil. During this time of stress the diaphragm was flattened, owing to increased muscular contraction and shortening. This phenomenon may be responsible for symptoms such as inability to draw a full breath, a substernal tightness or cramp, and a sensation of breathing only with the top of the chest. An additional factor was demonstrated by George Wolf in a young woman with nocturnal dyspnea (15). In this patient the stress of unexpressed anger and hostility caused an exaggerated pressor response, hyperventilation, and decreased ventilatory efficiency. An interview which brought these feelings to the surface caused a circulatory and ventilatory response similar to that produced by strenuous muscular work. These were the basis of the nocturnal dyspnea. The dyspnea diminished after the patient was given an opportunity freely to discuss these feelings.

Thus with such dyspnea not only are the rate, depth, and muscular pattern of respiration appreciably modified, but the rhythm is also disorganized: slow, deep, sighing respiration alternates with apnea and rapid, shallow, ineffective movements.

Cerebral anoxia attendant upon diminished venous return to the heart may give rise to feelings of giddiness and faintness. But the latter feelings may also result from hyperventilation, which is followed by cerebral vasoconstriction, impaired dissociation of oxyhemoglobin, and cerebral anoxia. Both types of cerebral anoxia occur in response to stress-producing life situations in association with feelings of desperation, defeat, exhaustion, anxiety, and fear, and during the early part of convalescence. Fatigue, prostration, and asthenia, as experienced by patients, are a complex state dependent upon emotional attitude, the absence of a dominant motivation, and the presence of a stress-producing life situation, with accompanying inefficiency of cardiovascular and respiratory function.

Substernal and precordial pain and discomfort result not only from reduced myocardial circulation but also from sustained contractions of the diaphragm, as mentioned above, and the sustained and forceful contraction of the intercostal, pectoral, and shoulder muscles. Such sustained contractions of the skeletal muscles are a common accompaniment of prolonged emotional tension and conflict in both those with and without structural defects of the heart and with or without arterial hypertension.

Moreover, ventilatory function is dramatically modified and ventilatory efficiency impaired. Changes in the visceral parenchymal circulation, notably in the kidney, may affect other vital functions, further jeopardizing the health and survival of the organism (16). Many of these alterations give rise to sensations and complaints and may cause the heart to work uneconomically. This becomes of special importance if the myocardium or the valves are already damaged; it leads on the one hand to a faulty appraisal of the heart's potential effectiveness and on the other to an extra burden upon an already heavily laden organ.

In subjects with structural heart disease, with or without hypertension, similarly studied, the same relationship was found between emotional disturbances and the occurrence of symptoms and signs of effort intolerance. The symptoms themselves were similar to those associated with cardiac failure. Changes in the emotional state were accompanied by changes in exercise tolerance (17). Also, dramatic alterations in exercise tolerance were observed during a period of less than an hour. During sustained periods of stress, the resting cardiac indices were commonly normal values, while the indices after exercise became abnormal. As improvement in the feeling state progressed, a complete return of the cardiac indices to normal after exercise was repeatedly noted.

In a group of unselected patients with paroxysmal auricular and nodal tachycardia and auricular fibrillation, certain life situations and emotional states were found to be most significant factors in the occurrence of attacks (18). When the emotional reaction to an incident was intense, the attack was usually precipated at the time of the associated event; when the reaction was less severe, the attack was initiated some time later, after an intervening period of mounting tension.

During interviews involving topics of great personal significance, electrocardiograms were recorded on a group of patients with precordial complaints. They demonstrated not only changes in rate and rhythm but alterations in the configuration of the action potential itself (19). In one half of the patients the electrocardiographic changes found during an ostensibly basal state could have been interpreted as abnormal had they occurred during or after standard exercise tests. Prolonged and moderately severe tachycardia with associated T wave changes were most commonly observed. In contrast, standard exercise tests performed during periods of relative tranquillity produced little increase in the heart rate or change in the electrocardiogram and were followed by rapid recovery.

CONSTIPATION

Perhaps the most common gastrointestinal complaint among hypertensives is constipation. This has been shown to be commonly encountered among patients who are grimly depressed but are continuing to strive in the face of adversity. Such constipation is associated with a hypodynamic state of the colon in which there is an absence of contractile activity in the cecum and ascending colon, resulting in a failure to propel the fecal contents (20).

THE MEANING OF SYMPTOMS IN PATIENTS WITH ESSENTIAL HYPERTENSION UNCOMPLICATED BY CARDIAC OR RENAL FAILURE

It would appear from this review of symptoms and bodily disorders that hypertensive persons exhibit a variety of adaptive and protective reactions evoked during stress, among which perhaps the most important, and certainly for this conference the most interesting, is the hypertension.

It is clear, however, that the hypertension is in no sense causative and is in most instances an entirely independent manifestation of the accompanying disturbance.

Elsewhere in this volume* the evidence is reviewed which indicates the pertinence of life situation and emotion to the hypertensive process. It follows that such considerations must inevitably apply to the management of hypertensive patients and of the symptoms of which they complain. The hypertensive person, as we have shown, has a capacity to develop and sustain anger, coupled with a fear of expressing it. His reaction in this situation is not one of feeling overwhelmed or defeated. He shows no tendency to withdraw. Instead he keeps his anger alive, though he represses and suppresses it so deeply that it may be unrecognized by him and is commonly associated with efforts at placation or the maintenance of peaceful relations (21). It has been noted that despite his repression of hostile expression, he appears to be mobilized as regards his circulatory apparatus. Thus he is poised, ready, alert, but reined in (22). These proclivities of hypertensive patients were taken into account by the physicians in their management.

---

*Stewart Wolf and Harold G. Wolff, "A Summary of Experimental Evidence Relating Life Stress to the Pathogenesis of Essential Hypertension in Man," p. 288.

Method

A group of 90 patients who came to the hospital with a variety of complaints were selected for study on the basis of their having essential hypertension. With few exceptions those selected did not exhibit major defects in cardiac or renal functions; they were able to speak English fluently; and they lived near enough to the hospital to be able to attend at frequent intervals as ambulatory patients if necessary. No patients known to have developed hypertension as a complication of pregnancy or renal disease or to have adrenal or pituitary neoplasms were included in the study. In one group (Group 1) there were a few patients with cardiovascular disease as indicated by retinopathy, cardiac enlargement, or electrocardiographic changes. In Groups 2, 3, and 4 no such changes were noted except for slight 0–1 retinopathy in a few. The patients were assigned to one of 16 physicians at random. Appointments were made according to the need of the patient. The duration of the interviews was usually one hour, although an occasional one was as short as a few minutes. During the early weeks of the study the time interval between visits was short, usually a week or less. After a certain point the interval between visits became greater.

The orientation of the various physicians and the methods they utilized in dealing with these patients were similar, differing only in that the special personality features of the individual hypertensive patient were taken into consideration. The procedure followed that outlined by Ripley, Wolf, and Wolff (23).

In addition to the usual medical history and examination with appropriate laboratory tests, the personality was studied. Special note was made of the family and cultural background. The state of the patient's health was correlated with events, overt activities, attitudes, and emotional responses. The object was to understand the motivations and mechanisms of disturbed function. Attempts were made to alter the disordered pattern, so that the patient might achieve a more adequate utilization of his capacities toward a greater satisfaction and a more salutary integration. Insofar as was possible, physiologic changes, qualitative and quantitative, were correlated with the emotional reactions and behavior pattern of the patient under varying life situations. Then an attempt was usually made to explain to the patient what had been happening to him, in order that perplexity might be replaced by a grasp of the dynamic mechanisms at work. His past experiences and reactions were integrated with the present in order to increase insight into his life adaptation.

No absolute distinctions between procedures could be made, and no one method was administered in pure culture. Nevertheless, each physician delineated as far as was possible the treatments used and the value of each.

Giving reassurance and emotional support employed the human warmth of the physician and was helpful in enhancing the strength, faith, and determination of the patient as well as in releasing his inhibitions and repressions. It implied an understanding and tolerant attitude on the part of the physician and included recognition and praise of the assets and achievements of the patient. It also involved an unswerving interest in and concern for whatever problem or question the patient brought to the doctor. In short, without becoming too identified with the patient's problems, the physician attempted to play the role of a strong, thoroughly dependable, authoritative, but not authoritarian, fellow man.

The free expression of conflicts and feelings through verbalization promoted a release of tension and often resulted in relief from anxiety and resentment and in less need to act out emotional conflicts in a socially undesirable manner. Patients repeatedly stated that the free expression of their conflicts had given them a sense of relief and had aided in an understanding that was of the greatest help to them. Many complained of not having been previously permitted to talk, of having been told that there was nothing wrong, that they imagined they were ill, or that they should forget their symptoms.

There appeared to be no short cut in the method by which the patient was allowed to find out about himself by discussing himself frankly with a tolerant physician. When direct questions were asked bluntly, the patient often felt that he was being cross-examined, and an attitude of antagonism resulted. When he was allowed to talk at his own pace, however, relevant conflicts and significantly traumatic situations were relatively easily brought out.

The patients were encouraged to discuss the advantages and disadvantages of a given situation before making important decisions. Helping them to take independent action led to the development of a greater feeling of security and a greater capacity to deal with ensuing problems. However, at certain times, when the psychodynamics had been clarified, direct practical advice was helpful in enabling them to break away from unhealthy, fixed habit patterns. Such advice, coming from a physician, relieved the patient of responsibility and guilt, so that he could make constructive decisions which might otherwise have been delayed indefinitely.

The patient's emotional development during infancy, childhood, and adult life was appraised by eliciting from him a biographic review and also by allowing him to express freely his associations with significant life events and his reactions to them. The recall and interpretation of dreams through spontaneous association facilitated the uncovering of his emotional conflicts. The feeling of security engendered and the release of emotional repression aided in establishing healthier patterns of bodily function and in the development of more mature attitudes and behavior.

Intravenously administered "sodium amytal" was of value in the alleviation of troublesome symptoms, through aiding in the elucidation of dynamic mechanisms and the gaining of therapeutic leverage.

Considerable improvement was frequently achieved without the verbal expression of insight. Many patients who appeared to have developed some comprehension of the dynamics of their illness expressed it rarely or not at all. In some of these pride and a need of feeling self-sufficient interdicted an admission of improved integration. However, it was often conveyed indirectly to the physician.

The process of recording and measuring the patient's physiologic disturbances and correlating them with his emotional reactions and behavior in varying life situations served to promote an understanding of the total biologic response and was often followed by improvement. It was especially helpful to patients who came to the clinic perplexed about the nature of their disorder or apprehensive of its being a serious or perhaps fatal disease.

Interviews with other members of the family led to an improvement in interpersonal relationships and a decrease in anxieties and resentments at home. These were usually carried out by the physician, but sometimes by the social service worker. The Social Service Department was also helpful in obtaining employment, arranging for convalescent care, making plans for the children of the patients, and carrying out follow-up studies.

Occasionally barbiturates were used to give symptomatic relief. They were usually employed to tide the patient over a difficult period in his illness, and their use was discontinued as soon as possible.

The depth or significance of the change effected depended on the ability of the patient to use his resources in developing improved patterns of reaction rather than on the frequency of the interviews or the over-all duration of the patient-physician relationship.

The most powerful constructive force stemmed from the ability of the physician and the clinic to inculcate in the patient faith in himself and the capacity to recognize and deal constructively with his problems. This usually involved a reorientation of attitude and entailed far more than a personal attachment to the physician. Only when he had acquired such faith and confidence was it possible for him to abandon costly inappropriate emergency patterns and deal more directly and constructively with the threats and challenges of day-to-day living.

Thus although a variety of therapeutic instruments were knowingly or unknowingly used, their effectiveness appeared to be basically dependent upon what might be loosely called a constructive patient-physician relationship. This assumed that the two persons involved were able to establish contact, that the physician was capable of disinterested affection, and that he was able to share the anxieties of the patient without adding to them, to tolerate his dissatisfactions and hostilities, and by virtue of his own developed personality and stable life orientation to impart confidence that there was a way of life that was both satisfactory and relatively secure. It was also important that he be able to convince the patient he would not abandon him during an insecure moment and that he would by virtue of his training not wrongly direct him or give him improper counsel concerning his bodily dysfunctions.

It should perhaps be stated in passing that the physician did not have to allow a consciously or unconsciously erotic relationship to develop with the patient in order to effect a suitable influence. The patient, however, had to feel he could completely express his fears and guilt and discuss freely his twisted or confused drives, sexual as well as other. It was essential that he feel permitted to divulge fantasies, and it was often necessary for the physician to help him become articulate about an aspect of his behavior which never before had been given voice.

Since hostility, suspicion, guilt, and anger were exhibited in subtle and multitudinous ways, the physician had to become familiar with their indirect manifestations. The commonest were such as being late for appointments, breaking appointments, making sarcastic remarks, misquoting the physician's words from a previous interview, denying that anything was being accomplished, refuting what had seemed apparent to him at an earlier visit, or disapproving of some personal mannerism of the physician or article of his clothing. Perhaps the most frequently encountered evidence of unexpressed hostility during an interview consisted in the patient's utterances' becoming laconic or in his finding any utterance extremely difficult. It became the rule of the physician then with caution to direct his attention to his attitudes and emotional state; if possible to indicate their genesis in past experiences and to suggest how common they were in his day-to-day life pattern; to point out their relevance to his illness; and occasionally to make suggestions as to their management and alteration for the better.

The patient was thus given an opportunity for fuller expression that was of major value. Without fear of punishment or the evil effects of a show of rage or hostility, he could speak out to a physician who not only was tolerant but occupied an authoritative position. It was unnecessary for the patient to "act out" in a histrionic way the full force of his feeling. Rather the physician tried to release tension bit by bit, to assure the patient that it was safe to release it, to instruct him piecemeal as to the meaning of the tension, and to educate him as to his own nature and how and why he had developed the pattern of repressing hostility.

Because of the patient's tentative and noncommittal ways, the desirability of making commitments was emphasized. Efforts were made to show him that there was safety in such commitments and in the spontaneous exhibition of feelings as they arose. In recognition of the special problem presented by his control of, and fear of releasing aggressive drives, certain things were emphasized. Spontaneous and free discussion were encouraged, the aim being the recognition and acceptable expression of hostility. Such encouragement in the expression of hostile feelings often involved interviews with an associate or another member of the family, as mentioned earlier, in order to get the patient properly to appreciate his problems. The explanation of the importance of such assertiveness for the patient, especially when the other person interviewed was the target of the aggression, proved to be, when sympathetically received, of great importance. The development also of all possible means of suitably though vicariously expressing aggression was encouraged, including sports involving vigorous or even violent activity, such as hunting, shooting, and boxing.

The successful demonstration by the physician that certain tentative efforts in assertive activity in a pertinent direction were safe and unaccompanied by untoward effects was especially effective when the patient could rely on the physician's standing by to lend support during possible crises or feelings of panic. Because of his suspiciousness and sensitivity to symbols of being "pushed around," encouragement and support had to be tendered with great circumspection. Hence he was allowed more than usual latitude in the matter of appointments, and to initiate the progressive steps in his retraining was left up to him. Perhaps most was gained from the physician's assuring the patient at appropriate moments that the management of his anger was within his grasp and capacity, that his assets as well as those contained in the whole life situation were such as to allow of a more constructive attitude, that he had less need to feel resentful of deprivation, rejection, indifference, and other threats, and that hence he could feel relatively more safe and secure.

For a time the patient's security stemmed largely from the crutch that the physician afforded him during his vulnerability, but the physician gradually denied the use of this crutch as the patient's needs became less prominent and his strength and conviction of safety increased. The degree to which the patient needed to assert his independence would in large measure guide the manner in which support was offered.

In brief, the aims in the management of the hypertensive person in this study became threefold: (1) to help him feel more secure, (2) to enable him to recognize that he felt threatened and hence angry and anxious, and (3) to indicate how, when he did feel threatened, he might deal with the danger by more direct and appropriate action rather than by repression.

Results

The changes effected in 90 subjects with hypertension are presented in Tables 1 and 2. In Table 1 all the subjects are appraised regardless of the level of their blood pressure at the time they were initially studied. In Table 2 are presented data on only those patients (39) whose blood pressure at the time they first presented themselves was 170/100 or below, so that all patients in all four groups may be the more appropriately compared. The group designated "no change" includes a few who either developed more symptoms and more cardiovascular changes or died. The tables have been so arranged as to indicate the changes from the initial state. These are expressed in terms of (1) sphygmomanometer readings taken under similar conditions, (2) the alterations in basic attitudes or in life orientation and the appropriateness or inappropriateness of the methods of dealing with life circumstances, and (3) the effect of the physician-patient relationship upon symptoms, complaints, and a variety of other bodily changes which have been generally grouped under the category "other stress reactions." Included in this category are giddiness, headache, vertigo,

TABLE 1. Data on 90 Essential Hypertensives Divided into 4 Groups on the Basis of Changes during Periods of Consideration of Life Situations, Attitudes, and Feeling States

	1. No Change, 41%	2. Minor Change, 40%				3. Moderate Change, 9%	4. Major Change, 10%
		Subgroup A	Subgroup B	Subgroup C	Total A–C		
Definition*							
B. P.	Same	Same	Lower	Normal		Same or sl. altered	Normal
B. A.	Same	Sl. change or same	Same	Same		Mod. alt.	Much alt.
O. S. R.	Same	Reduced	Reduced	Reduced		Reduced	Much red.
Number							
Total	37	16	18	2	36	8	9
Men	11	5	7	1	13	5	9
Women	26	11	11	1	23	3	0
Age, in years							
Average	40	42	45½	35½	41	32½	32
Range	19–74	28–65	25–62	32–39	25–65	19–41	18–49
Duration of hypertension							
Average	6 yr.	5¼ yr.	3¼ yr.	2½ yr.	3½ yr.	2¼ yr.	1½ yr.
Range	1 mo.–28 yr.	1 mo.–10 yr.	1 mo.–10 yr.	2 mo.–5 yr.	1 mo.–10 yr.	3 mo.–7 yr.	1 mo.–6 yr.

* B. P.—blood pressure; B. A.—basic attitudes; O. S. R.—other stress reactions and symptoms.

TABLE 1—*continued*

	1. No Change, 41%	2. Minor Change, 40%				3. Moderate Change, 9%	4. Major Change, 10%
		Subgroup A	Subgroup B	Subgroup C	Total A–C		
Initial B. P.							
Average	176/108	187/116	187/109	153/98	176/108	177/113	159/100
Range	140/80–260/200	150/100–255/135	135/100–270/180	150/100–155/95	135/100–270/180	150/110–200/120	150/100–170/90
Final B. P.							
Average	169/106	179/120	152/89	128/78	151/96	160/99	128/82
Range	130/95–220/170	155/90–220/190	130/80–195/95	110/75–135/80	110/75–220/120	140/80–190/95	110/80–140/90
No. of visits							
Average	16	18	20½	26	21½	23½	12
Range	3–65	4–54	3–44	5–47	3–54	3–63	5–24
Period of consideration, in months							
Average	11	14	12¼	8	11½	12	7
Range	2–29	2–50	2–44	4–12	2–50	2–22	2–15
Duration of change, in months							
Average	0	22½	12½	21	19	20½	26
Range	0	6–48	2–32	18–24	2–48	5–45	8–40
Prognosis rating, per cent							
Average	51.8	63.3	62.7	63	63	76	82.5
Range	25–62	57–70	58–71	61–65	57–71	69–88	80–89

TABLE 2. Data on 39 Essential Hypertensives with Initial Blood Pressures Not above 170/100, Divided into 4 Groups on the Basis of Changes during Periods of Consideration of Life Situations, Attitudes, and Feeling States

	1. No Change, 38%	2. Minor Change, 31%				3. Moderate Change, 8%	4. Major Change, 23%
		Subgroup A	Subgroup B	Subgroup C	Total A–C		
Definition*							
B. P.	Same	Same	Lower	Normal		Same or sl. altered	Normal
B. A.	Same	Sl. change or same	Same	Same		Mod. alt.	Much alt.
O. S. R.	Same	Reduced	Reduced	Reduced		Reduced	Much red.
Number							
Total	15	3	7	2	12	3	9
Men	4	1	3	1	5	2	9
Women	11	2	4	1	7	1	0
Age, in years							
Average	37	32	47½	35½	38	26	32
Range	23–54	28–39	36–57	32–39	28–57	19–34	18–49
Duration of hypertension							
Average	6 yr.	4 yr.	2½ yr.	2½ yr.	3 yr.	1¼ yr.	1½ yr.
Range	1 mo.– 12 yr.	1 yr.– 7 yr.	1 mo.– 6 yr.	2 mo.– 5 yr.	1 mo.– 7 yr.	3 mo.– 2 yr.	1 mo.– 6 yr.

* B. P.—blood pressure; B. A.—basic attitudes; O. S. R.—other stress reactions and symptoms.

474

Table 2—continued

	1. No Change, 38%	2. Minor Change, 31%				3. Moderate Change, 8%	4. Major Change, 23%
		Subgroup A	Subgroup B	Subgroup C	Total A–C		
Initial B. P.							
Average	157/94	160/102	164/88	153/98	159/96	162/100	159/100
Range	140/80– 170/100	150/100– 170/100	135/100– 165/100	150/100– 155/95	135/100– 170/100	150/110– 175/85	150/100– 170/90
Final B. P.							
Average	155/94	155/97	138/80	123/78	139/85	153/102	128/82
Range	140/75– 170/110	155/90– 160/95	120/95– 150/70	110/75– 135/80	110/75– 160/95	150/90– 160/105	110/80– 140/90
No. of visits							
Average	12	6	21	26	18	19	12
Range	3–23	5–9	3–44	5–47	3–47	9–31	5–24
Period of consideration, in months							
Average	11	5	17	8	10	10	7
Range	1–29	2–7	1–44	4–12	1–44	4–18	2–16
Duration of change, in months							
Average	0	12	9	21	14	22	26
Range	0	1–18	2–32	18–24	1–32	5–45	8–40
Prognosis rating, per cent							
Average	55	64	62	63	63	79	82.5
Range	48–61	62–66	58–70	61–65	58–70	73–88	80–89

palpitations, dyspnea, muscle pains and aches, constipation, and obesity. Also included, but obviously less numerous, are peptic ulceration, dyspepsia, hyperthyroidism, and asthma. It has been possible to group patients, as indicated in the chart, according to whether their blood pressures were the same or lower, whether basic attitudes were the same, slightly altered, or fundamentally altered, and whether symptoms and "other stress reactions" were reduced or greatly diminished.

From Tables 1 and 2 it is clear that the possibilities of change are intimately related to the duration of hypertension. This probably reflects not only a lack of flexibility in the vasomotor or neurohumoral equipment but also a fixity in life orientation. The amount of change did not appear to be intimately related to either the number of visits or the time over which the visits were spread. Finally, though less striking, there is the relation of modifiability to age. Greater modification was associated with younger age, especially when the duration of the symptoms and complaints had not been long. In the last entry a roughly appraised "prognosis rating," based on the work of Berle (24) discussed in detail below, is given; it is expressed as a percentage of the possible top score of 88.

It would appear that some alteration could be anticipated as a result of a constructive physician-patient relationship in approximately 60 per cent of patients with essential hypertension and symptoms. The bulk of these, or about 40 per cent of the total, were those changed in the sense that they presented fewer symptoms, less outward expression of anxiety, and greater tranquillity than before the experience, although in most of these the blood pressure was not appreciably lowered. However, even in this group, a slight lowering of the blood pressure was associated with a decline in symptoms and a restitution of some degree of tranquillity. In 2 persons of this second group the change in the blood pressure was striking, although it is the opinion of the patients' physician that despite the fact that the duration of this change has been 2 years, the patients will probably again develop hypertension or some other stress response in an adverse situation. The patients in the fourth group, or those referred to as exhibiting major change, had been hypertensive for relatively few years. In one instance, however, the hypertension had been present for as long as 6 years, and the readings seemed to be fairly predictable at all times during that period. In terms of the total number of patients in Table 1, those that fall into Groups 3 and 4 constitute not more than one fifth. But in Table 2, the analysis of the segment with lower blood pressures, Groups 3 and 4 constitute approximately one third of the total. If one includes the patients in categories B and C of Group 2, the number improved exceeds one half.

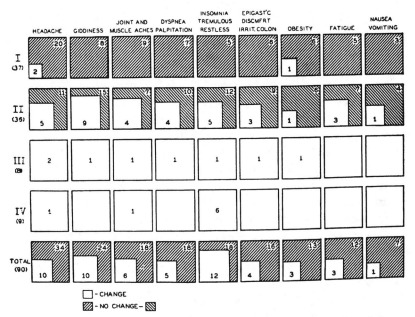

FIGURE 1. The changes in symptoms and in other reactions effected in 90 hypertensive patients during a period of intervention.

An inspection of Figure 1, based on a study of 90 patients, reveals the changes brought about during the period of intervention. The severity and number of symptoms and other bodily changes associated with stress were independent of the level of the blood pressure. The patients in Group 1 were modified minimally or not at all, and those in Groups 3 and 4 lost their symptoms completely. The symptom loss was not directly related to a change in the blood pressure level, although in Group 4 the loss of symptoms was accompanied by a lowering of the blood pressure. Tremulousness, insomnia, and restlessness were most readily modified. Headache, mainly related to more or less superficially suppressed anger or frustration and to fatigue, was also modifiable and, as mentioned elsewhere, was not related to the level of the blood pressure. These reactions were far more manipulatable than the blood pressure elevation, which was associated with more deeply repressed anger or frustration. Thus a consideration of life situations, attitudes, and feeling states reduced or eliminated symptoms and other stress reactions in the majority of those with essential hypertension and in a few reduced the blood pressure to normotensive levels.

Comment

It would appear that although the experiences of these patients with their physicians yielded changes which often were superficial and less commonly were fundamental, the return on energy expended was reasonably high. It might be claimed that those in Group 4 had never really been hypertensive persons. No evidence, however, opposes the view that among this group are persons who had they not had this medical experience would have continued to have elevated blood pressures and would gradually have become hypertensive. Perhaps some patients in Group 3, despite a basic reorientation and a reduction of symptoms, had irreversible bodily change already established either in the kidney or blood vessel walls in general or in the endocrine structures. Even in these, however, the blood pressure during this period of intervention did not rise further.

Garb (25) has observed in the course of a study of the effects of pharmacologic agents on the blood pressure the effects of placebo administration on a group of 44 patients with hypertension. He emphasizes that this was not a balanced statistical study since it was not primarily concerned with placebo action. During the placebo administration, however, and for various periods of time thereafter, 80 per cent of the patients exhibited a decrease in the systolic and diastolic blood pressures. In one half of the patients the reduction was statistically significant. Nineteen per cent of the group exhibited an elevation in the blood pressure during the period of placebo administration. A few patients responded with strikingly lowered levels of the systolic and diastolic pressures, which remained low not only during the administration of the placebo but for several weeks thereafter. Moreover, a substantial number of patients reported a marked reduction in symptoms. One patient known to have had hypertension for 15 years, with blood pressure readings as high as 210/135, had an average pressure of 161/97 during the last week of placebo administration. Subsequently the pressure remained low and averaged 143/84, when the patient had already been two weeks without "medication." With the placebos were given words of encouragement and reassurance concerning the efficiency of the substances administered. In addition the patients were encouraged to discuss their complaints fully.

Thus in appraising the results of the role of the physician, it is important to recall that only gradually and painfully has it become obvious from the study of so-called placebo action that often the major bodily changes following upon the administration of a substance have been falsely ascribed to its chemical and physical nature whereas, indeed, they were in no way related to it (26).

It is equally fallacious, out of partiality for some aspect of the patient-physician relationship, to attribute to it and to manipulations of the patient's personality specific effects which may be based on some entirely different or even unrecognized component of this important period in the patient's life, both within and without the protected area created by the physician.

Hence it is recognized that the factors offered in this study as most pertinent to the genesis of essential hypertension and its prognosis may indeed be subordinate in significance to other aspects of the patient's experience.

The method being approximately the same with all patients, why, then, was more change achieved in some than in others? It has already been suggested that a variety of factors operate in the potential profitableness of such an interchange. Where in a larger series it might have become evident that greater skill, experience, and penetration on the part of the physician made for greater success, it is doubtful whether any in the "no change" group could have been shifted to the "major change." It is possible that some might have been moved from the "moderate change" to the "major change" group. Those in the major change group, it is apparent, were ready for such an experience as they encountered.

A small number of patients in the moderate change group exhibited a striking lowering of the blood pressure but no appreciable change in basic attitudes, symptoms, or other stress reactions. These patients became far more aggressive, expressing freely their hostility, but were in no sense more secure, and they exhibited through other reactions their own dissatisfaction and tension. They became generally unattractive, unlikable, uncooperative persons—changed, but even less able to operate effectively. They could recognize no assets in their life situations and make no basic commitments. As an example of another variant of this phenomenon, take a patient who at one time presented migraine as a major disability, had peptic ulceration as a dominant feature at another, Graves disease at still another, and gradually developed hypertension throughout. At no time did his over-all adjustment improve or his health and satisfaction in life basically alter.

It is evident that the largest group of patients were those who changed to no remarkable degree (about 50 per cent). The change was featured mainly by fewer stress manifestations and a slight fall in the blood pressure. There was little evidence that the efforts of the physician modified the basic attitudes, although the relief of much anxiety about the complaints and a slight lowering of the blood pressure were achieved. The impression was that the patients felt comfortable because of the attention of a capable physician, felt less anxious about their hypertension, were able to talk more freely and more frequently to an understanding person; yet their hostility remained deeply repressed and their understanding of their pattern of behavior remained essentially unaltered. But though through long habit and the fixity of old-established human relationships, little change was effected, a reduction in the amount of headache, giddiness, and fatigability added to the satisfaction of living.

As mentioned above, the achievement of an adequate understanding of their situation as shown by an ability to be vocal about it was not striking in even the most satisfactorily altered patients. Yet the new manner in which they faced their problems, the altered pattern of their human relations, and their ability to get satisfaction and make commitments were evidence of change often absent in the spoken word. The discrepancy is not without precedent, however, for the ability to formulate often lags far behind a changed behavior. Indeed, the facile statement of understanding was sometimes so conspicuous in those without changed patterns that we came to attribute small significance to articulate expression.

The evidence also suggests that many of the stress accompaniments in hypertensive patients are the manifestation of more or less overt anxiety. This not uncommonly arises from the fact that in their hypertension they believe they have a dangerous disorder. For the most part, because these anxieties and tensions are accessible, symptoms arising from them are more readily modified than the conflicts and attitudes related more fundamentally to the arterial hypertension itself. The comparative ease with which "other stress reactions" are reduced or eliminated contrasts with the difficulty of modifying the basic attitudes of the patients and hence their arterial hypertension. The latter, as emphasized above, is usually associated with more or less deeply repressed conflicts or more fixed attitudes.

Prognosis

The person with hypertension has many features which he shares in common with other hypertensives regardless of whether his prognosis is good or poor. It is quite likely that he comes of a family in which arterial hypertension occurs in one or more members. Also he comes of a stock in which certain bodily features may be notable, such as stockiness, muscularity, "energy," love of activity, lusty appetite, and obesity. He also exhibits in a somewhat emphasized form certain traits of personality such as the ready development of anger, the fear to assert or express hostility and the capacity to repress it, the need to placate, to maintain poise, to "rein in" or "sit on the lid," and wariness and readiness for action. It is likely that at the time of his hypertension he is involved in a situation which makes him feel threatened.

Yet despite the fact that these features are exhibited by those who present the pattern of essential hypertension for longer or shorter periods, in some persons with the same features there are counterbalancing ones or because of good fortune they have not been forced to fall back upon the hypertensive pattern.

It becomes understandable that even though two persons are as similarly equipped as identical twins with proclivities toward hypertension, one may be more fortunate in his life experience and hence seldom or rarely call upon this reaction (27). Though both can be demonstrated to react similarly during stress, they are not equally threatened by the same circumstances. One may have become "sensitized" to threats through experience and may by long habit view with alarm lesser and more commonplace threats and assaults. Hence it should be possible to pick out from the data about hypertensives facts that are specially relevant to whether a given individual will continue to exhibit this protective reaction or, conversely, regain his tranquillity and maintain homeostasis at a lower cost.

Following the analysis of hundreds of items gleaned from the study

TABLE 3. Prognosis Rating Chart I, Based on Objective Details of the Patient's History

Prognostically Significant Details	Maximum Possible Points	Score of Patient
Under 40 years of age	2	....
Not divorced or separated	2	....
Third generation, American, white, Gentile, non-minority	2	....
High school education completed	2	....
Both parents at home until the patient reached age 12	4	....
No previous formal psychiatric care	2	....
Steady employment	2	....
Duration of present illness under 5 years	2	....
Total	18	....

TABLE 4. Prognosis Rating Chart II, Based on the Patient's Appraisal of
His Own Past History

Factors Subjectively Appraised	Maximum Possible Points	Score of Patient
Past medical history: healthy	1	....
Some religious education	1	....
Emotional support from both parents	4	....
Congenial siblings	2	....
Emotional support from spouse	2	....
Sexual compatibility with spouse	2	....
Spouse an adequate economic provider (if patient is a woman)	2	....
No problem of sexual deviation or appetite	3	....
Satisfactory relations with children	2	....
No housing problem	2	....
Occupational satisfaction	2	....
Congenial working conditions	2	....
Moderately adequate salary	2	....
"Success," financial or social	3	....
Total	30	....

TABLE 5. Prognosis Rating Chart III, Based on the Physician's Appraisal of the
Patient's History and Personality Structure

Factors in the Physician's Appraisal	Maximum Possible Points	Score of Patient
Evidence from past performance	10	....
No exaggerated sensitivity to traumatic situations		
Good interpersonal relations (including sexual)		
Evidence that the activities, achievements, and other experiences of life have afforded satisfaction		
Evidence from the personality structure	10	....
Moderate flexibility		
Minimal or short-lived repressed hostility		
Capacity to face and solve personal problems		
Active participation in the give-and-take of daily affairs		
Moderate orderliness and reliability		
Good judgment and evidence of adequate discrimination regarding human values and goals		
Prevailing attitudes of the patient toward his illness and his problems at the time of his admission to the clinic	10	....
Recognition of the failure of present patterns of adjustment and willingness to adopt others		
Willingness to consider the possibility that life stress, attitudes, and feeling states are relevant to his illness		
Confidence in the physician, the hospital, and its methods		
Capacity and willingness to assume responsibility in therapy		
The extent to which a specific aspect of the life situation was a factor in precipitating the patient's illness; the extent to which this specific feature is modifiable with regard to the involved individual, other persons, and circumstances	10	....
Total	40	....

of the 90 patients discussed here and of several hundred other patients treated by the group of 16 physicians, the factors that appeared relevant to prognosis were grouped together. In collaboration with Dr. Beatrice Berle, a prognosis scale, to be presented in a final form elsewhere, was constructed. No single factor appeared determinative, but different weights were assigned to various ones the relevance of which to prognosis had been established by a comprehensive review of the patient's previous life experience, his personality structure, his attitudes at the time of admission to the clinic, and the circumstances precipitating the illness, and by the physician's clinical appraisal of the situation. In Tables 3, 4, and 5 are listed the items selected and their relative weights. These present briefly, and with good approximation, the probable prognosis in terms of the blood pressure level, symptoms, and ultimate capacity for a good life adjustment. From these it has been possible to indicate the features favorable or less favorable to a good prognosis. The most dramatic changes occurred in those with scores of over 80 per cent; the least in those with scores under 50 per cent. The patients with a good prognosis obviously had more of the following features than did those who did not do well.

FAVORABLE RESULTS

The patients who changed most were likely to be those who were under 35 years of age, who had had hypertension for less than 2 years, with a systolic pressure not over 180 and a diastolic not over 110, who were white, Protestant, third generation Americans, and who had both parents living at home until they were at least 12 years old.

Most of them also had had, in their own estimation, healthy and satisfactory lives—perhaps until recently. They indicated that they had had good emotional support from their parents and later from their spouses, with whom they were sexually compatible. They considered themselves well married and, as far as they knew, had no serious sexual deviation or "appetite." They wanted, loved, and enjoyed their children. They had work which they viewed as agreeable and steady, with relatively adequate salaries, and they considered that they were "doing well." All these favorable features were not found in any one patient, but in every patient that did well, the favorable items predominated. The same qualification applies to the following findings.

Upon examination it was the physician's opinion that the patients had not overreacted to the common traumatic life experiences and had actually shown, by past performance, evidence of good interpersonal relations, including those involving sexual intimacies. There was also evidence that their activities, achievements, and other life experiences had afforded them satisfaction, and they had made a few major commitments.

The personality structures of the patients, according to the physicians, exhibited considerable flexibility, not too long-lasting or deeply repressed hostility, and the ability to take steps to "get out of a hole" and to take part in life activities. Furthermore, they were moderate and reliable people and appeared to have made adequate discriminations regarding human values and goals.

The patients who did well showed a willingness to accept the possibility that their attitudes, feelings, and life situations might be relevant to their illness. Moreover, they were willing to recognize the failure of their present way of dealing with their problems and to adopt others. They expressed feelings of confidence in the physician, the hospital, and its methods.

The life situations that formed the settings for their illness, and perhaps precipitated it, were, in the physician's opinion, capable of modification.

The favorable progress of one illustrative patient is detailed below and graphically represented in Figure 2.

An 18-year-old boy of Greek parentage came to the clinic complaining of having had palpitations, insomnia, and loss of energy for the past 6 months, despite a remarkable increase in appetite and a gain in weight of 10 pounds. Nothing remarkable appeared in the general examination except for a blood pressure of 162/105. The boy was the third of four sons in a turbulent family, where the parents had been in continual dispute. Ultimately they had been divorced when he was 11. He remained with his mother, and his father remarried and moved to another city. He preferred his father's new wife to his mother, whom he considered cold and difficult to please. The following year his mother also remarried and thereafter displayed even less interest in him than before. He became increasingly dependent upon his mother, however, and felt guilty because of his resentful attitude toward her. In school he was shy and wary, and he avoided commitments with his schoolmates at play or in school activities. He even abandoned religious observances—"I adopted a scientific attitude." By this he meant that he was detached and suspicious in all his dealings but never self-assertive or combative. In the clinic he was given quiet approval and was encouraged to discuss his family difficulties at his own pace. Arrangements were made for him to visit his father in Chicago, where he enjoyed a complete remission of symptoms. Before he left Chicago, his blood pressure had fallen to 118/65. Shortly after his return his diastolic pressure was still low, although the systolic reading was slightly elevated, 140/65.

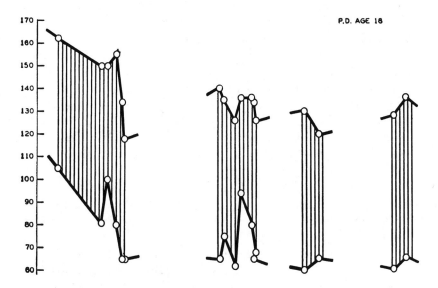

Figure 2. The blood pressure changes over a period of 2 years in an 18-year-old boy who initially displayed evidences of hypertension.

During subsequent visits to the clinic his growing inclination to emancipate himself from his mother was endorsed. With encouragement he got a job. At first there was considerable inner conflict about whether or not he was justified in withholding a part of his salary from his mother, but gradually he felt able to discuss this point and other problems with her, vigorously asserting his own position. "If you keep everything inside you, you don't feel right; if you let some of it out, you feel better." Finally, with his mother's approval, he was able to move away from home and share an apartment with a friend. His blood pressure remained low, 120/65, and he was free of symptoms.

Concerning his experience at the clinic he said, "I've been helped a lot here by talking things over. I feel surer of myself."

UNFAVORABLE RESULTS

On the other hand, the patients who changed little or not at all were likely to be persons who had most of the following characteristics: they were over 40 years of age, members of a minority group, had one or both parents missing before they reached the age of 12, and were themselves separated or divorced. They had had hypertension 7 or more years, the systolic blood pressure at the time of presentation being over 180 and the diastolic over 110.

In addition they had various combinations of the following items in their background: They had had relatively unhealthy and unsatisfactory lives. Their parents had been exceedingly strict or had given them no emotional support. Later they had not got this support from their spouses, to whom they were not well married, often not being sexually compatible. Many had had frequent extramarital sexual relationships or were promiscuous. They had poor relations with their children, whom they often rejected. Most of them were dissatisfied with their working conditions, having changed jobs frequently, the salary being, in their estimation, inadequate. They considered that they were not "doing well" or at least had gained no satisfaction from their place in work or society.

Upon examination it was the physician's opinion that the patients had overreacted to the usual vicissitudes of life or had experienced unusually severe traumatic situations. Interpersonal relations, according to the physician, including those involving sexual intimacies, were usually poor, being superficial and fleeting, though perhaps numerous. Most of them also gave evidence that their activities, achievements, and other life experiences had afforded them little or no satisfaction and that they had made no commitments or dedications.

The personalities of the patients were relatively rigid and inflexible, and deeply repressed hostilities had been present since childhood or early adult life. Although often exceedingly active, the patients exhibited little evidence of ability to deal with the basic difficulties or major problems of life, and their failure to have made commitments or the absence of satisfactions interfered with suitable life participations. Furthermore, though often excessively meticulous and compulsive, they were unsteady and unreliable and made poor discriminations regarding human values and goals.

Finally, the prevailing attitudes of the patients at the time they presented themselves to the physician were those of skepticism, suspicion, and lack of confidence in him and the hospital, often despite opposite protestations. There was little evidence that they recognized the failure of their present way of dealing with problems or that they were genuinely willing to adopt others. They also exhibited a reluctance to consider the possibility that attitudes, feelings, and life situations might be relevant to their illness.

The life situations that formed the settings for their illness were, in the opinion of the physician, immutable, or if changed would recur soon in slightly altered form.

The unfavorable progress of one illustrative patient is detailed below and graphically represented in Figure 3.

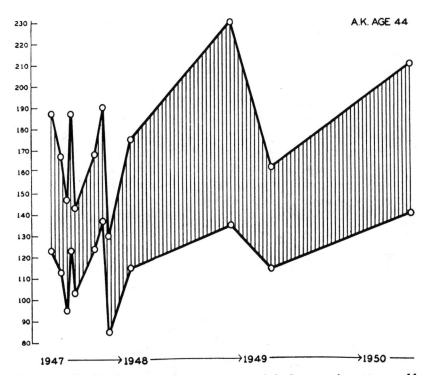

FIGURE 3. The blood pressure changes over a period of 3 years in a 44-year-old man who improved briefly but whose blood pressure was ultimately higher than when he was first seen.

A 44-year-old assistant superintendent of public schools had been discovered to have hypertension in a routine examination 9 years before. During the interval he had had no symptoms, but finally consulted the hospital because concerned over the implications of continuous high blood pressure.

At the time he was first seen at the New York Hospital his blood pressure was 190/122. He was a moderately obese, ruddy-faced man and did not appear ill. His manner was superficially casual and friendly, but also wary, noncommittal, and suspicious. The general examination showed nothing remarkable except for his blood pressure. His heart size and EKG were normal, and detailed studies of renal function were negative.

The patient had spent his childhood with his orthodox Jewish parents, from whom he was never able to get adequate approval. He reacted by rejecting the forms of the church and at 26 eloped with a Jewish girl of a more "worldly" family. He found her to be a highly materialistic, independent, and self-sufficient woman who was also difficult to please. She did not support his aspirations to become a psychologist, but was slightly contemptuous of his activities in that direction because of the comparatively poor financial return. She herself continued working and ultimately became an "executive" with an income larger than her husband's. He found her cold sexually, and despite almost daily intercourse he found it necessary to masturbate to reach adequate sexual gratification. He nevertheless became increasingly dependent upon his wife and frequently doubted his own values and aspirations and tended to adopt those of his wife.

His physician, on the other hand, encouraged his efforts in psychology and supported his plan to write a thesis on some of his work. When finally, late in 1947, he was at work on his thesis, his blood pressure was normal. Shortly thereafter, however, his blood pressure rose again in a setting of conflict about an extramarital relationship with a woman who he felt possessed all the warmth and understanding his wife lacked. Hereafter his contacts with the hospital diminished to visits only once or twice a year. He was especially reluctant to pay for his treatment, since this would reduce an income his wife already considered inadequate. His tentative and wary attitude could not be successfully modified; it was clear that his relationship with the clinic was a limited commitment. He clung to the reassurance that his kidney function was adequate, and he persistently implied that the clinic was doing nothing for him.

Over the course of the ensuing two years he virtually abandoned his aims and interests in psychology and in an effort to placate and "win over" his wife took on numerous extracurricular jobs for pay. As will be noted in Figure 3, his blood pressure over this period was consistently high on the occasions when he was seen.

Conclusion

It would appear justifiable from the above to infer that an interest by the physician in the feelings, attitudes, and life situations of patients with essential hypertension reduced or eliminated symptoms in about two thirds. In a few, between one tenth and one fifth, the blood pressure was lowered to normotensive levels for significantly, if not indefinitely long periods.

Questions and Discussion

DR. GEORGE A. PERERA: May I just ask Dr. Wolff one question? I noticed that he corrected his group with reference to the initial blood pressure level. However, his most favorable responses were among younger subjects—those in whom one might expect greater lability and more adaptability to psychiatric suggestion. I wonder if he has re-analyzed his data so that comparable age groups have been compared?

DR. WOLFF: The 9 patients in the group that were seemingly most altered by the described management to which they were exposed are even younger than those in the other group. Their ages ranged from 18 to 49 as follows:

Hypertensives (9), Group 4

Name	Age	Initial Blood Pressure	Final Blood Pressure	Prognosis, Per Cent
D.	18	160/105	120/65	89
J.	23	160/90	130/80	81
G.	25	150/100	138/88	83
R.	29	170/90	125/80	81
S.	29	150/110	130/80	88
R.	31	160/100	120/90	80
D.	38	160/95	140/90	80
D.	47	160/110	110/80	80
M.	49	160/100	140/90	80

But there were 2 patients over 40. On the other hand, there were 5 patients under 25 in Groups 1 and 2. Hence what you imply is correct, namely, that younger persons with hypertension are on the whole better candidates for such management than older persons. But exceptions are striking.

I should like to add a few words. It is quite possible that what I have exhibited this afternoon in the way of alterations in the blood

490

pressure in those with hypertension represents nothing more than spontaneous variations constituting the natural history of the disorder. But my guess is that we have been dealing with the group that Dr. Hines has brought into focus. He indicated that among persons with the proclivity to develop hypertension when examined after 20 years only about 80 per cent get sustained hypertension and the other 20 per cent do not. What is it that makes the latter group more or less large?

Is it possible that we can make that group larger by introducing ourselves, our good will, our values, and our attitudes and by helping the patient better to understand and more suitably to express himself?

· · · · · · · · · · · · · · · · *by* ROBERT W. WILKINS

Recent Experiences with the Pharmacologic Treatment of Hypertension

THERE is no satisfactory pharmacologic treatment for hypertension. In part this is because we do not understand the etiology of the disease and therefore do not know how to attack it at the source. In part it is because essential hypertension, instead of being resistant, usually is susceptible to treatment, at least temporarily, by many different agents and procedures. But chiefly it is because we still have no agent that will persistently lower the blood pressure without undesirable side effects. For example, the available sympatholytic drugs are neither persistent in action nor free from unpleasant side effects such as postural hypotension. And though Veratrum viride will lower the blood pressure, it does so only in a dose range extremely close to that causing nausea and vomiting. Nevertheless, since Veratrum from the experimental and also from the clinical point of view has appeared to produce a higher proportion of favorable to unfavorable effects than any other available hypotensive agent, it has been given in severe cases of essential hypertension in an attempt to modify the natural course of the disease. Experience with it now is extensive enough to warrant a preliminary discussion.

The Parenteral Administration of Veratrum Viride
Although pure alkaloids of Veratrum viride with potent hypotensive effects have been prepared, they are as yet of little practical importance because they are so enormously difficult and expensive to make. Moreover, preliminary trial has indicated that they are in no way superior to or essentially different in action from the less refined preparations. Recently, highly purified extracts suitable for both parenteral and oral use have been prepared in amounts and at costs feasible for clinical trial. These are Veriloid (Riker Laboratories, Inc.) and Anatensol (E. R. Squibb & Sons). The action of these two agents given intra-

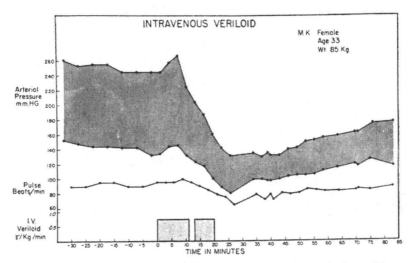

FIGURE 1. A chart of the arterial pressure and the pulse rate (taken with an intra-arterial needle and a Sanborn electromanometer) in a hypertensive patient receiving an intravenous infusion of Veriloid, as noted.

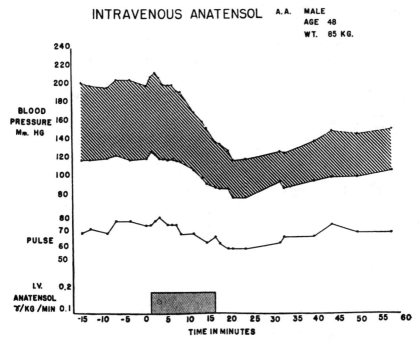

FIGURE 2. A chart of the arterial pressure and the pulse rate in a hypertensive patient receiving an intravenous infusion of Anatensol, as noted.

493

venously is essentially the same. They are best given by slow infusion at a constant rate (based on the weight of the patient). The average dose of Veriloid is from 0.75 to 1.0 microgram and of Anatensol from 0.08 to 0.2 microgram per kilogram per minute (Figs. 1 and 2). With this dose there is usually a striking hypotensive effect within from 8 to 15 minutes, commonly but not invariably associated with bradycardia. The infusion is then interrupted or retarded so that the hypotension may be maintained or allowed to moderate.

During the hypotensive response to intravenous Veratrum the patient may remain entirely asymptomatic, or may, if the drug is carried too far, complain of burning in the throat or epigastrium, and even of nausea and vomiting. However, with careful regulation of the dose it is usually possible to avoid or minimize such unpleasant side effects and still obtain a hypotensive response. In 45 acute administrations of Veratrum, carried out as just described, the blood pressure was lowered in all but 1 (a patient in the terminal malignant phase), without vomiting in all but 3, and without nausea in all but 10. In 28 of the 45 experiments (62 per cent) the lowering of the arterial pressure was 50 mm. Hg or more systolic, and 20 mm. Hg or more diastolic (Fig. 3).

The results so far with the intravenous and intramuscular administration of Veratrum viride indicate that the drug may be useful paren-

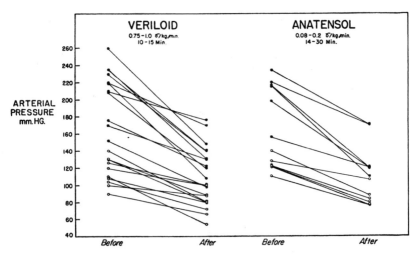

FIGURE 3. A composite chart of the systolic (upper group, indicated by solid bars) and diastolic (lower group, indicated by open bars) arterial pressures in 10 hypertensive patients before and after intravenous Veriloid, and in 6 patients before and after intravenous Anatensol, as noted.

terally, at least for the treatment of acute hypertensive crises and of pre-eclampsia, and particularly when it seems desirable to reduce the arterial pressure quickly. The hypotensive action and symptomatic improvement in such cases may be very striking indeed.

The Oral Administration of Veratrum

Parenteral administration, no matter how effective, is obviously impracticable for the routine therapy of a chronic and frequently asymptomatic disease like essential hypertension. Both crude Veratrum and its various extracts are effective by mouth. However, since different batches of the natural drug vary so markedly in potency, it is desirable to have a chemically pure or a biologically standardized preparation. Of the commercially available oral extracts, Vertavis (Irwin, Neisler & Company) is standardized in daphnia, while Veriloid (Riker Laboratories, Inc.) is standardized in dogs. The acute action of Veratrum viride on oral administration is quite similar to that on parenteral injection. Of course, the dose cannot be gauged so nicely by the oral as by the intravenous route, so that there is a somewhat higher incidence of nausea and vomiting (Fig. 4). However, in from 50 to 60 per cent of cases on acute oral administration it is possible to achieve a significant lowering of the arterial pressure without untoward symptoms.

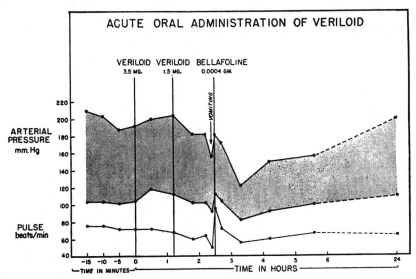

FIGURE 4. A chart of the arterial pressure and the pulse rate in a hypertensive patient receiving oral Veriloid, as noted. As the patient became nauseated and vomited, Bellafoline was given, with complete relief of all symptoms thereafter.

By significant lowering is meant a decrease in pressure of at least 30 mm. Hg systolic and 15 mm. Hg diastolic.

In an attempt to prolong the hypotensive effects of Veratrum viride over a period of days, weeks, or months the drug has been given four times a day (after meals and at bedtime) for periods up to three years. Even with highly purified and biologically standardized extracts such as Veriloid, the effective maintenance dose varies considerably from patient to patient. In addition, in any one patient the dose is highly critical because the differences between the non-hypotensive, the hypotensive, the emetic, and the excessively hypotensive doses are small. Therefore, the proper dose can be determined only by cautious clinical trial. Obviously this would be done best in a hospital where the blood pressure can be measured frequently and the factors enhancing "spontaneous" variations usually are minimized. However, it often has been necessary to institute the drug in ambulatory patients with observations only at weekly or even at monthly intervals.

Using Veriloid, the ordinary hypertensive patient is started on 2.0 mg. four times a day with instructions to increase two of the doses (after breakfast and before bedtime) to 3.0 mg. unless burning, nausea, or vomiting appears, in which case two of the doses (at noontime and after supper) should be reduced to 1.0 mg. A dose of Veriloid of less than 6.0 mg. a day is usually completely ineffectual in lowering the blood pressure. As time goes on, it may be necessary to increase the dose after breakfast, lunch, supper, and at bedtime respectively to 4.0, 3.0, 3.0, and 4.0 mg., or even to 5.0, 4.0, 4.0, and 5.0 mg. A dose in excess of this amount, even when tolerated by the patient, usually is not more effective in lowering the blood pressure.

Given in this way, oral Veratrum causes significant hypotensive effects initially (for a period of from days to a few weeks) in at least 50 per cent of patients. This was to have been expected from the preliminary observation that on acute administration the drug caused hypotensive effects without symptoms in about 50 per cent of cases. Thus the usual experience with oral Veriloid, for example, is that on a total daily dose of from 10.0 to 18.0 mg. there is a definite hypotensive effect for a period of weeks, as compared with the control period. During this time the physician, as well as the patient, may feel very much encouraged about the treatment.

As the oral administration of Veratrum for the treatment of essential hypertension is prolonged over a period of several months, the clinical results may become less, rather than more, satisfactory. Thus if the physician critically reviews the records of his patients from six months to one year after the beginning of oral treatment, he may be considerably less certain than he was initially that the drug is lowering the patient's blood pressure. There are at least several reasons for this. First, the natural course of the blood pressure in hypertensive disease is so variable that the longer the period of observation the more unequivocal must be any lowering of the blood pressure to insure that it was not due to chance. A preliminary trial of frequent (at least daily) home blood pressure measurements has indicated that this method of study may show more clear-cut results with Veratrum therapy than are obtainable by the usual method of weekly or monthly office measurements. Second, continuous oral Veratrum at best has only a moderating, not a curative, effect on hypertension, allowing the blood pressure to vary over ranges as wide as, even if lower than, before. Third, Veratrum does not maintain a significantly lower pressure in many patients, particularly those with chronic severe hypertension, without causing at least occasional nausea, vomiting, or collapse, side reactions which to many patients are intolerable. Fourth, as time progresses some patients apparently become more rather than less susceptible to the nauseating, as compared with the hypotensive, effects of the drug, requiring a reduction in the dose to below the effective hypotensive range.

The substitution of placebos after several weeks or months of therapy has been made with a number of persons and with most has resulted in a rapid rise of the blood pressure to, or above, the pretreatment control levels. Occasionally, however, the blood pressure has not returned immediately (within 48 hours) to its previous levels, so that now it is considered necessary to allow at least one week on placebo therapy before judgment is made as to the effects of this regimen compared with the treatment by the potent drug. Such observations, preferably made by means of frequent home blood pressure measurements, must be continued and enlarged before final judgment is made as to the long-term effectiveness of continuous oral Veratrum treatment in hypertensive disease.

Symptoms during Veratrum Therapy

The unpleasant symptoms caused by oral Veratrum treatment commonly are related to the upper gastrointestinal tract and consist of a peppermint taste in the mouth, salivation, burning in the throat, the substernum, or the epigastrium, and nausea and vomiting. These symptoms are the most frequent causes of limitation of the dose. When the drug is given intravenously these symptoms almost invariably follow, rather than precede, some lowering of the blood pressure. The same is true on acute oral administration. However, on chronic oral administration these symptoms may appear without any appreciable lowering in the blood pressure or may occur suddenly on the same dose schedule that previously had caused no difficulty. Furthermore, on continued oral administration, as already mentioned, such symptoms may become more rather than less annoying and require reduction of the dose to below an effective therapeutic level.

Attempts to reduce the gastrointestinal side effects of Veratrum have been only partly successful. The use of slow-dissolving preparations orally appears to be definitely helpful. Dramamine in a dose of 50 mg. three times a day has seemed of mild benefit in some patients, but of none in others. Atropine is sometimes effective in lessening the nausea if given before vomiting occurs. The initial trial of Banthine in oral doses of 50 mg. three times a day has been helpful in allowing certain patients to take Veriloid in larger doses than was otherwise possible and so to achieve hypotensive effects that previously had not been obtained. Work is continuing on this problem.

A second group of symptoms that may appear on Veratrum therapy seem to be related directly to its hypotensive effects. Thus dizziness or weakness and a sense of tingling, numbness, stiffness, fatigue, or coldness of the extremities may come on at the peak of the drug's action. Although postural hypotension is not a usual accompaniment, it has been observed with excessive doses of the drug. If the hypotensive effects of Veratrum are too great, they may progress to actual syncope or collapse. By this time the patient is almost invariably vomiting and is extremely distressed. However, such reactions appear more alarming than dangerous, and to date, so far as is known, none has resulted fatally.

The most common symptomatic improvement noted by hypertensive patients on continuous oral Veratrum therapy is a feeling of increased strength and endurance. For example, a woman may clean her house for the first time in months, or a man may go back to work. Indeed, it is possible that such increased activities may account for the equivocal hypotensive effects obtained in some patients. Explosive headaches of a throbbing character have been relieved or abolished, and facial flushing and blotchiness of the neck have disappeared. Symptomatic improvement, when it occurs, is not always associated with an appreciable lowering of the blood pressure and, therefore, is difficult to evaluate. For example, there are a group of patients who refuse to take the drug in doses sufficient to cause significant hypotensive effects because of the associated unpleasant side effects, but continue to take it in reduced doses, insisting that they have symptomatic improvement. Finally, a good proportion of patients have no symptoms whatever, either off or on the therapy and whether or not their blood pressure is changed.

Combinations of Therapy

Efforts in this laboratory have been directed chiefly at determining the efficacy of Veratrum viride alone as a therapeutic agent in hypertension. Therefore, patients have been instructed to continue their ordinary diets and not to take any other form of treatment while on the drug. However, a few patients have been carried on with combinations of therapy. For example, the drug has been given along with a salt-free diet and has also been used after a surgical sympathectomy which has not had the desired hypotensive effects. In addition, combinations with other drugs, especially sympatholytic agents, have been tried with Veratrum. To date, the drug has not seemed incompatible; on the contrary has seemed, if anything, to be more effective when used with these other forms of treatment. The drug has also been given freely to patients who have been digitalized with no untoward effects. Further experience with combinations of therapy is urgently needed and is being sought in our own as well as in other laboratories.

A Case History

A brief case history is given to illustrate a long-term clinical trial of Veratrum in a hypertensive patient and some of the difficulties that may be encountered (Fig. 5). Mrs. R. W., a Jewish housewife, aged 51, had had known arterial hypertension for 8 years when she was first seen in the Hypertension Clinic complaining of marked fatigue, nervousness, and frontal headache. Physical examination revealed moderate obesity, Grade 1 hypertensive retinopathy, and a blood pressure of 240/120, but no other abnormalities.

Roentgenographic and electrocardiographic examinations of the heart and laboratory studies of the blood, urine, and renal function gave results all within normal limits. Her blood pressure responses to cold and postural stimuli were abnormally exaggerated.

During a 6-months' control period on symptomatic therapy the blood pressure remained elevated between 240/130 and 200/110. She was then started on increasing doses of Veriloid up to 10.0 mg. a day. During the first 3 months of this treatment the blood pressure moderated until it ranged between 200/100 and 170/85. The patient reported

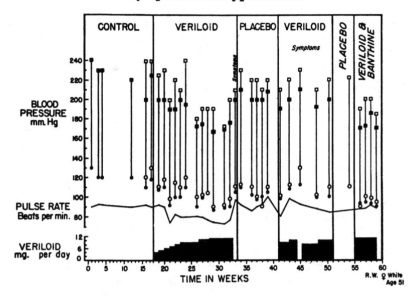

FIGURE 5. A chart of the course of the systolic (squares) and diastolic (circles) arterial pressures (casual, open symbols; resting, solid symbols) in patient R. W., treated intermittently with Veriloid, placebos, and a combination of Veriloid and Banthine, as noted.

marked symptomatic relief, with freedom from headache, fatigue, and nervousness. However, because of one episode of vomiting she voluntarily discontinued the therapy, and her blood pressure rose to from 200/105 to 210/110.

She was promptly placed on placebos, but her blood pressure remained elevated between 230/110 and 200/100. She then reported a gradual return of her previous complaints of fatigue, headache, and nervousness, along with episodes of flushing. After 7 weeks on placebos, Veriloid therapy was resumed without her knowledge, but with a prompt return of gastrointestinal symptoms and no relief of her complaints. In spite of encouragement, she took the drug irregularly, and the blood pressure showed no further change. Therefore, after 10 weeks, placebos were again given, with relief of the gastrointestinal symptoms but with an increase in fatigue and nervousness. At the end of 1 month, Veriloid therapy was resumed in a dose of 11.0 mg. a day, along with Banthine 200 mg. a day. There was prompt relief of her original complaints without any gastrointestinal symptoms. The blood pressure ranged between 200/100 and 170/90. Efforts will now be made to increase the dose of Veriloid.

Comment

With the information presently available no one can predict with certainly the ultimate place of Veratrum viride in the therapy of hypertension. However, one can state that until something with superior pharmacologic properties appears, Veratrum will be tried parenterally or even orally in a number of patients with acute hypertensive crises when it seems desirable to lower the blood pressure quickly. The situation with regard to the chronic oral use of the drug is considerably less clear than with the parenteral, and much more work is needed. In its present forms oral Veratrum viride is a tricky and troublesome drug. This seems to be chiefly because of the critical dose necessary to obtain hypotensive, without nauseating or collapsing, effects. Patients at best have to reconcile themselves to occasional unpleasant symptoms; indeed, some patients use these symptoms as a gauge of dosage. In those who have severe hypertensive disease, especially with serious symptoms, the occasional side effects of the drug seem definitely preferable to the symptoms of the untreated disease.

Our experience so far with Veratrum has convinced us that it is the most effective pharmacologic agent now available for lowering the blood pressure of hypertensive patients. There is no question, however, that in its present forms the drug leaves considerable to be desired. Of course, there is always the hope that pure alkaloids or new derivatives will be made which have a smoother and wider range of hypotensive activity without unpleasant side effects. Also it is possible that certain agents used in conjunction with Veratrum will be found to block its unpleasant effects or to enhance its favorable ones. Until that time or until a better agent appears, it seems likely that Veratrum will continue to be used, at least for experimental studies and the clinical relief of severe cases of hypertension.

Questions and Discussion

DR. MARK NICKERSON: In connection with the use of drugs in the management of hypertension, the primary objective is to determine the etiology of the disease, a problem which we discussed in detail on the first day of this symposium, and then to develop agents to combat the basic physiological derangement. We have not reached this goal as yet. A secondary, empirical approach is to reduce sympatho-adrenal activity. This is the basis of the surgical treatment of hypertension. Dr. Smithwick has presented evidence indicating that sympathectomy will ameliorate the condition and prolong the life span.

As I mentioned earlier, there are a number of ways in which drugs may reduce sympatho-adrenal activity. I think we should not neglect the basic pharmacological and physiological information regarding the mechanisms by which various agents produce this effect.

The veratrum alkaloids act reflexly. They stimulate receptors located primarily in the left ventricle and lungs. From these receptors afferent impulses are carried to the brain stem. We must not forget that the parasympathetic and the sympathetic pathways are interrelated within the central nervous system. Thus in reducing sympathetic activity by a reflex mechanism, the veratrum alkaloids almost inevitably also increase parasympathetic activity. The latter accounts for the decreased heart rate and the nausea and vomiting which commonly accompany the administration of effective doses of the veratrum alkaloids. It is perhaps too much to expect of an agent acting reflexly that it should differentiate between the parasympathetic and sympathetic systems. Consequently, we may anticipate that separation of the undesirable side effects of such agents from their therapeutic action will be difficult if not impossible.

Agents which act within the central nervous system have the same disadvantage, I believe. The ergot alkaloids fall into this category. They may inhibit sympathetic vasoconstrictor reflexes by their action

502

on the brain stem. However, they also stimulate the vagal nuclei and the emetic center. This accounts for the reduced heart rate as well as the nausea and vomiting seen in patients given the ergot alkaloids. If the dose of either the natural or dihydrogenated ergot alkaloids is increased in an effort to produce a more complete inhibition of sympathetic reflexes, the direct stimulant action on the hypothalamus brings about a rise in the blood pressure which may be most disconcerting.

Blockade at sympathetic ganglia has similar limitations of specificity in that most ganglionic blocking agents inhibit transmission through both the sympathetic and parasympathetic systems. This leads to a decreased gastric secretion, a decrease in intestinal motility, etc., as well as to peripheral vasodilatation.

On the basis of the above considerations I would make a strong plea that current studies be particularly directed to those agents which act peripherally. It is only at the peripheral neuro-effector junctions that the sympathetic nervous system differs sufficiently from other divisions of the nervous system to allow a good possibility of blocking sympathetic activity, vasoconstriction in particular, without complicating cross reactions involving the central nervous system and the parasympathetic division of the autonomic nervous system.

DR. SIBLEY W. HOOBLER (ANN ARBOR): In regard to Dr. Nickerson's remarks and to shed some ray of hope on the situation as far as drug therapy is concerned, we have studied protoveratrin, a derivative of Veratrum album prepared and originally studied by Dr. Krayer and Dr. Meilman, which appears to be without any nauseating or emetic effects. When given intravenously, it has about the same circulatory effects as Dr. Wilkins has described for the other types of veratrum alkaloids. I don't know the pharmacologic explanation for the absence of emetic properties, but I do know clinically it is quite effective on the blood pressure and has not in any of our cases—we have given more than 50 or 60 injections—caused any nausea or vomiting, so there may be some hope of developing a veratrum derivative without this very disturbing side effect.

• • • • • • • • • • • • • • • *by* CARLETON B. CHAPMAN

Some Effects of the Rice-Fruit Diet in Patients with Essential Hypertension

THE belief that restriction of the salt intake is beneficial to patients suffering from various types of cardiovascular-renal disease is by no means new. The lineage of this notion, with special reference to the treatment of hypertension, goes back at least to the first half of the nineteenth century. Table 1 shows the developments that probably influenced Ambard and Beaujard (1), who were the first to observe that salt deprivation may produce a decline in the blood pressure in hypertensive patients. The most direct line of reasoning began with Redtenbacher (2), who in 1850 observed that the excretion of urinary chloride was markedly diminished in patients suffering from febrile diseases. Salkowski's work (3) brought the sodium ion onto the scene, and von Korányi (4) established the fact that there is retention of chloride in patients with cardiac failure. One of the most significant experimental contributions of the period lies buried in the voluminous French medical literature of the late nineteenth century. Scarcely two paragraphs long, the report by Carrion and Hallion (5) presents proof that the injection of small quantities of concentrated salt solution may produce severe peripheral and pulmonary edema, and even death, in experimental animals. Several years later Widal and Lemierre (6) in effect confirmed Carrion and Hallion's results by adding salt to the diets of patients with Bright's disease. This and other work by French workers led directly to the study by Ambard and Beaujard. The therapeutic emphasis was placed on restriction of the chloride, and not the sodium, intake. Parallel developments, proceeding concurrently all this time, included the concept of essential hypertension and the use of the skimmed milk diet. The latter measure was, in fact, the first attempt to limit the intake of salt and fluids as a therapeutic adjunct, although its originators had little or no understanding of its effective feature.

TABLE 1. The Origins of the Concept

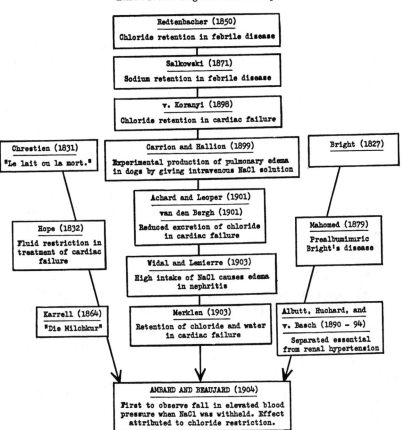

Redtenbacher (1850)
Chloride retention in febrile disease

Salkowski (1871)
Sodium retention in febrile disease

v. Koranyi (1898)
Chloride retention in cardiac failure

Chrestien (1831)
"Le lait ou la mort."

Carrion and Hallion (1899)
Experimental production of pulmonary edema in dogs by giving intravenous NaCl solution

Bright (1827)

Achard and Leoper (1901)
van den Bergh (1901)

Hope (1832)
Fluid restriction in treatment of cardiac failure

Reduced excretion of chloride in cardiac failure

Mahomed (1879)
Prealbuminuric Bright's disease

Vidal and Lemierre (1903)
High intake of NaCl causes edema in nephritis

Karrell (1864)
"Die Milchkur"

Merklen (1903)
Retention of chloride and water in cardiac failure

Albutt, Huchard, and v. Basch (1890 - 94)
Separated essential from renal hypertension

AMBARD AND BEAUJARD (1904)
First to observe fall in elevated blood pressure when NaCl was withheld. Effect attributed to chloride restriction.

Sixteen years after the work by Ambard and Beaujard, Allen and co-workers (7) found a low-salt diet to be effective in lowering the blood pressure of some hypertensive patients. Like the French workers, they thought that the effective feature of the regimen was chloride restriction. Subsequently other workers failed to confirm Allen's results, but none of the studies was extensive enough or well enough controlled to confirm or deny Allen's views.

The introduction of the rice-fruit diet in 1944 by Kempner (8) constitutes the latest attempt to control hypertension by dietary means. By the use of the diet, its originator obtained a significant lowering of the blood pressure in 62 per cent of 500 patients with essential hypertension; he also reported marked improvement in the eyegrounds, reversal of abnormal electrocardiographic patterns, and diminution in the size of the heart in many of his patients (9). The diet caused loss of body weight in most of the patients, mainly, according to Kempner, because of diminution in "visible and invisible edema." In his hands the diet did not induce negative nitrogen balance, although it provides a daily intake of only 20 gm. of protein, all of which is from vegetable sources.

Since Kempner's earlier articles appeared, almost all of his claims for the diet have been questioned by other investigators. Some observers doubt that the diet exerts a specific depressor effect on the blood pressure in patients with hypertension. It has been shown that in some patients, at least, the diet induces negative nitrogen balance (10), and the suggestion that the diet is, in reality, a semistarvation regimen has been made repeatedly. The occurrence of the salt depletion syndrome in some patients receiving the rice-fruit diet has recently been held to indicate a need for discrimination in the therapeutic use of the measure.

A final evaluation of the rice-fruit regimen is not yet possible partly because of the lack of basic information concerning its effect on the human body. To limit inquiry to the effect of the regimen on the blood pressure alone is, for purposes of evaluation, obviously inadequate. Such drastic dietary limitation is almost certain to produce important changes in body composition which, in turn, may determine whether or not the diet is therapeutically practicable. The following work, done in collaboration with Drs. Thomas Gibbons and Austin Henschel, was undertaken in an effort to throw light on some of the changes the diet may induce.

Method

Eight male patients with well-established, moderately severe essential hypertension were selected for the study (Table 2). All had more or less incapacitating symptoms, of which headache was the most frequent, but none had an elevated blood urea nitrogen or other signs of renal insufficiency. Four of the 8 men complained of dyspnea on exertion (in 2 it was the chief complaint), but none had frank congestive failure.

Basically, two diets were employed. The standard hospital diet provided 3000 calories, 100 gm. of protein, and 8 to 12 gm. of salt per day. The rice-fruit diet as used in the study supplied slightly more than 2000 calories, 22 gm. of vegetable protein, and about 20 mg. of sodium per day.

For the measurement of the specific gravity and of the total fat of

TABLE 2. General Data on 8 Male Hypertensive Subjects at the
Time of Their Selection for Study

Subject Age	Resting Blood Pressure	Duration of Hypertension, in Years	Eyegrounds	Symptoms
L. A. 46	166/110	6	I	Headaches, dizziness
K. M. 40	186/136	6	I	Headaches, dyspnea, and weakness
H. H. 58	190/120	9	II	Headaches, dyspnea on exertion
A. B. 44	180/106	4	II	Headaches, dyspnea on exertion
C. M. 32	198/132	4	III	Headaches, numbness in right arm and leg
J. M. 53	224/134	3	II	Headaches, dyspnea on exertion
C. P. 31	190/120	3	III	Headaches, dizziness, loss of vision O.S.
G. R. 34	196/132	4	I	Headaches

the body, the methods described by Behnke et al. (11), Rathbun and Pace (12, 13), and Morales et al. (14) were employed in 6 of the subjects. These methods require measurement of the weight of the body in air, on the one hand, and the weight of the body under water, on the other. From these values the volume displacement of the body can be calculated if the amount of residual air in the lungs is known. The latter was measured by means of the open-circuit technique. Since the specific gravity of the body (body weight/volume displacement) varies inversely with its fat content, an approximation of the weight of the total body fat can be made once the specific gravity has been determined. The extracellular fluid volume and plasma volume were estimated by the thiocyanate method and the Evans blue-dye technique, respectively.

From these key measurements it is possible to calculate the approximate composition of the body in terms of weight. The bones are known to account for about 4 per cent of the normal adult body weight, and this figure was used in the present calculations. It is assumed, on reasonably good evidence, that under the conditions of these experiments, any change in body weight that may have occurred as a result of demineralization of the bones was relatively insignificant. The weight of the inactive tissue compartment is calculated as follows: weight of fat + weight of bones + weight of extracellular fluid (including plasma volume). When the weight of the inactive compartment is subtracted from the total body weight, one obtains an approximate value for the weight of active body tissue. This compartment is composed mainly of muscle tissue, but includes small amounts of other tissue components (for example, fibrous and glandular tissue) as well.

The order of the experiments was not constant in all the subjects, but invariably included a prolonged control period, during which the standard hospital diet was given, and a test period, during which the unmodified rice-fruit diet was employed. The effect of adding sodium-free protein to the rice-fruit diet was studied in 5 subjects, and the effect of salt supplements (10 gm. daily) in 3 subjects. In 4 of the patients, the extreme monotony of the rice-fruit diet necessitated the substitution of a less rigid low-salt diet during a 40-day furlough from the hospital. This low-salt diet provided 2000 calories, 70 gm. of protein, and about 400 mg. of sodium per day. When the patients returned to the hospital for the final phases of the study, the standard rice-fruit diet was reinstituted for a period of 20 days before the use of salt supplements began.

Results

All the subjects complained of the extreme dietary restrictions made necessary by the regimen, but in general there was surprisingly little evidence of discontent during the experiments. One subject (C. M.) deviated slightly from the diet, which may or may not account for the fact that his blood pressure remained unchanged throughout the experiments. The effect of the rice-fruit diet on the symptoms of which the subjects complained initially was salutary. Headache was markedly diminished or abolished in 6 of the 8 patients. There was less impressive improvement in symptoms other than headache. In Figure 1, a dramatic fall in the systolic and diastolic blood pressures when the rice-fruit diet was administered is seen. During the 44-day control period, the patient's blood pressure was quite labile, but at no time did it approach the upper limits of normal. The addition of salt-free protein (Lonolac) to the diet had no effect on the blood pressure. Following this, the patient was maintained on the low-salt diet (supplying about 0.5 gm. of sodium per day) for 42 days. The rice-fruit

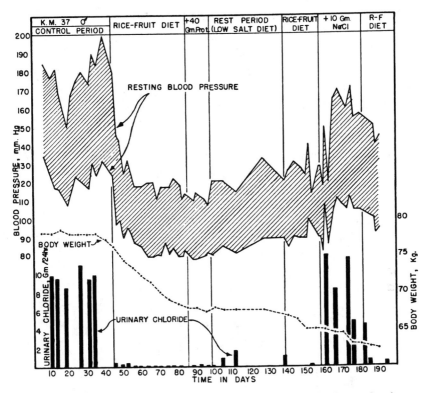

FIGURE 1. The course of the blood pressure, total body weight, and urinary chloride excretion in subject K. M.

FIGURE 2. Changes in the composition of the body in subject K. M.: March 30, end of control period; May 11, after 38 days of treatment with the rice-fruit diet; July 21, after furlough from the hospital (40 days) and reinstitution of the rice-fruit diet (18 days); August 17, after the addition of salt to the rice-fruit diet.

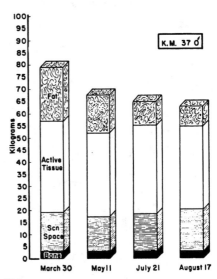

diet was then reinstituted for a 3-week period, at the end of which time salt was added to the diet. The blood pressure promptly rose, and severe headache returned. The weight curve is of greatest interest; it steadily declined during the rice-fruit diet periods, but was held constant by the addition of protein to the diet.

Figure 2 shows the changes that took place in the same patient's body composition. A comparison of the second column with the first shows what happened after the patient had received the rice-fruit diet for about 40 days. He lost 8.3 kg. of body weight; of this loss, 6.14 kg. was in the form of fat, 1.78 kg. in thiocyanate space, and 0.4 kg. in active body tissue (mainly muscle). The addition of protein and small amounts of salt to the diet stopped the loss of active tissue, but the loss of fat continued. Use of the rice-fruit diet plus 10 gm. of salt a day brought a return of the symptoms and an increase in the thiocyanate space.

Figure 3 is very similar to Figure 1, although the drop in the blood

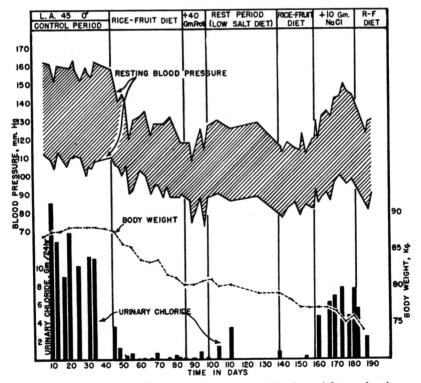

FIGURE 3. The course of the blood pressure, total body weight, and urinary chloride excretion in subject L. A.

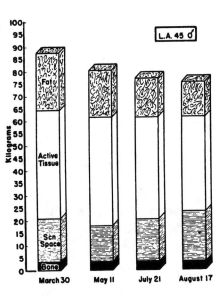

Figure 4. Changes in the composition of the body in subject L. A. Significance of dates same as in Figure 2.

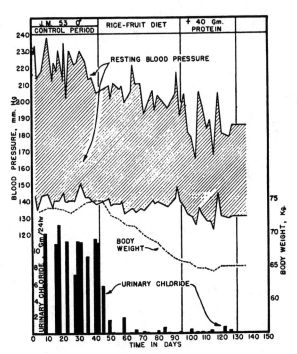

Figure 5. The course of the blood pressure, total body weight, and urinary chloride excretion in subject J. M.

511

pressure was less dramatic than in the previous instance. It did, however, reach the upper limits of normal after the patient had been on the rice-fruit diet for about 40 days. The changes in body composition (Figure 4) were similar to those in the previous patient, although the loss of fat was less marked.

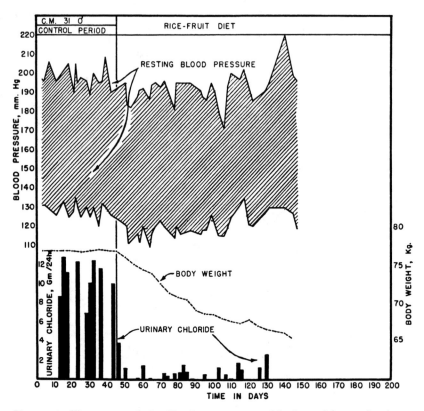

FIGURE 6. The course of the blood pressure, total body weight, and urinary chloride excretion in subject C. M.

In a third patient the blood pressure did not decline significantly, although the weight curve was almost identical with that of the other 2, as was the effect of the administration of salt. The changes in body composition were identical, qualitatively, with those previously shown.

In patient J. M. (Figure 5) there was a decline in the systolic pressure, but little change in the diastolic. The loss of body weight was at about the same rate as in the other patients and was halted by the addition of salt-free protein. Figure 6 shows a complete failure in that the blood pressure was unaffected. Judging from the excretion of urinary chlorides, however, there is reason to believe that the patient did not adhere strictly to the diet. Finally, 2 shorter experiments are depicted in Figure 7. In both subjects, the blood pressure declined almost, but not quite, to normal values. Again one sees definite and

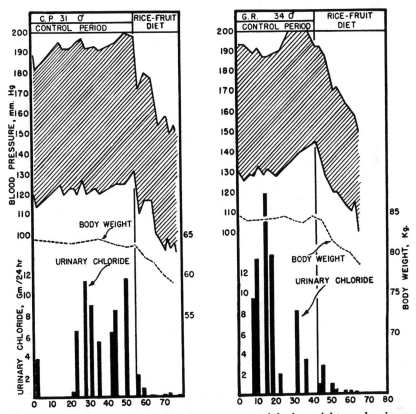

FIGURE 7. The course of the blood pressure, total body weight, and urinary chloride excretion in subjects C. P. and G. R.

continuing loss of weight as long as the unmodified rice-fruit diet is employed. In the eighth subject, the blood pressure was unaffected although there was some relief of symptoms (Table 3).

Discussion

There can be no doubt that the rice-fruit diet produces a decrease in the blood pressure of some hypertensive patients. It is known, of course, that hospitalization itself frequently causes a decline in the

TABLE 3. Changes in the Composition of the Body in 7 Male Hypertensive Subjects
Attributable to the Rice-Fruit Diet

Subject	Total Body S. G. of Weight, Kg.	Body	Weight in Kilograms Body Fat	SCN Space	Dry Bone	Total Inactive	Active
L. A.							
Control 87.7		1.045	23.24	17.33	3.51	44.08	43.62
RF 38 .... 80.3		1.050	19.27	13.35	3.51	36.13	44.17
K. M.							
Control 75.9		1.048	18.98	16.13	3.04	38.15	37.75
RF 38 .... 67.6		1.060	12.84	14.35	3.04	30.23	37.37
H. H.							
Control 75.1		1.080	7.36	22.83	3.00	33.19	41.91
RF 38 .... 67.6		1.088	4.06	18.52	3.00	25.58	42.02
A. B.							
Control 77.2		1.059	15.05	17.90	3.09	36.04	41.16
RF 38 .... 68.4		1.064	11.63	15.12	3.09	29.84	39.36
C. M.							
Control 78.7		1.048	19.68	17.55	3.15	40.38	38.32
RF 46 .... 68.4		1.057	14.02	16.45	3.15	33.62	34.78
J. M.							
Control 76.2		1.044	20.57	19.25	3.05	42.87	33.33
RF 46 .... 66.4		1.052	15.30	17.05	3.05	35.40	31.00
C. P.							
Control 63.3		1.085	4.43	16.40	2.53	23.36	39.94
RF 23 .... 60.6		...	...	14.50	2.53	...	...
Average change in kg., total ..... −8.55		...	−4.63	−2.69	...	−7.32	−1.23
Average change in kg/week ..... −1.47		...	−0.80	−0.47	...	−1.28	−0.19

NOTE. The symbols RF 38, RF 46, etc., indicate the number of days after the institution of the rice-fruit diet. S. G. refers to specific gravity, SCN to thiocyanate.

blood pressure of such patients, but in the present study there was no
decrease in the resting blood pressure of the 8 hypertensive subjects
after the first few days of the control periods. Day-to-day variations
in the blood pressure, some of which were relatively large, were noted
throughout the experiments, but such changes were not systematic.
Coincident with the institution of the rice-fruit diet there was an impressive decrease in the blood pressure of 4 of the 8 subjects. In 2 of
the 4, the blood pressure returned to normal levels, and in the other
2 the levels were approaching normal when the experiments had to be
discontinued. The addition of 40 gm. of sodium-free animal protein
to the daily diet (in 5 subjects) did not affect the blood pressure. The
depressor effect of the rice-fruit regimen was neither abolished nor
enhanced by the measure, considerable doubt thus being cast on the
justification of the low-protein feature of the rice-fruit regimen. On

the other hand, the addition of 10 gm. of salt to the daily diet in 3 subjects produced a prompt rise in the systolic and diastolic blood pressures as well as a prompt return of unusually severe headache and other symptoms.

Common to all 8 subjects was a steady loss of weight, which began immediately after institution of the rice-fruit diet and continued at the rate of about 1.5 kg. per week until the diet was abandoned or modified. None of the subjects in the present study had visible edema, and determination of the thiocyanate space during the control period indicated that only 1 of the subjects (H. H.) had a significant increase in the volume of extracellular fluid. Judging from measurements on 6 of the subjects, the rice-fruit diet invariably produced a relatively marked decline in the extracellular fluid volume. Just as striking was the loss of body fat. In addition 3 of the subjects lost significant amounts of active body tissue. These findings are similar to those obtained in normal young men by the use of a semistarvation diet (15) in that body fat and probably active tissue were consumed for the production of energy. They differed from those due to semistarvation in that the rice-fruit diet produced a definite decline in the thiocyanate space, a phenomenon that is doubtless attributable to the low sodium content of the diet. The loss of significant amounts of active tissue by 3 of our subjects suggests that in some, if not in all, of the 8 subjects a negative nitrogen balance prevailed. The abrupt cessation of weight loss when salt-free protein was added to the diets lends credibility to this view. Furthermore, it is not unreasonable to believe that any human subject receiving the rice-fruit diet begins to lose active body tissue in significant amounts if the diet is continued long enough.

Also common to all 8 of the subjects was a decline in serum cholesterol levels. This result, which was noted previously by Kempner and by Schwartz and Merlis, is at variance with the claim that serum cholesterol levels in the human being cannot be influenced by dietary means.

Summary

The rice-fruit diet induces a lowering of the blood pressure and an amelioration of symptoms in some hypertensive patients. It also induces a rapid loss of body weight, a result that may be desirable in some patients. In the earlier phases of the treatment, the loss of weight is attributable to a loss of extracellular fluid and of fat. Later there is probably a significant loss of active body tissue as well. The semistarvation feature of the rice-fruit diet may be significantly modified by the addition of an adequate amount of protein, which, if provided in a sodium-free form, does not interfere with the depressor effect of the regimen. Finally, the use of the rice-fruit diet does not, in all probability, constitute a therapeutic weapon against the cause or causes of essential hypertension. The diet is of importance in that it provides the investigator with a relatively safe means of lowering the blood pressure for fairly long periods of time in some hypertensive patients. To the clinician it provides a temporary means of relieving symptoms attributable to hypertension, but it is a measure that is dangerous in some patients and is curative in none.

Questions and Discussion

DR. IRVINE MCQUARRIE (MINNEAPOLIS): My research associates and I are greatly interested in the data presented by Dr. Chapman and his colleagues because they are consistent with the results of experiments of another type which we obtained some years ago. I take the liberty of presenting here some of the latter which demonstrate the hypertensive effect of an excessive intake of sodium and the antagonistic role of potassium. This study, which I wish to report very briefly, grew out of the chance observation that one of our 14-year-old boys, L. R., after being brought out of a precomatose state, manifested an inordinate craving for salt. He said, "I don't want any more sugar with the insulin, I want salt."

At first, while on ward rounds, I explained his craving for salt very glibly as being due most likely to the fact that he had vomited an undetermined number of times and had thereby lost hydrochloric acid. He had not perspired excessively and had no signs whatever of adrenal insufficiency. After his diabetes was under good control, it became apparent that a loss of chloride from vomiting was not an adequate explanation. He still craved salt and so was admitted to the metabolic ward for investigation into the cause of this craving. When allowed to consume from a weighed container what salt he required to satisfy his abnormal taste, it was found that he ingested as much as from 80 to 90 gm. a day, and, of course, drank extra water also. Special clinical tests for adrenal insufficiency were found to be quite negative, and the craving for salt was unassuaged by the administration of adrenal cortical extract.

Throughout the period of study the basic diet, which contained slightly more than 1 gm. of sodium and 1 gm. of potassium in 24 hours, was kept constant. The insulin dose, likewise kept constant, was set at a level that would permit continuous mild glycosuria, for our interest at the time centered largely on the effect that variations in the electrolyte intake might have on the diabetic glycosuria. I will not go into that aspect of the study here, except to say that the degree

517

of glycosuria was significantly decreased by the excessive ingestion of salt. Our exhilaration over this latter observation was dampened, however, when it was found that coincidental with the apparent improvement in the carbohydrate metabolism, the patient's blood pressure had increased from average basal values of 114 mm. Hg systolic and 75 diastolic to 185 systolic and 110 diastolic. The results of one such study are presented in Figure 1. You will note that the hypertension induced by this high-sodium, low-potassium regimen disappeared following withdrawal of the extra sodium chloride. This fall in pressure coincided with excretion of the extra sodium chloride and water, which had been retained during the period of excessive intake.

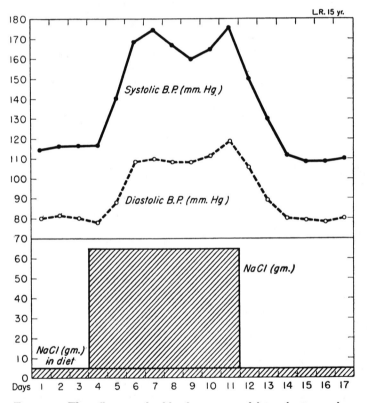

FIGURE 1. The effect on the blood pressure of ingesting excessive amounts of sodium chloride (64 gm. daily) together with a low-potassium diet. Subject: L. R., an insulin-treated, diabetic boy, aged 15 years. (The data represented in this figure and in the three following are taken from I. McQuarrie, W. H. Thompson, and J. A. Anderson: J. Nutrition 11:77, 1936.)

An adequate explanation of the craving was never found, but its intensity is known to have decreased somewhat at a later time. A point in the family history which was revealed belatedly may be significant. The patient's older brother was reported to be a salt craver, and was said to have been under medical care for high blood pressure at the Veterans' Hospital.

That the effect of an excessive intake of sodium chloride on the blood pressure is not peculiar to persons afflicted with an abnormal craving for salt is indicated by less dramatic data from studies on other diabetic patients treated similarly (Figs. 2, 3, and 4). These latter figures

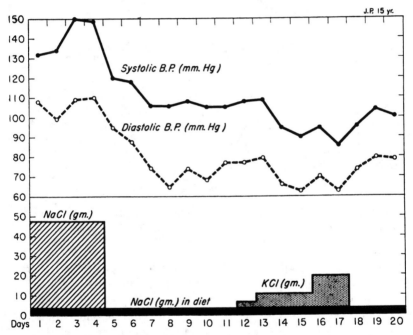

FIGURE 2. A comparison of the effect on the blood pressure of a high-potassium, low-sodium intake with that of a high-sodium, low-potassium intake. Subject: J. P., a 15-year-old girl with insulin-treated diabetes.

likewise show the antagonistic effect of the potassium ion, so far as the blood pressure response is concerned. Hypertension was not induced by an excessive intake of sodium chloride unless the potassium intake was minimal. One part of potassium appears to be sufficient to nullify the hypertensive effect of several chemically equivalent amounts of sodium. We believe, therefore, that the role of potassium

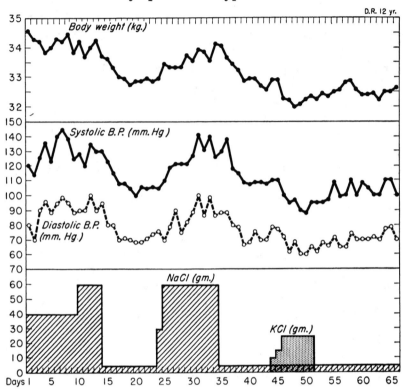

FIGURE 3. The effect on the blood pressure of a high-sodium, low-potassium regimen compared with that of a high-potassium, low-sodium intake. Subject: D. R., a 12-year-old girl with mild diabetes; no insulin used.

as well as that of sodium must be taken into account in studies relating to the effects of electrolytes on the arterial pressure.

DR. M. JAY FLIPSE (MIAMI): It was a pleasure to hear Dr. Chapman report his results on 8 patients treated for hypertension with a low-salt diet and to note the careful controls carried out on his study.

In a publication* we described 32 cases treated with a rice-fruit routine, of which group 20 obtained a successful reduction in the blood pressure. Subsequently 14 of the 32 patients were given a modification of the rice diet with the addition of meat and vegetables. Of the 14 given this modified diet, 10 maintained a successful result.

In 1950 we presented an additional 64 cases before the Florida Medical Association at their April meeting and our over-all results were better than in our initial study. Forty-eight cases obtained successful

*South. M. J. 40: 721–728 (September) 1947.

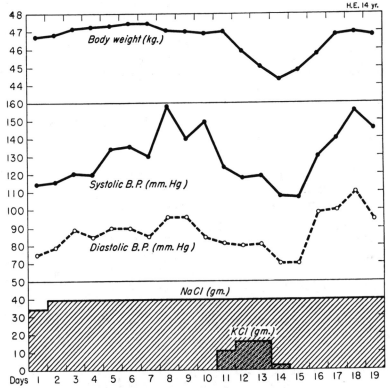

FIGURE 4. The antagonistic effect of potassium on arterial hypertension induced by a high-sodium, low-potassium regimen. Subject: H. E., a 14-year-old, insulin-treated, diabetic girl.

results in reducing a previously elevated blood pressure under the rice-fruit diet. We later modified the diet in 37 of these patients by the addition of meat and vegetables, with successful maintenance of the blood pressure levels in 23.

We have had no difficulty with excessive weight loss in our patients on our low-salt routines. In some instances it has been necessary to devise methods to insure an adequate intake of food. One such method was to prepare the food with a blender and reduce it to liquid form. We found that patients who were not able to eat sufficient rice to maintain body weight could be persuaded to drink the concoction and thus avoid weight loss. We also modified our rice-fruit diet as soon as possible and thus avoided the tendency toward weight loss on the strict routine. Since our patients were ambulatory, private patients, it was impossible to follow them up with complete laboratory studies.

Nevertheless, in the studies that were made we noted a reduction in the blood cholesterol to normal levels, a return of excessive non-protein nitrogen to normal levels, and no tendency toward anemia.

From the standpoint of clinical evaluation, in our successful cases there were improvement in the subjective symptoms, improvement in the vascular changes noted in the eyegrounds, improvement in electro-cardiographic abnormalities, a loss of edema, and in general a better physical condition in the patients after treatment than before the institution of dietotherapy.

Some of our earliest cases have now been followed for 5 years and have maintained improvement. It is noteworthy that on the basis of mortality only 2 of our patients have succumbed, both of these from causes unrelated to cardiovascular renal pathology. Three of our unsuccessful cases have succumbed, 1 from malignant disease, 1 from coronary disease, and 1 from a cerebral vascular accident.

During the last year we have deviated from the strict rice routine and have been utilizing the 200 mg. sodium diets recommended by Drs. Grollman and Harrison and others. Our primary difficulty with these diets has been the maintenance of a sodium content low enough to obtain results, particularly since we have been dealing with private ambulatory patients who are compelled to supervise their own diets at home.

In regard to the danger of our low-sodium dietotherapy in hypertension, we have noted only 1 patient who showed evidence of sodium deprivation. This patient was taking mercurials and ammonium salts in an attempt to increase his elimination of sodium. In the majority of instances we have avoided the use of these medications and believe that the diet is safe for use in private practice.

It is recognized that perhaps some of our patients cheat from time to time and that their sodium intake is somewhat higher than the previous 200 mg. which we have specified in our routine. However, in many persons an intake of 400 or even 500 mg. daily does not produce an increase in the pressure after the hypertension has once been controlled by the more rigid routines.

Some of our patients have had pressures of 250 systolic and 150 diastolic mm. Hg. We have found that in many such cases an ultimate result of 150 systolic and 90 diastolic can be obtained with the low-sodium diets. In others, while the pressure may not return to the normal level, benefits accrue in both subjective and objective findings that make the routine well worth while.

DR. JOHN W. GOFMAN: Inasmuch as I was the only one who spoke this morning about the effect on serum cholesterol levels, I must presume that it is I that am being misquoted by Dr. Chapman to the effect that the blood cholesterol does not drop on a diet of this type. This is not what I said, to set the record straight. I said one can put patients on a low fat, low cholesterol diet and the blood cholesterol may or may not drop.

In many cases, even though the blood cholesterol does not drop, the level of molecules in the S_f 10–20 class will show a significant reduction. What I pointed out was that since these molecules represent a very small fraction of the total cholesterol, even though this level of the molecules drops in half, one may not see it in a total cholesterol determination.

But there *are* many, many cases on a low fat diet, nothing like the Kempner rice diet, that according to the routine techniques show very marked and significant drops in the blood cholesterol.

DR. CHAPMAN: I merely wish to set the record further right; there was no misquotation at all. I did not attribute to Dr. Gofman the notion that it is impossible to influence serum cholesterol levels by dietary means. That is a statement that has appeared in the literature over and over again. It was my impression that that notion was alluded to this morning.

As regards the other material that was presented, I do think it ought to be pointed out again that extreme limitations of the salt intake are still potentially dangerous, particularly in patients who have elevated BUN's or other signs of compromised renal function. As to Dr. McQuarrie's material, I have no comment to make, mainly because we have no information on the potassium intake of our patients.

...... *by* IRVINE H. PAGE, ROBERT D. TAYLOR,

and A. C. CORCORAN

Pyrogens in the Treatment of
Malignant Hypertension

MALIGNANT hypertension is a disease which seriously endangers life and usually runs its fatal course within two years. The urgency of treatment is therefore understandable. Measures become acceptable to the patient and the physician which under less trying circumstances would not be entertained. It is in this light that we view the treatment of malignant hypertension with pyrogens.

But first I want to define what we mean by the malignant syndrome, or malignant hypertension. It is a syndrome usually engrafted upon pre-existing essential hypertension, although it may appear without prior cardiovascular disease. Arterial pressure is persistently greatly elevated, especially the diastolic. The eyeground changes are usually characteristic, consisting of papilledema, exudates, hemorrhages, vascular sclerosis, and constriction and edema of the retina. Exceptional cases occur in which the eyegrounds are not involved. Hematuria is usually present at some stage, as well as proteinuria. Renal blood flow and renal excretory function may be almost normal at the outset, but become impaired at an extraordinarily rapid rate. There is electrocardiographic and roentgenologic evidence of progressive hypertensive heart disease. The beta globulin fraction of the plasma proteins is relatively and absolutely elevated even after extraction of lipids. The ultracentrifuge pattern shows a high incidence of the supposedly atherogenic S_f 10–20 lipoprotein molecules in the plasma. An example of these abnormal Tiselius and ultracentrifuge patterns is shown in Figure 1.

The loss of body weight is progressive and striking. While the course of the disease is irregular, most patients die within 2 years, though some have been known to live as long as 11. Spontaneous remission has occurred in a very few, but the number is altogether too scant.

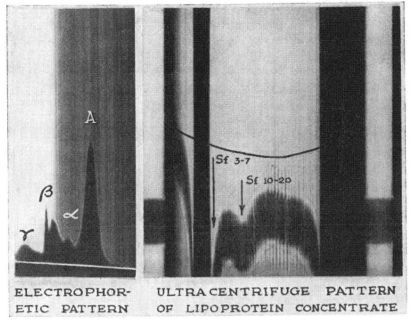

ELECTROPHOR-   ULTRA CENTRIFUGE   PATTERN
ETIC PATTERN   OF LIPOPROTEIN CONCENTRATE

FIGURE 1. This figure illustrates the large beta globulin peak in the electrophoresis pattern and the large number of S_f 10–20 molecules described by Gofman in the ultracentrifuge pattern.
Electrophoretic studies carried out in phosphate buffer, pH 7.8, ionic strength μ-0.16. Ultracentrifuge studies carried out using density of 1.0623. (Density adjusted with NaCl, 5 times the concentration present in serum.)

Treatment until the past 15 years was almost entirely expectant. In 1934 Dr. George Heuer performed anterior nerve root sections on 6 of my malignant hypertensive patients (1). Dr. E. V. Allen had told me about the preliminary results of operations that had been initiated by Dr. Alfred Adson, Dr. G. E. Brown, Dr. W. M. Craig, and Dr. Allen on patients with essential hypertension. Theirs was surely pioneer work.

At that time we were blissfully unaware that malignant hypertension later was to be made a contraindication to operation. I think the reason we chose the malignant hypertensives was chiefly my fear. But Dr. Heuer, who had never done the operation or seen it done, had not the slightest qualms about his ability to perform it without mishap. And this proved to be the right view. After operation, to my great surprise, a reversal of the eyeground changes occurred rapidly, the blood pressure fell, and no significant deterioration in renal function was observed (2). For a while it seemed as though this operation were the answer to the problem of malignant hypertension. But with further experience it became evident that not all patients responded and that after one to several years, many had reverted to the pre-operative state, and the disease pursued its inexorable course.

With the introduction of the surgical procedures of Dr. Smithwick and the late Dr. Peet, the operative risk was reduced and the operation re-established as a treatment for malignant hypertension with hopes of success. Indeed, Dr. Smithwick's figures show some of the best results in this group, so that it might well be debated whether sympathectomy should not be tried as the first assault on the disease. Currently our opinion is that pyrogen should be tried initially, but this is contingent on the assumption that the results with pyrogen will be as good as or better than those we have already obtained.

Kempner's retinal photographs convinced us that the rice diet also had to be considered a possible treatment. We, among others, have duplicated Kempner's results in a few patients. Unfortunately, there is a large residue of patients, including 6 we studied in 1944–1945, who do not respond to the rice diet and go on to death without remission of vascular disease. Our own experience has been considerably greater with the drastic low-salt diets because of our belief, and we think partial proof (Corcoran et al., 3), that the chief merit of the rice diet is its extremely low salt content. Undoubtedly some striking results are obtained with these low-salt diets, but again there is a goodly residue of failures and, so far as we know, no way short of trial to separate the potential failures from successes. And it must not be forgotten that diet requires several weeks' trial before the outcome can be predicted. These weeks may be crucial ones, and if failure is the verdict, there may be little renal function or time left for trial of other methods of treatment.

Ten years or more ago, with Dr. A. C. Corcoran, Dr. Robert Taylor, and Dr. O. M. Helmer, we were led to approach the problem from still another angle, namely, the injection of extracts of kidneys. Most of you know that we held, and still hold, the view that there is contained in the kidneys an antipressor of inhibitory substance which lowers the blood pressure. You also know that we have still not been able to prove this, though much suggestive evidence has been accumulated. One of the main sources of confusion was the occurrence of so-called "re-actions" to the injected kidney extract, consisting chiefly of backache, fever, and severe hypotension.

Since it was well known that fever lowers the blood pressure, the results with kidney extract could never be convincingly attributed to anything other than its fever-producing qualities. We were, however, able to show that the blood pressure fell in some cases even when fever was blocked by antipyretics. It was also known from the studies of Chasis *et al.* (6) that the renal vascular bed dilated when fever was elicited and that antipyretics did not prevent the dilatation.

Measurements of renal function in both hypertensive patients and dogs with experimental perinephric hypertension (Corcoran and Page, 4) showed that the injection of these kidney extracts over long periods of time caused an increase of diodrast clearance and a decrease in the ratio inulin/diodrast clearance, which persisted long after the last elevation of body temperature. These changes were interpreted as due to increased renal blood flow and a decrease in the proportion of water removed from the plasma by glomerular filtration. The mechanism of the change seems to be relaxation of the tone of the glomerular arterioles, both afferent and efferent.

In the past week, an excellent study by Stamler *et al.* (5) of the effects on circulatory dynamics of abscess formation in dogs has appeared. The authors show that this acute inflammation causes no change in the cardiac output and blood volume, concluding therefore that the sustained fall in the blood pressure is due to a decrease in the total peripheral resistance. They too find an increase in the renal blood flow which may account for a significant portion of the decreased peripheral resistance. A change in the cardiac output does not seem important under these particular circumstances as it does in patients given pyrogen. It is evident that more work is required before the mechanism of the hypotensive action of pyrogens and inflammation is known.

The careful work of Bradley *et al.* (7) has shown that pyrogenic inulin, in brief experiments in both normal and hypertensive patients given amidopyrine to prevent fever, causes profound hemodynamic changes. The cardiac output was increased as the result of an increase in both the pulse rate and stroke volume, as Grollman (8) had found in patients given typhoid vaccine. The total peripheral resistance decreased. In normal subjects and in some hypertensives, reciprocal changes in the peripheral resistance and cardiac output resulted in an adequate maintenance of the arterial pressure. In other hypertensives the arterial pressure fell, owing to a fall in the cardiac output. The renal vascular bed exhibited relatively greater vasodilatation than the rest of the circulatory system. Whether the same changes occur in our patients after prolonged treatment with pyrogen has not been determined.

Dr. Taylor and I (9) studied a wide variety of proteins injected into renal hypertensive dogs in the hope that further light might be thrown on the subject. When fever and leucocytosis occurred, the arterial pressure usually fell. Attempts were then made to extract hypotensive substances from pus and leucocytes, but with indifferent success. The reaction of the body to the pyrogenic substance seemed to be a necessary prerequisite to its hypotensive action. This is illustrated by the well-known fact that an abscess, no matter what the infecting organism, in both patients and dogs, is one of the most effective ways of lowering the blood pressure known. We therefore tried a number of ways of producing abscesses in patients. True, they lowered the pressure, but the whole thing had to be abandoned as impracticable. But we came away with a healthy respect for the hypotensive qualities of tissue reaction to irritants of the fever-producing sort.

The next step obviously was the use of bacterial pyrogens given by vein. A number of these were tried without its being demonstrated that one had any great superiority over another. An unfortunate outcome of intravenous treatment with killed typhoid bacilli led us away from the injection of particulate pyrogens. At that time Pyromen, an experimental water-soluble pyrogen, was being prepared by the Baxter Laboratories and was made available to us. This extract is the one subsequently employed by us and has proved to be quite satisfactory.

Let me describe to you how the pyrogen is used in a typical patient who responds, and then we shall be in a position to discuss its difficulties and shortcomings.

After as long a control period in the hospital as can be safely tolerated by the patient—and this is usually about 1 month—single intravenous injections 5 or 6 days weekly are given in amounts sufficient to cause a rise in temperature to 101°–103° F. each day. The first dose is 0.5 cc. of a solution containing 50 gamma of solid per cc. Thereafter, the amount is determined by the temperature response of the previous day. If tolerance does not develop, treatment is continued as long as improvement is observed. The average length of time before a change in the patient may be noted is from 2 to 3 weeks, and treatment is usually continued for from 6 weeks to 3 months.

The retinae first show improvement, especially papilledema, followed by resorption of hemorrhage and much of the exudate (Fig. 2).

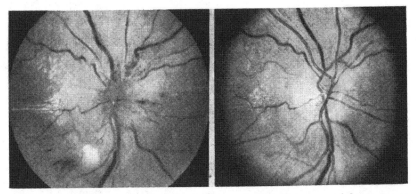

FIGURE 2. Eyeground photographs before and after the successful treatment of malignant hypertension with pyrogen.

Vision may be greatly improved. Hematuria and proteinuria may lessen sharply or disappear. The ability to concentrate urine and the renal blood flow may be temporarily depressed, but later may be restored not only to control levels but toward normal. "Tubular mass," as measured by para-aminohippurate, changes but little. The arterial pressure slowly falls and may reach normal levels, but after a period of weeks, it tends to rise again. After the discontinuance of treatment, it may even return to its pretreatment level without the reappearance of the signs of the malignant phase of the disease (Fig. 3).

The selection of patients for pyrogen therapy depends chiefly on a careful appraisal of renal function. This must be adequate to excrete para-aminohippurate at a rate of at least 35 mg. per minute per 1.73 sq. m. of body surface or to concentrate urine to a specific gravity of 1.020 or above. If the functional values exceed these, the widespread vascular disease is more likely to be reversed by prolonged pyrogen treatment, and a recurrence of the malignant syndrome is unlikely. Cardiac decompensation is no contraindication, as some patients have done well on pyrogen who failed to respond satisfactorily to digitalis, sodium restriction, and diuretics (Fig. 4).

In addition to the physical requirements, there are psychological ones as well. The patient must be intelligent enough to appreciate the significance of his disease and hence willingly adjust to the inconvenience of prolonged treatment and to the discomfort of repeated febrile reactions. If he lacks this willingness, sympathectomy or drastic low-sodium diets may be tried.

The best type of pyrogen to employ has not been established. We have used a variety of them and come only to very preliminary con-

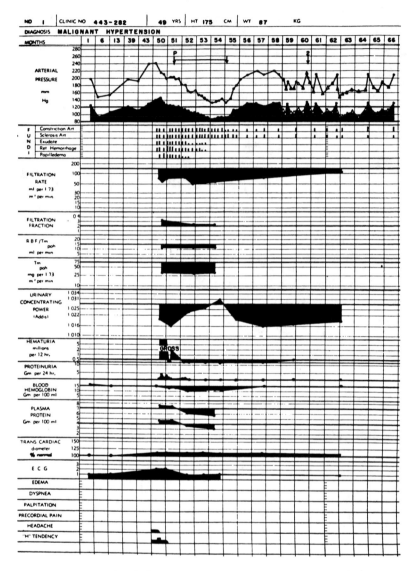

FIGURE 3. An example of the successful treatment with pyrogen of a patient with malignant hypertension. The solid dots on the arterial pressure scale represent weekly averages of blood pressure measurements taken twice daily; the triangles represent single measurements as an outpatient. The eyegrounds are graded on a + to 4+ scale. The remainder of the scales are self-explanatory. Between the two arrows from the 51st to 55th month, pyrogen was given.

clusions. The coccal organisms were discarded as a source because patients felt excessively ill following their injection. Killed tubercle bacilli often induced chronic draining abscesses when injected intramuscularly. Typhoid bacilli induced hematuria and possibly focal nephritis in 2 patients and hence was not further used. The need is for a powerful pyrogen which does not produce tolerance.

In patients with moderate signs of the syndrome and where a long period of hospitalization is impossible for whatever reason, lumbodorsal sympathectomy is our choice. This offers a reasonable chance that the disease will be arrested for from 2 to 3 years.

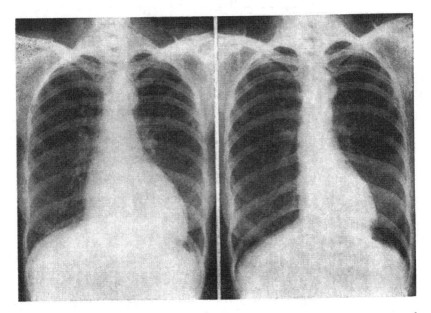

FIGURE 4. X-rays of the heart before and after the successful treatment of malignant hypertension with pyrogen.

If hospitalization is impossible or the response to pyrogen unsatisfactory, severe sodium restriction may be added to the program. I should point out that it is seldom our practice to combine these treatments for the reason that no clear evaluation of the separate treatments would thus be possible. But where a therapeutic goal is the only factor involved, there would seem to be no reason why a drastic low-sodium diet, pyrogen, and such drugs as Veriloid should not be given concurrently (Fig. 5).

Among the first group of our patients (10), 19 with malignant

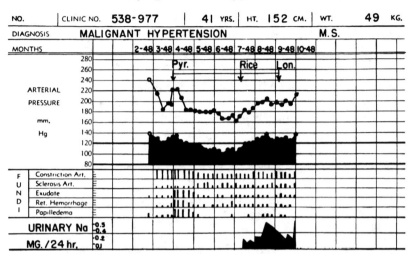

FIGURE 5. An example of a partially successful treatment with pyrogen. At Pyr., pyrogen was given. Three months later it was stopped and a rice diet was given, followed 2 months later by a drastic low-sodium diet.

hypertension were treated. Most of these had been in the hospital for 3 weeks or more before treatment was started. In some cases we should have preferred longer control periods, as in our management of essential hypertensives, but the downhill progress of the disease precluded it. The blood pressure averages in these patients did not show so great a fall in the control period as is common in patients with essential hypertension.

Nine of this original group are still alive, an average of 44 months since treatment was stopped. Five discontinued treatment against advice and have since died of cerebral hemorrhage; the other five died of cerebral hemorrhage 10 to 37 months after treatment was stopped (11).

In a later group of 10 patients, 6 did not respond well to treatment. This is a higher proportion of non-responders than in the former group. The pyrogen used had been changed and did not seem satisfactory, but we cannot be sure of this. Some patients show only small rises in temperature, even at the beginning of treatment, and these are least likely to do well.

Treatment should be continued as long as the signs of malignancy continue to regress. These are usually in the following order: papilledema, hemorrhages and exudates, poor vision, hematuria, proteinuria, decrease in renal blood flow and decrease in concentrating power, hypertensive heart disease. The major changes for the better in the eyegrounds and heart occur more gradually, from 2 to 4 months usually being required. The patient is then treated as though one with essential hypertension.

I need hardly say this is an unpleasant treatment. It is expensive of bed space in the hospital and of the patient's time. The degree of fever elicited is a helpful guide to treatment, and unless extremely distressing, which it seldom is, it need not be suppressed by antipyretics. But considering the danger of the disease to the life of the patient, it is a small price to pay for its benefits.

With this record in the past, what then of the future? Clearly, the problem of tolerance to exogenous pyrogens of the type used must somehow be solved. Not only does the development of tolerance gradually interfere with the clinical response, but its existence increases the patient's discomfort by making it necessary to avoid the use of antipyretics until the day's maximum fever has been recorded. What is required is a stable, soluble pyrogen of known composition and indefinitely reproducible efficacy. There are various evidences that the pyrogenic agents formed at the sites of exudation in the body differ from exogenous pyrogens in that they do not elicit tolerance. Consistent with this view were the prolonged clinical responses we observed in patients with cold abscesses or with empyemas. Unfortunately these materials are difficult to prepare, most of the preparations are grossly impure and relatively insoluble, and their study is only beginning. However, as they become better characterized, it may be that pyrogenic preparations of stable, reproducible fever-producing qualities can be prepared, and, should this be the case, treatment with pyrogens can be robbed of many of its discomforts and uncertainties by the simultaneous use of pyrogen and antipyretic.

To recapitulate: Our current views on the management of malignant hypertension are: If renal tubular excretory capacity is above 50 per cent of normal, regardless of the severity of the necrotizing arteriolitis, pyrogen is to be tried. If the renal reserve is more severely reduced, it may still be tried, since occasionally some patients do surprisingly well.

Questions and Discussion

DR. ARLIE R. BARNES: You know, as I listen to this discussion, I am reminded of the old saying that a medical man is a physician who knows a lot about diseases but knows little to do about them, and a surgeon is a physician who doesn't know much about diseases but could do a lot about them. In this discussion it looks to me as though the surgeons have the advantage so far.

DR. REGINALD H. SMITHWICK: I know I have already said too much but I can't help taking this occasion to disagree with my good friend Dr. Page a little bit regarding the treatment of malignant hypertension.

If the diagnosis is based primarily upon eyeground changes and if the patient still has good renal function, I certainly would urge that that patient be operated on as the treatment of first choice. These operated cases have really done very well. In the survival curves that I have shown you, about 50 per cent of our patients with malignant hypertension were alive from 5 to 10 years after the operation. They are composed of the group that still had satisfactory renal function as well as those that had very poor renal function to begin with. If I should separate the cases according to the status of the kidney at the time they were operated on, the survival rate would be very, very high—from 80 to 90 per cent, I believe, for patients with satisfactory renal function. On that ground, I should feel that one certainly ought not to waste any time operating on these patients.

I should like to ask Dr. Page one question about the potential hazard of these febrile episodes. Years ago I had a little experience with pyrogens. At one time I wrote a couple of articles about the treatment of peripheral vascular disease by intermittent injections of typhoid vaccine. We found after a while we had some catastrophes in the nature of coronary thromboses and cerebral vascular accidents and

534

even massive thromboses of the iliac and femoral vessels. We had these complications even in middle-aged persons.

Of course, they had vascular disease, but as we studied the response to fever, we found that in the prechill stage, if one watches the capillaries in the nail-bed and the corpuscles going through them, there is a period where circulation virtually ceases. It was presumably at this point that the thromboses occurred. In the febrile stages the circulation increases tremendously. Therefore I should think that with this form of treatment if a person did have a good deal of vascular disease here, there, or elsewhere, he would be subject to the hazard of serious thrombosis at a certain phase of the reaction.

DR. WILLIAM KUBICEK (MINNEAPOLIS): I certainly enjoyed Dr. Page's complete frankness in this discussion. I was reminded in the course of it of a few points that might be of interest concerning the question of the mechanism of the changes in the renal circulation. The question is whether the pyrogen itself or the increase in temperature causes the increase in the renal circulation.

Dr. Kottke and I took some interest in this problem some time ago, and being in the Department of Physical Medicine, we of course thought of the diathermy machine to increase the temperature.

We applied diathermy heat to hypertensive patients by various types of diathermy machines. We noted either no change or a decrease in the renal circulation. This result caused us eventually to stop the experiments, for we feared we might be causing damage to the kidney tissue. Inasmuch as it was already somewhat damaged and the increase in temperature would increase the metabolism, and accompanying decrease in the circulation would probably be dangerous.

We tried conventional diathermy, which is by means of the older type of diathermy machine where large pads are placed on the skin and an electrical current is passed directly through the body. We applied a pad over the abdomen and one over the back and increased the body temperature, and we noted a decrease in the circulation in the kidneys.

Then we tried the short-wave diathermy, with an induction coil in various positions; again we produced the same decrease in the renal circulation. We wrapped the coil around the neck of the patient, thinking that we could possibly increase the temperature of the vital centers without increasing the temperature directly over the kidney. This again decreased the circulation through the kidney.

My primary concern here is the possible danger of increasing the temperature and consequently the metabolism of damaged kidney tissue without increasing the renal blood flow in proportion.

DR. PAGE: In response to Dr. Smithwick, I think it is fair to say that surgeons always want to get their fee before medical men do.— In seriousness, though, I think that until more evidence is available, it is premature to say whether surgery or treatment with pyrogens should be undertaken first. If you are a medical man, you will probably give pyrogen first. If you are surgically inclined, you will probably operate first. I think that Dr. Smithwick's point is well taken.

Now, as regards Dr. Kubicek, I am going to put my long gray beard on and say that a quarter of a century ago, when I was in Germany, the Germans had an idea that if you put a patient with acute Bright's disease on a diathermy machine and gave him a good cooking, it relaxed the blood vessels in his kidneys and that that was very good for him.

Well, after seeing a number of the patients being well cooked over there, I was not convinced. One of the first things I did when I got back to this country was to see if the blood flow in the kidneys could be raised by means of diathermy. Later we tried the same by means of inductothermy. We found that inductothermy didn't do any better than diathermy. In fact, just as Dr. Kubicek said this afternoon, it slightly lowers the blood flow.

I think his point is well taken, that the pyrogen itself has quite a different effect, and indeed, as Drs. Chasis and Goldring have shown, one can block the febrile response with amidopyrine and still get a marked increase in the renal blood flow. In practice, with the use of pyrogens other than typhoid vaccine, we have produced no bad effects on the renal blood flow in what is already a very bad situation.

DR. GEORGE N. AAGAARD: On behalf of the University, I should like to thank our distinguished speakers and those who have entered into the discussion. I should also like to thank our presiding chairmen and those of you who have made up such a large and interested audience for joining us during these three days in our efforts to honor Dr. Bell, Dr. Clawson, and Dr. Fahr.

BIBLIOGRAPHY

Bibliography

Anatomical Considerations of Hypertension, by Harry Goldblatt

1. R. Bright: Cases and observations illustrative of renal disease accompanied with the secretion of albuminous urine, Guy's Hosp. Rep. 1:339–379, 1836.

2. George Johnson: I. On certain points in the anatomy and pathology of Bright's disease of the kidney. II. On the influence of the minute blood vessels upon the circulation, Med.-Chir. Tr. (London) 51:57–78, 1868.

3. Sir William W. Gull and Henry G. Sutton: On the pathology of the morbid state commonly called Bright's disease with contracted kidney ("arterio-capillary fibrosis"), Med.-Chir. Tr. (London) 55:273–329, 1872.

4. Geoffrey Evans: A contribution to the study of arteriosclerosis, with special reference to its relation to chronic renal disease, Quart. J. Med. 14:215–282, 1921.

5. James W. Kernohan, Edward W. Anderson, and Norman M. Keith: The arterioles in cases of hypertension, Arch. Int. Med. 24:395–423, 1929.

6. Roy W. Scott, David P. Seecof, and Albert A. Hill: Arteriolar lesions of skeletal muscles in hypertension, Tr. A. Am. Physicians 48:283–288, 1933.

7. Frank C. Andrus: The relation of age and hypertension to the structure of the small arteries and arterioles in skeletal muscles, Am. J. Path. 12:635–654, 1936.

8. Leonhard Jores: Uber die Arteriosklerose der kleinen Organarterien und ihre Beziehungen zur Nephritis, Virchows Arch. f. path. Anat. 178:367–406, 1904.

9. Franz Volhard: The Kidney in Health and Disease, Philadelphia, Lea & Febiger, 1935.

10. Arthur M. Fishberg: Anatomic findings in essential hypertension, Arch. Int. Med. 35:650–668, 1925.

11. E. T. Bell and B. J. Clawson: Primary (essential) hypertension: A study of 420 cases, Arch. Path. 5:939–1002, 1928.

12. Alan R. Moritz and M. R. Oldt: Arteriolar sclerosis in hypertensive and non-hypertensive individuals, Am. J. Path. 13:679–728, 1937.

13. Harry Goldblatt, James Lynch, Raymon F. Hanzal, and Ward W. Summerville: Studies on experimental hypertension: I. The production of persistent elevation of systolic blood pressure by means of renal ischemia, J. Exper. Med. 59:347, 1934.

14. Harry Goldblatt: The Renal Origin of Hypertension (Monograph in American Lectures in Pathology), Springfield, Ill., Charles C. Thomas, 1949.

15. W. Stanley Hartroft and Charles H. Best: Hypertension of renal origin in rats following less than one week of choline deficiency in early life, Brit. Med. J. 1:423, 1949.

16. Sidney Sobin and Eugene Landis: Blood pressure of the rat during acute and chronic choline deficiency, Am. J. Physiol. 148:557–562, 1947.

17. John W. Gofman, Frank Lindgren, Harold Elliott, and William Mantz: The role of lipids and lipoproteins in atherosclerosis, Science 111:166, 1950.

18. H. Selye: Textbook of Endocrinology, ed. 2, Montreal, Acta Endocrinologica Inc., Medical Publishers, 1949.

19. Dorothy Loomis: Hypertension and necrotizing arteritis in the rat following renal infarction, Arch. Path. 41:231, 1946.

20. R. L. Holman: Acute necrotizing arteritis and auriculitis following uranium nitrate injury in dogs with altered plasma proteins, Am. J. Path. 17:359, 1941.

21. R. Dominguez: Effect on the blood pressure of the rabbit of arteriosclerosis and nephritis caused by uranium, Arch. Path. 5:577, 1928.

22. William J. Cromartie: Arteritis in rats with experimental renal hypertension, Am. J. Med. Sc. 206:66, 1943.

23. Talia Bali and Harry Goldblatt: Unpublished.

24. Eli Moschcowitz: The pathology of hypertension, J. A. M. A. 79:1196–1200, 1922.

25. C. Wilson and G. W. Pickering: Acute arterial lesions in rats with experimental renal hypertension, Clin. Sc. 3:343, 1938.

26. C. Wilson and F. D. Byrom: Renal changes in malignant hypertension, Lancet, 1939, p. 136.

27. F. D. Byrom and L. F. Dodson: The mechanism of the vicious circle in chronic hypertension, Clin. Sc. 8:1, 1949.

28. F. J. Kottke, W. G. Kubicek, and M. B. Visscher: Production of arterial hypertension by chronic renal artery nerve stimulation, Am. J. Physiol. 145:37–47, 1945.

29. M. C. Winternitz, D. Mylon, L. L. Waters, and R. Katzenstein: Studies on the relation of the kidney to cardiovascular disease, Yale J. Biol. & Med. 12:623, 1940.

30. Russell R. Holman: Experimental necrotizing arteritis in dogs: III. Bilateral nephrectomy as effective as heavy metal injury in its production, Am. J. Path. 19:147, 1943.

31. Arthur Grollman, E. E. Muirhead, and John Vanatta: Role of the kidney in pathogenesis of hypertension as determined by a study of the effects of bilateral nephrectomy and other experimental procedures on the blood pressure of the dog, Am. J. Physiol. 157:21, 1949.

32. J. F. Rinehart, D. D. Williams, and W. S. Cappeller: Adenomatous hyperplasia of the adrenal cortex associated with essential hypertension, Arch. Path. 32:169, 1941.

33. William S. Dempsey: The adrenal cortex in essential hypertension, Arch. Path. 34:1031, 1942.

34. I. Mark Scheinker: Hypertensive disease of the brain, Arch. Path. 36:289–296, 1943.

35. I. Mark Scheinker: Changes in cerebral veins in hypertensive brain disease and their relation to cerebral hemorrhage, Arch. Neurol. & Psychiat. 54:395–408, 1945.

36. I. Mark Scheinker: Alterations of cerebral capillaries in the early stage of arterial hypertension, Am. J. Path. 24:1, 211–221, 1948.

37. Arthur Lack et al.: Biomicroscopy of conjunctival vessels in hypertension, Am. Heart J. 38:5, 654–664, 1949.

Experimental Studies on Hypertension, by Arthur Grollman

1. E. T. Bell: Renal Diseases, Philadelphia, Lea & Febiger, 1946.

2. E. T. Bell and A. H. Pedersen: Causes of hypertension, Ann. Int. Med. 4:227, 1930.

3. A. Chanutin and E. B. Ferris, Jr.: Experimental renal insufficiency produced by partial nephrectomy; controlled diet, Arch. Int. Med. 49:767, 1932.

4. H. Goldblatt, J. Lynch, R. F. Hanzal, and W. W. Summerville: Studies on experimental hypertension; production of persistent elevation of systolic blood pressure by means of renal ischemia, J. Exper. Med. 59:347, 1934.

5. A. Grollman and J. R. Williams, Jr.: Experimental chronic hypertension in rat, Am. J. M. Sc. 204:73, 1942.

6. A. Grollman: Simplified procedure for producing chronic renal hypertension in mammal, Proc. Soc. Exper. Biol. & Med. 57:102, 1944.

7. J. R. Williams, Jr., T. R. Harrison, and A. Grollman: Simple method for determining systolic blood pressure of unanesthetized rat, J. Clin. Investigation 18:373, 1939.

8. B. W. Zweifach and E. Shorr, eds.: Transactions of the Third Conference on Factors Regulating Blood Pressure, Josiah Macy, Jr., Foundation, New York, 1949.

9. A. Grollman: Experimental hypertension in dog, Am. J. Physiol. 147:647, 1946.

10. L. McGregor: A new indirect method for taking blood pressure in animals, Arch. Path. 5:630, 1938.

11. R. Tigerstedt and P. G. von Bergmann: Niere und Kreislauf, Skandinav. Arch. f. Physiol. 8:223, 1898.

12. A. Grollman: Experimental chronic hypertension: Its mechanism and amelioration by use of various blood-pressure reducing substances, Special Publications, New York Acad. Sc. 3:99, 1946.

13. A. Grollman: in Recent Progress in Hormone Research 1:371, 1947.

14. A. Grollman: in Transactions of the First Conference on Factors Regulating Blood Pressure, Josiah Macy, Jr., Foundation, New York, 1947, p. 20.

15. A. Grollman: Experimental chronic hypertension in rabbit, Am. J. Physiol. 142: 666, 1944.

16. A. Grollman and B. Halpern: Renal lesions in chronic hypertension induced by unilateral nephrectomy in the rat, Proc. Soc. Exper. Biol. & Med. 71:394, 1949.

17. A. Grollman and C. Rule: Experimentally induced hypertension in parabiotic rats, Am. J. Physiol. 138:587, 1943.

18. A. Grollman, E. E. Muirhead, and J. Vanatta: Role of the kidney in pathogenesis of hypertension as determined by a study of the effects of bilateral nephrectomy and other experimental procedures on the blood pressure of the dog, Am. J. Physiol. 157:21, 1949.

19. A. Grollman et al.: Unpublished observations.

20. E. E. Muirhead, A. Grollman, and J. Vanatta: Hypertensive cardiovascular disease (malignant hypertension), Arch. Path. 50:137, 1950.

21. C. G. Child: Observations on pathological changes following experimental hypertension produced by constriction of renal artery, J. Exper. Med. 67:521, 1938.

22. H. Goldblatt: Studies on experimental hypertension; production of malignant phase of hypertension, J. Exper. Med. 67:809, 1938.

23. A. R. Moritz and M. R. Oldt: Arteriolar sclerosis in hypertensive and nonhypertensive individuals, Am. J. Path. 13:679, 1937.

24. E. E. Muirhead and A. Grollman: Am. J. Med., in press.

25. A. Grollman, T. R. Harrison, et al.: Sodium restriction in diet for hypertension, J. A. M. A. 129:533, 1945.

26. C. B. Chapman and T. B. Gibbons: The diet and hypertension, Medicine 29:29, 1950.

27. A. Grollman and T. R. Harrison: Effect of rigid sodium restriction on blood pressure and survival of hypertensive rats, Proc. Soc. Exper. Biol. & Med. 60:52, 1945.

28. G. A. Perera and D. W. Blood: Disturbance in salt and water metabolism in hypertension, Am. J. Med. 1:602, 1946.

29. M. E. Ellis and A. Grollman: The antidiuretic hormone in the urine in experimental and clinical hypertension, Endocrinology 44:415, 1949.

30. L. Eichelberger: Distribution of water and electrolytes between blood and skeletal muscle in experimental hypertension, J. Exper. Med. 77:205, 1943.

31. D. C. Laramore and A. Grollman: Am. J. Physiol. 161:278, 1950.

32. A. Grollman and A. Konnerth: In press.

33. A. Grollman, T. R. Harrison, and J. R. Williams, Jr.: Therapeutics of experimental hypertension, J. Pharmacol. & Exper. Therap. 69:76, 1940.

34. A. Grollman and T. R. Harrison: Further studies on separation from kidney tissue of substance capable of reducing blood pressure in experimentally induced hypertension, J. Pharmacol. & Exper. Therap. 78:174, 1943.

35. A. Grollman: Preparation of extracts from oxidized marine and other oils for reducing blood pressure in experimental and human chronic hypertension, J. Pharmacol. & Exper. Therap. 84:128, 1945.

36. F. Reichsman: Survival time of hypertensive rats receiving fish-oil extracts, Science 104:64, 1946.

37. K. S. Grimson: Sympathetic nervous system in neurogenic and renal hypertension; experimental correlation and clinical considerations, Arch. Surg. 43:284, 1941.

38. E. J. Farris, E. H. Yeakel, and H. S. Medoff: Development of hypertension in emotional gray Norway rats after air blasting, Am. J. Physiol. 144:331, 1945.

39. A. Grollman, J. A. McLean, and A. Konnerth: Unpublished observations.

40. E. O. Wheeler, P. D. White, E. W. Reed, and M. E. Cohen: Neurocirculatory asthenia (anxiety neurosis, effort syndrome, neurasthenia), J. A. M. A. 142:878, 1950.

41. A. Dubois: Note sur la tension artérielle chez les indigènes congolais, Ann. Soc. belge de méd. trop. 12:133, 1932.

42. W. G. Hartnett and H. E. Ratcliffe: Study in hypertension on southern Negroes, South. M. J. 41:847, 1949.

Experimental Hypertension in the Rabbit, by George W. Pickering

1. R. B. Blacket, A. DePoorter, G. W. Pickering, A. L. Sellers, and G. M. Wilson: Hypertension produced in the rabbit by long continued infusions of renin, Clin. Sc. 9:223, 1950.

2. R. B. Blacket, G. W. Pickering, and G. M. Wilson: The effects of prolonged infusions of noradrenaline and adrenaline on the arterial pressure of the rabbit, Clin. Sc. 9:247, 1950.

3. R. B. Blacket and A. L. Sellers: Unpublished observations, 1950.

4. A. Blalock: Experimental hypertension, Physiol. Rev. 20:159, 1940.

5. A. Blalock and S. E. Levy: Studies on etiology of renal hypertension, Ann. Surg. 106:826, 1937.

6. E. Braun-Menendez, J. C. Fasciolo, L. F. Leloir, and J. M. Muñoz: Substance causing renal hypertension, J. Physiol. 98:283, 1940.

7. A. Grollman: Experimental hypertension in dog, Am. J. Physiol. 147:647, 1946.

8. O. M. Helmer and I. H. Page: Purification and some properties of renin, J. Biol. Chem. 127:757, 1939.

9. G. Hessel: Uber Renin, Klin. Wchnschr. 17:843, 1938.

10. J. R. Hill and G. W. Pickering: Hypertension produced in rabbit by prolonged renin infusion, Clin. Sc. 4:207, 1939.

11. E. M. Landis, H. Montgomery, and D. Sparkman: Effects of pressor drugs and of saline kidney extracts on blood pressure and skin temperature, J. Clin. Investigation 17:189, 1938.

12. G. W. Pickering: Role of kidney in acute and chronic hypertension following renal artery constriction in rabbit, Clin. Sc. 5:229, 1945.

13. G. W. Pickering and M. Prinzmetal: Some observations on renin, pressor substance contained in normal kidney, together with method for its biological assay, Clin. Sc. 3:211, 1938.

14. G. W. Pickering, M. Prinzmetal, and A. R. Kelsall: Assay of renin in rabbits with experimental renal hypertension, Clin. Sc. 4:401, 1942.

15. R. E. Shipley, O. M. Helmer, and K. G. Kohlstaedt: Presence in blood of principle which elicits sustained pressor response in nephrectomized animals, Am. J. Physiol. 149:708, 1947.

16. R. Tigerstedt and P. G. von Bergmann: Niere und Kreislauf, Skandinav. Arch. f. Physiol. 8:223, 1898.

The Renin-Angiotonin Pressor System, by Irvine H. Page

1. R. Tigerstedt and P. G. von Bergmann: Niere und Kreislauf, Skandinav. Arch. f. Physiol. 8:223, 1898.

2. A. Bingel and E. Strauss: Uber die blutdrucksteigernde Substanz der Niere, Deutsche Arch. f. klin. Med. 96:476, 1909.

3. R. M. Pearce: An experimental study of the influence of kidney extracts and the serum of animals with renal lesions upon the blood pressure, J. Exper. Med. 11:430, 1909.

4. S. Vincent and W. Sheen: The effects of intravascular injections of extracts of animal tissues, J. Physiol. 29:242, 1903.

5. J. B. Collip: A non-specific pressor principle derived from a variety of tissues, J. Physiol. 66:416, 1928.

6. G. Hessel and A. Hartwick: Chemische Eigenschaften des blutdrucksteigernden Prinzips in Niernautolysaten, Zentralbl. f. inn. Med. 53:626, 1932.

7. A. Hartwick and G. Hessel: Experimentelle Untersuchungen zur Kreislaufwirkung körpereigene Stoffe: I. Die Wirkung frischer und autolysierte Organpressäfte auf den Blutdruck, Zentralbl. f. inn. Med. 53:612, 1932.

8. G. Hessel: Uber Renin, Klin. Wchnschr. 17:843, 1938.

9a. O. M. Helmer and I. H. Page: Purification and some properties of renin, J. Biol. Chem. 127:747, 1939.

9b. W. D. Collings, J. W. Remington, H. W. Hays, and V. A. Drill: A modified method for the preparation of renin, Proc. Soc. Exper. Biol. & Med. 44:87, 1940.

9c. O. Schales: Preparation and properties of renin, J. Am. Chem. Soc. 64:561, 1942.

9d. Y. T. Katz and H. Goldblatt: Studies on experimental hypertension: XXI. The purification of renin, J. Exper. Med. 78:67, 1943.

9e. T. Astrup and A. Birch-Andersen: Purification of renin by means of protein precipitating agents, Nature, London 160:570, 1947.

9f. J. Marshall and G. E. Wakerlin: Purification of renin, Federation Proc. 7:78, 1948.

10. K. G. Kohlstaedt, O. M. Helmer, and I. H. Page: Activation of renin by blood colloids, Proc. Soc. Exper. Biol. & Med. 39:1214, 1938.

11. I. H. Page and O. M. Helmer: A crystalline pressor substance, angiotonin, resulting from the reaction between renin and renin-activator, Proc. Central Soc. Clin. Research 12:17, 1939.

12. I. H. Page and O. M. Helmer: A crystalline pressor substance (angiotonin) resulting from the reaction between renin and renin-activator, J. Exper. Med. 71:29, 1940.

13. J. M. Muñoz, E. Braun-Menendez, J. C. Fasciolo, and L. F. Leloir: Hypertensin; the substance causing renal hypertension, Nature, London 144:980, 1939.

14. A. A. Plentl and I. H. Page: On the enzymatic specificity of renin: I. The proteinase components of renin preparations and their relation to renin activity, J. Biol. Chem. 155:363, 1944.

15. O. Schales, M. Holden, and S. S. Schales: Renin and kidney cathepsins, Arch. Biochem. 6:165, 1945.

16. J. C. Fasciolo, L. F. Leloir, J. M. Muñoz, and E. Braun-Menendez: On the specificity of renin, Science 92:554, 1940.

17. A. A. Plentl, I. H. Page, and W. W. Davis: The nature of renin-activator, J. Biol. Chem. 147:143, 1943.

18a. I. H. Page, B. McSwain, G. M. Knapp, and W. D. Andrus: The origin of renin-activator, Am. J. Physiol. 135:214, 1941.

18b. K. G. Kohlstaedt, I. H. Page, and O. M. Helmer: The activation of renin by blood, Am. Heart J. 19:92, 1940.

19. L. F. Leloir, J. M. Muñoz, A. C. Taquini, E. Braun-Menendez, and J. C. Fasciolo: La formación del hipertensión ogeno, Rev. argent. de cardiol. 9:269, 1942.

20. J. Taggart and D. R. Drury: The action of renin on rabbits with renal hypertension, J. Exper. Med. 71:857, 1940.

21. W. Dock: Vasoconstriction in renal hypertension abolished by pithing, Am. J. Physiol. 130:1, 1940.

22. F. Glenn, C. G. Child, and I. H. Page: The effect of destruction of the spinal cord on the artificial production of hypertension in dogs, Am. J. Physiol. 122:506, 1938.

23. P. Edman: On the purification and chemical composition of hypertensin (angiotonin), Ark. f. Kuni, Mineral. voch. Geo. 22A:1, 1945.

24. O. M. Helmer: A simple chromatographic procedure for the separation of angiotonin from crude mixtures, Proc. Soc. Exper. Biol. & Med. 74:642, 1950.

25. A. A. Plentl and I. H. Page: The action of crystalline proteolytic enzymes on angiotonin, J. Exper. Med. 79:205, 1944.

26a. A. A. Plentl and I. H. Page: A kinetic analysis of the renin-angiotonin pressor system and the standardization of the enzymes renin and angiotonase, J. Exper. Med. 78:367, 1943.

26b. A. A. Plentl and I. H. Page: The purification of angiotonin, J. Biol. Chem. 158:48, 1945.

27a. E. Braun-Menendez, J. C. Fasciolo, L. F. Leloir, and J. M. Muñoz: The substance causing renal hypertension, J. Physiol. 98:283, 1940.

27b. J. M. Muñoz, E. Braun-Menendez, J. C. Fasciolo, and L. F. Leloir: The mechanism of renal hypertension, Am. J. M. Sc. 200:608, 1940.

28. O. M. Helmer, K. G. Kohlstaedt, and I. H. Page: Destruction of angiotonin by extracts of various tissues, Federation Proc. 1:114, 1942.

29. L. Dexter, F. W. Haynes, and W. C. Bridges: The renal humoral pressor mechanism in man: I. Preparation of assay of human renin, human hypertensinogen and hypertensin, J. Clin. Investigation 24:62, 1945.

30. J. C. Fasciolo, L. F. Leloir, J. M. Muñoz, and E. Braun-Menendez: La hipertensinasa, su dosaje y distributión, Rev. Soc. argent. de biol. 16:643, 1940.

31. L. A. Sapirstein, R. K. Reed, and E. W. Page: The site of angiotonin destruction, J. Exper. Med. 83:425, 1946.

32a. H. Croxatto, R. Croxatto, H. Manriquez, and B. Valuezuela: Destrucción de la hipertensina por la aminopolipeptidasa, Rev. de med. y aliment. 5:137, 1942.

32b. R. Croxatto and H. Croxatto: Destruction of hypertensin and pepsitensin by an amino peptidase obtained from yeast, Science 96:519, 1942.

33. F. Gollan, E. Richardson, and H. Goldblatt: Studies on plant hypertensinase, J. Exper. Med. 87:29, 1948.

34. E. W. Page: Plasma angiotonase concentration in normal and toxemic pregnancies, Am. J. M. Sc. 213:715, 1947.

35. O. M. Helmer, K. G. Kohlstaedt, G. F. Kempf, and I. H. Page: The assay of anti-pressor extracts of kidney by in vitro destruction of angiotonin, Federation Proc. 1:114, 1942.

36. H. Croxatto and R. Croxatto: "Pepsitensin"—a hypertensin-like substance produced by peptic digestion of proteins, Science 95:101, 1942.

37. O. M. Helmer and I. H. Page: Formation of angiotonin-like pressor substance from action of crystalline pepsin on renin-activator, Proc. Soc. Exper. Biol. & Med. 49:389, 1942.

38. O. Alonso: Estudio comparativo de las propiedades de la hipertensina y de la pepsitensina, Tesis, Univ. Catolica, Santiago de Chile, 1942.

39. E. Braun-Menendez, J. C. Fasciolo, L. F. Leloir, J. M. Muñoz, and A. C. Taquini: Relaciones entre hipertensina y pepsitensina, Rev. Soc. argent. de Biol. 19:304, 1943.

40. U. S. von Euler and T. Sjöstrand: Factors influencing renin pressor action, Acta physiol. Scandinav. 2:264, 1941.

41. I. H. Page and A. C. Corcoran: Arterial Hypertension: Its Diagnosis and Treatment, ed. 2, Chicago, Year Book Publishers, 1949.

42. I. H. Page: On the nature of the pressor action of renin, J. Exper. Med. 70:521, 1939.

43. I. H. Page: On certain aspects of the nature and treatment of oligemic shock, Am. Heart J. 38:161, 1949.

44. J. W. Bean: Specificity in the renin-hypertensinogen reaction, Am. J. Physiol. 136:731, 1942.

45. A. C. Corcoran, O. M. Helmer, and I. H. Page: The renal pressor system as an index of species relationship, Federation Proc. 1:17, 1942.

46. G. M. C. Masson, A. C. Corcoran, and I. H. Page: Vascular diseases due to desoxycorticosterone acetate and anterior pituitary extract: I. Comparison of functional changes, J. Lab. & Clin. Med. 34:1416, 1949.

47. G. M. C. Masson, J. B. Hazard, A. C. Corcoran, and I. H. Page: Experimental vascular disease due to desoxycorticosterone and anterior pituitary factors: II. Comparison of pathologic changes, Arch. Path. 49:641, 1950.

48. D. C. Laramore and A. Grollman: Water and electrolyte content of tissues in normal and hypertensive rats, Am. J. Physiol. 161:278, 1950.

49. N. C. Hughes-Jones, G. W. Pickering, P. H. Sanderson, H. Scarborough, and J. Vandenbroucke: The nature of the action of renin and hypertensin on renal function in the rabbit, J. Physiol. 109:288, 1949.

The Participation of Hepatorenal Factors in Experimental Renal Hypertension, by Ephraim Shorr

1. R. Chambers and B. W. Zweifach: Topography and function of the mesenteric capillary circulation, Am. J. Anat. 75:173, 1944.

2. B. W. Zweifach: Basic mechanisms in peripheral vascular homeostasis, in Transactions of the Third Conference on Factors Regulating Blood Pressure, Josiah Macy, Jr., Foundation, New York, 1949, p. 13.

3. E. Shorr, B. W. Zweifach, and R. F. Furchgott: Hepatorenal factors in circulatory homeostasis: III. The influence of humoral factors of hepatorenal origin on the vascular reactions to hemorrhage, Ann. New York Acad. Sc. 49:571, 1948.

4. B. W. Zweifach: Microscopic observations of circulation in rat mesoappendix and dog omentum: Use in study of vasotropic substances, in Methods in Medical Research, ed. V. R. Potter, Chicago, Year Book Publishers, 1948, vol. 1, p. 131.

5. A. Mazur and E. Shorr: Hepatorenal factors in circulatory homeostasis: IX. The identification of the hepatic vasodepressor substance, VDM, with ferritin, J. Biol. Chem. 176:771, 1948.

6. A. Mazur, I. Litt, and E. Shorr: The relation of the sulfhydryl groups in ferritin to its vasodepressor activity, J. Biol. Chem. 187: Dec. 1950, in press.

7. R. F. Furchgott and E. Shorr: Physiological and chemical characteristics of a renal vasoexcitor (VEM) involved in circulatory regulation, in Transactions of the First Conference on Factors Regulating Blood Pressure, Josiah Macy, Jr., Foundation, New York, 1947, p. 60.

8. A. Mazur, I. Litt, and E. Shorr: The relation of sulfhydryl-disulfide groups in ferritin to the hepatic activation and inactivation of its vasodepressor properties, J. Biol. Chem. 187: Dec. 1950, in press.

9. B. W. Zweifach, S. Rosenfeld, and E. Shorr: Hepatorenal factors in circulatory homeostasis: XVI. Vascular changes in mesentery in renal hypertension in rats, Federation Proc. 7:139, 1948.

10. B. W. Zweifach and E. Shorr: Hepatorenal factors in circulatory homeostasis: XXVI. Effect of adrenalectomy on renal VEM system and hypertension, Federation Proc. 8:175, 1949.

11. B. W. Zweifach and E. Shorr: Desoxycorticosterone hypertension in relation to hepatorenal mechanisms, Federation Proc. 9:141, 1950.

Blood Volume and Extracellular Fluid Volume in Experimental
Hypertension, by Eduardo Braun-Menendez

1. Abrams, M., A. I. C. De Friez, D. C. Tosteson, and E. M. Landis: Self-selection of salt solutions and water by normal and hypertensive rats, Am. J. Physiol. 156:233, 1949.

2. Backman, E. L.: Effet sur la pression artérielle de la néphrectomie et rôle probable des reins dans le système endocrine, Compt. rend. Soc. de biol. 68:406, 1916.

3. Beckwith, J. R., and A. Chanutin: Blood volumes in hypertensive partially nephrectomized rats, Proc. Soc. Exper. Biol. & Med. 46:66, 1941.

4. Blalock, A., and S. E. Levy: Studies on etiology of renal hypertension, Ann. Surg. 106:826, 1937.

5. Boycott, A. E., and R. A. Chisolm: The influence of underfeeding on the blood, J. Path. & Bact. 16:263, 1911.

6. Braun-Menendez, E.: (a) Metabolismo del agua y de los electrólitos e hipertensión arterial experimental, Cien. e invest. 6:35, 1950; (b) Modificaciones del metabolismo del agua y de la sal en las ratas hipertensas, Rev. Soc. argeₐt. de biol. 26:16, 1950.

7. ————, and M. R. Covián: Mecanismo de las hipertensión de las ratas totalmente nefrectomizadas, Rev. Soc. argent. de biol. 24:130, 1948; Compt. rend. Soc. de biol. 142:1569, 1948.

8. ————, and U. S. von Euler: Hypertension after bilateral nephrectomy in rat, Nature, London 160:905, 1947.

9. ————, and C. Martínez: Mayor frecuencia de hipertensión por perinephritis o desoxicorticosterona en ratas diabéticas, Rev. Soc. argent. de biol. 25:162, 1949.

10. ————, and C. Martínez: Aumento del volumen sanguíneo y del líquido extracelular en ratas diabéticas e hipertensas, Rev. Soc. argent. de biol. 25:168, 1949.

11. Cash, J. R.: Further studies of arterial hypertension, Proc. Soc. Exper. Biol. & Med. 23:609, 1926.

12. Chanutin, A., and E. B. Ferris: Experimental renal insufficiency produced by partial nephrectomy; control diet, Arch. Int. Med. 49:767, 1932.

13. Chisolm, R. A.: Experimental anaemic plethora (chlorotic anemia), J. Path. & Bact. 15:358, 1911.

14. Dicker, E.: Recherches sur le pathogénie de l'hypertension; une lésion rénale peut déterminer une élévation de la pression sanguine, Acta med. Scandinav. 93:265, 1937.

15. Eichelberger, L.: Distribution of water and electrolytes between blood and skeletal muscle in experimental hypertension, J. Exper. Med. 77:205, 1943.

16. Ellis, M. E., and A. Grollman: The antidiuretic hormone in the urine in experimental and clinical hypertension, Endocrinology 44:415, 1949.

17. von Euler, U. S., and E. Braun-Menendez: Hipertensión arterial en ratas nefrectomizadas en parabiosis, Rev. Soc. argent. de biol. 24:362, 1948.

18. Foglia, V. G.: Características de la diabetes en la rata, Rev. Soc. argent. de biol. 20:21, 1944.

19. ————: El peso de los órganos de la rata diabética, Rev. Soc. argent. de biol. 21:45, 1945.

20. ————, R. E. Mancini, and A. F. Cardeza: Esclerosis glomerular del riñón de la rata diabética por pancreatectomia subtotal, Rev. Soc. argent. de biol. 24:114, 1948.

21. Freeman, N. E., and I. H. Page: Hypertension produced by constriction of renal artery in sympathectomized dogs, Am. Heart J. 14:405, 1937.

22. Friedman, S. M., and C. L. Friedman: Observations on the role of the rat kidney in hypertension caused by desoxycorticosterone acetate, J. Exper. Med. 89:631, 1949.

23. Gaudino, M., and M. F. Levitt: Influence of the adrenal cortex on body water, J. Clin. Investigation 28:1487, 1949.

24. Gibson, J. G., and R. W. Robinson: Blood volume, cardiac size and renal function in dogs with hypertension produced by Goldblatt technique, Proc. Soc. Exper. Biol. & Med. 39:497, 1938.

25. Goldblatt, H.: Studies on experimental hypertension; pathogenesis of experimental hypertension due to renal ischemia, Ann. Int. Med. 11:69, 1937.

26. Grant, H., and F. Reichsman: The effects of the ingestion of large amounts of sodium chloride on the arterial and venous pressures of normal subjects, Am. Heart J. 32:704, 1946.

27. Griffith, J. Q., and D. J. Ingle: Blood volume in experimental hypertension following subtotal nephrectomy: Effect of posterior pituitary lobectomy, Proc. Soc. Exper. Biol. & Med. 44:538, 1940.

28. Grollman, A., E. E. Muirhead, and J. Vanatta: Role of the kidney in pathogenesis of hypertension as determined by a study of the effects of bilateral nephrectomy and other experimental procedures on the blood pressure of the dog, Am. J. Physiol. 157:21, 1949.

29. ———, and C. Rule: Experimentally induced hypertension in parabiotic rats, Am. J. Physiol. 138:587, 1943.

30. Hall, C. E., and O. Hall: Persistence of desoxycorticosterone-induced hypertension in the nephrectomized rat, Proc. Soc. Exper. Biol. & Med. 71:690, 1949.

31. Harrison, T. R., M. F. Mason, H. Resnik, and J. Rainey: Changes in blood pressure in relation to experimental renal insufficiency, Tr. A. Am. Physicians 51:280, 1936.

32. Hartwich, A.: Der Blutdruck bei experimenteller Urämie und partieller Nierenausscheidung, Ztschr. f. d. ges. exper. Med. 69:462, 1930.

33. Houssay, B. A., and A. C. Taquini: Especificidad de la acción isquemiado, Rev. Soc. argent. de biol. 14:86, 1938.

34. Jeffers, W. A., M. A. Lindauer, P. H. Twaddle, and C. C. Wolferth: Experimental hypertension in nephrectomized parabiotic rats, Am. J. M. Sc. 199:815, 1940.

35. Kimmelstiel, P., and C. Wilson: Intercapillary lesions in the glomeruli of the kidneys, Am. J. Path. 12:83, 1936.

36. Kruhoffer, P.: Inulin as indicator for extracellular space, Acta physiol. Scandinav. 11:16, 1946.

37. Laramore, D. C., and A. Grollman: Water and electrolyte content of tissues in normal and hypertensive rats, Am. J. Physiol. 161:278, 1950.

38. Lippman, R. W.: Effects of protein and fluid consumption upon plasma volume and circulating protein in rat, Proc. Soc. Exper. Biol. & Med. 67:196, 1948.

39. Lyons, R. H., S. D. Jacobson, and N. L. Avery: Increases in plasma volume following administration of sodium salts, Am. J. M. Sc. 208:148, 1944.

40. Metcoff, J., C. B. Favour, and F. J. Stare: Plasma protein and hemoglobin in protein-deficient rat; 3-dimensional study, J. Clin. Investigation 24:82, 1945.

41. Millard, E., and H. Root: Degenerative vascular diseases and diabetes mellitus, Am. J. Digest. Dis. 15:41, 1948.

42. Mosler, E.: Uber Blutdrucksteigerung nach doppelseitiger Nierenextirpation, Z. klin. Med. 74:297, 1912.

43. Newman, W., and L. Fishel: Circulation 1:706, 1950.

44. Ogden, E.: Extra-renal sequel to experimental renal hypertension, Bull. New York Acad. Med. 23:643, 1947.

45. Oppenheimer, B. S., S. S. Rosenak, and G. D. Oppenheimer: Abst. III Interamer. Cardiol. Congr., 1948, p. 72.

46. Oster, K., and O. Martínez: Water metabolism in hypertensive rats, J. Exper. Med. 78:477, 1943.

47. Overman, R. Q.: Permeability alterations in disease, J. Lab. & Clin. Med. 31:1170, 1946.

48. Perera, G. A.: Effect of continued desoxycorticosterone administration in hypertensive subjects, Proc. Soc. Exper. Biol. & Med. 68:48, 1948.

49. ———: The adrenal cortex and hypertension, Bull. New York Acad. Med. 26: 75, 1950.

50. ———, and D. W. Blood: Pressor activity of desoxycorticosterone acetate in normotensive and hypertensive subjects, Ann. Int. Med. 27:401, 1947.

51. ———, A. I. Knowlton, A. Lowell, and R. F. Loeb: Effect of desoxycorticosterone acetate on blood pressure of man, J. A. M. A. 125:1030, 1944.

52. Pickering, G. W.: Role of kidney in acute and chronic hypertension following renal artery constriction in rabbit, Clin. Sc. 5:229, 1945.

53. Rodbard, S., and S. C. Freed: Effect of desoxycorticosterone acetate on blood pressure of dog, Endocrinology 30:365, 1942.

54. Scott, J. M. D., and J. Barcroft: The blood volume and the total amount of haemoglobin in anaemic rats, Biochem. J. 18:1, 1924.

55. Skahen, J. G., and D. M. Green: Mechanisms of desoxycorticosterone action: IV. Relationship of fluid intake and pressor responses to output of antidiuretic factor, Am. J. Physiol. 155:290, 1948.

56. Stewart, J. D., G. M. Rourke: Effects of large intravenous infusions on body fluid, J. Clin. Investigation 21:197, 1942.

57. Sunderman, F. W.: Water and electrolyte distribution in diabetes mellitus; dehydration in diabetes, Am. J. M. Sc. 205:102, 1943.

58. ———, and F. C. Dohan: Distribution of water and electrolytes in experimental diabetes mellitus, Am. J. Physiol. 132:418, 1941.

59. Swingle, W. W., W. M. Parkins, and J. W. Remington: Effect of desoxycorticosterone acetate and of blood serum transfusions upon circulation of adrenalectomized dog, Am. J. Physiol. 134:503, 1941.

60. Tharp, C. P.: Comparison of mannitol and thiocyanate volumes in several pathophysiological conditions, Federation Proc. 7:124, 1948.

61. Verney, E. B., and M. Vogt: Experimental investigation into hypertension of renal origin, with some observations on convulsive "uremia," Quart. J. Exper. Physiol. 28:253, 1938.

62. White, P., and E. Waskow: Arteriosclerosis in childhood diabetes, Proc. Am. Diabetes A. 8:141, 1948.

63. Winternitz, M. C., E. Mylon, L. L. Waters, and R. Katzenstein: Studies on relation of kidney to cardiovascular disease, Yale J. Biol. & Med. 12:623, 1940.

The Mechanism of Hypertension Due to Desoxycorticosterone, by Eduardo Braun-Menendez

1. Abrams, M., A. I. C. De Friez, D. C. Tosteson, and E. M. Landis: Self-selection of salt solutions and water by normal and hypertensive rats, Am. J. Physiol. 7:3, 1948.

2. Anslow, W. P., L. G. Wesson, A. A. Bolomey, and J. G. Taylor: Chlouretic action of pressor-antidiuretic fraction of posterior pituitary extract, Federation Proc. 7:1, 1948.

3. Bechgaard, P., and A. Bergstrand: Can the administration of desoxycorticosterone acetate give rise to nephrosclerosis? Acta Endocrinol. 2:61, 1949.

4. Blake, W. D., R. Wegria, R. P. Keating, and H. P. Ward: Effect of increased renal venous pressure on renal function, Am. J. Physiol. 157:1, 1949.

5. Braun-Menendez, E.: Rev. Soc. argent. de biol. 26: 1950, in press.

6. ———, and U. S. von Euler: Hypertension after bilateral nephrectomy in rat, Nature, London 160:905, 1947.

7. ———, and V. G. Foglia: Influencia de la hipófisis sobre la presión arterial de la rata, Rev. Soc. argent. de biol. 20:556, 1944.

8. ———, and C. Martínez: Mayor frecuencia de hipertensión por perinefritis o desoxicorticosterona en ratas diabéticas, Rev. Soc. argent. de biol. 25:162, 1949.

9. ———, and C. Martínez: Aumento del volumen sanguíneo y del líquido extracelular en ratas diabéticas e hipertensas, Rev. Soc. argent. de biol. 25:168, 1949.

10. ———, and J. L. Prado: Rev. Soc. argent. de biol. 26: 1950, in press.

11. Briggs, A. P., et al.: Renal and circulatory factors in edema formation of congestive heart failure, J. Clin. Investigation 27:810, 1948.

12. Briskin, H. L., F. R. Stokes, C. I. Reed, and R. G. Mrazek: Effects of vitamin D and other sterols on blood pressure in rat, Am. J. Physiol. 138:385, 1943.

13. Buell, M. V., and E. Turner: Cation distribution in muscles of adrenalectomized rats, Am. J. Physiol. 134:225, 1941.

14. Carnes, W. H., C. Ragan, J. W. Ferrebee, and J. O'Neill: Effects of desoxycorticosterone acetate in albino rat, Endocrinology 29:144, 1941.

15. Clinton, M., and G. W. Thorn: Effect of desoxycorticosterone acetate administration on plasma volume and electrolyte balance of normal human subjects, Bull. Johns Hopkins Hosp. 72:255, 1943.

16. ———, G. W. Thorn, H. Eisenberg, and K. E. Stein: Effect of synthetic desoxycorticosterone acetate therapy on plasma volume and electrolyte balance in normal dogs, Endocrinology 31:578, 1942.

17. Corey, E. L., and S. W. Britton: Antagonistic action of desoxycorticosterone and post-pituitary extract on chloride and water balance, Am. J. Physiol. 133:511, 1941.

18. Croxatto, H., and R. Croxatto: Corteza suprarenal y mecanismo humoral de la hipertensión: II. Estudio de la reacción renina-hipertensinógeno, Rev. Soc. biol. Chile 7:38, 1949.

19. Darrow, D. C., and J. Miller: Production of cardiac lesions by repeated injections of desoxycorticosterone acetate, J. Clin. Investigation 21:601, 1942.

20. ———, and H. Yannet: Changes in distribution of body water accompanying increase and decrease in extracellular electrolyte, J. Clin. Investigation 14:266, 1935.

21. Earle, D. P., S. J. Farber, J. D. Alexander, and L. W. Eichna: Effect of treatment on renal functions and electrolyte excretion in congestive heart failure, J. Clin. Investigation 28:778, 1949.

22. Farnsworth, E. B., and J. S. Krakusin: Electrolyte partition in patients with edema of various origins, J. Lab. & Clin. Med. 33:1534, 1545, 1948.

23. Ferrebee, J. W., D. Parker, W. H. Carnes, M. K. Gerity, D. W. Atchley, and R. F. Loeb: Certain effects of desoxycorticosterone; development of "diabetes insipidus" and replacement of muscle potassium by sodium in normal dogs, Am. J. Physiol. 135:230, 1941.

24. Friedman, S. M.: A comparison of the effects of desoxycorticosterone acetate in Sherman and Wistar rats, Rev. canad. de biol. 8:320, 1949.

25. ———, and C. W. Friedman: Observations on the role of the rat kidney in hypertension caused by desoxycorticosterone acetate, J. Exper. Med. 89:631, 1949.

26. ———, C. L. Friedman, and J. R. Polley: Potentiation of hypertensive effects of desoxycorticosterone acetate (DCA) by various sodium salts, Am. J. Physiol. 153:226, 1948.

27. ———, J. R. Polley, and C. L. Friedman: Effect of desoxycorticosterone acetate on blood pressure, renal function, and electrolyte pattern in intact rat, J. Exper. Med. 87:329, 1948.

28. Gaudino, N. M.: Acción de las glándulas suprarenales sobre el hipertensinógeno, Rev. Soc. argent. de biol. 20:529, 1944.

29. Gaudino, M., and M. F. Levitt: Influence of the adrenal cortex on body water distribution and renal function, J. Clin. Investigation 28:1487, 1949.

30. Green, D. M., D. H. Coleman, and M. McCabe: Mechanisms of desoxycorticosterone action: II. Relations of sodium chloride intake to fluid exchange, pressor effects and survival, Am. J. Physiol. 154:465, 1948.

31. ———, and A. Farah: Non-dependence of tubular sodium reabsorption upon glomerular function, Federation Proc. 8:60, 1949.

32. ———, A. Farah, A. D. Johnson, and W. C. Bridges: Renal excretion of sodium, Proc. 22d Scientific Sessions, Am. Heart A., 1949, p. 27.

33. ———, and M. Glover: Factors influencing the hypertensive action of desoxycorticosterone, Federation Proc. 7:224, 1948.

34. Grollman, A., T. R. Harrison, and J. R. Williams: Effect of various sterol derivatives on blood pressure of rat, J. Pharmacol. & Exper. Therap. 69:149, 1940.

35. Hall, C. E., and O. Hall: Persistence of desoxycorticosterone-induced hypertension in the nephrectomized rat, Proc. Soc. Exper. Biol. & Med. 71:690, 1949.

36. Harkness, D. M., E. Muntwyler, F. R. Mautz, and R. C. Mellors: Electrolyte and water exchange between skeletal muscle, "available (thiocyanate) fluid," and plasma in dog following administration of desoxycorticosterone acetate, J. Lab. & Clin. Med. 28:307, 1942.

37. Harned, A. S., and W. O. Nelson: The relation between desoxycorticosterone acetate and diabetes insipidus in the rat, Federation Proc. 2:19, 1943.

38. Houssay, B. A.: Advancement of knowledge of role of hypophysis in carbohydrate metabolism during last 25 years, Endocrinology 30:884, 1942.

39. Kattus, A., A. Genecin, J. H. Sisson, C. Monge, B. C. Sinclair-Smith, and E. V. Newman: Correlation of changes in the renal circulation with metabolic balances of electrolytes and nitrogen during recovery from congestive heart failure, J. Clin. Investigation 28:793, 1949.

40. Knowlton, A. I., E. N. Loeb, H. C. Stoerk, and B. C. Seegal: Desoxycorticosterone acetate; potentiation of its activity by sodium chloride, J. Exper. Med. 85:187, 1947.

41. ———, H. C. Stoerk, B. C. Seegal, and E. N. Loeb: Influence of adrenal cortical steroids upon blood pressure and rate of progression of experimental nephritis in rats, Endocrinology 38:315, 1946.

42. Kuhlman, D., C. Ragan, J. W. Ferrebee, D. W. Atchley, and R. F. Loeb: Toxic effects of desoxycorticosterone esters in dogs, Science 90:496, 1939.

43. Leathem, J. H., and V. A. Drill: Role of hypophysis and adrenals in control of systolic blood pressure in rat, Endocrinology 35:112, 1944.

44. Lenel, R., L. N. Katz, and S. Rodbard: Arterial hypertension in chickens, Am. J. Physiol. 152:557, 1948.

45. Little, J. M., S. L. Wallace, E. C. Whatley, and G. A. Anderson: Effect of pitressin on urinary excretion of chloride and water in human, Am. J. Physiol. 151:174, 1947.

46. Loeb, R. F.: Adrenal cortex and electrolyte behavior, Bull. New York Acad. Med. 18:263, 1942.

47. ———, D. W. Atchley, J. W. Ferrebee, and C. Ragan: Observations on effects of desoxycorticosterone esters and progesterone in patients with Addison's disease, Tr. A. Am. Physicians 54:285, 1939.

48. McCance, R. A.: Medical problems in mineral metabolism, Lancet 1:823, 1936.

49. Miller, H. C., and D. C. Darrow: Relation of serum and muscle electrolyte, particularly potassium, to voluntary exercise, Am. J. Physiol. 132:801, 1941.

50. Mrazek, R. G., C. R. Novak, and C. I. Reed: Further study of the influence of activated sterols on blood pressure, Federation Proc. 1:61, 1942.

51. Perera, G. A., and D. W. Blood: Pressor activity of desoxycorticosterone acetate in normotensive and hypertensive subjects, Ann. Int. Med. 27:401, 1947.

52. ———, A. I. Knowlton, A. Lowell, and R. F. Loeb: Effect of desoxycorticosterone acetate on blood pressure of man, J. A. M. A. 125:1030, 1944.

53. Prado, J. L.: Hipertensão por Esteróides, Ciencia e Cultura 2:10, 1950.

54. ———: Estudos söbre hipertensão hormonal experimental, Tesis, Escola Paulista de Medicina, Sao Paulo, 1950.

55. Ragan, C., J. W. Ferrebee, P. Phyfe, D. W. Atchley, and R. F. Loeb: Syndrome of polydipsia and polyuria induced in normal animals by desoxycorticosterone acetate, Am. J. Physiol. 131:73, 1940.

56. Rice, K. K., and C. Richter: Increased sodium chloride and water intake of normal rats treated with desoxycorticosterone acetate, Endocrinology 33:106, 1943.

57. Rodbard, S., and S. C. Freed: Effect of desoxycorticosterone acetate on blood pressure of dog, Endocrinology 30:365, 1942.

58. Sapirstein, L. A., W. L. Brandt, and D. R. Drury: Production of hypertension in the rat by substituting hypertonic sodium chloride solutions for drinking water, Proc. Soc. Exper. Biol. & Med. 73:82, 1950.

59. Selkurt, E. E., P. W. Hall, and M. P. Spencer: Response of renal blood flow and clearance to graded partial obstruction of the renal vein, Am. J. Physiol. 157:40, 1949.

60. ————, and R. S. Post: Mechanism for renal clearance of sodium in the dog; effect of decreased and increased load on reabsorptive mechanism, Abstract, Am. J. Physiol. 159:589, 1949.

61. Selye, H.: Production of nephrosclerosis by overdosage with desoxycorticosterone acetate, Canad. M. A. J. 47:515, 1942.

62. ————: Production of nephrosclerosis in the fowl by sodium chloride, J. Am. Vet. M. A. 103:140, 1943.

63. ————: Alarm reaction and diseases of adaptation, Ann. Int. Med. 29:403, 1948.

64. ————, and C. Dosne: Changes produced by desoxycorticosterone overdosage in rat, Proc. Soc. Exper. Biol. & Med. 44:165, 1940.

65. ————, and C. E. Hall: Pathologic changes induced in various species by overdosage with desoxycorticosterone, Arch. Path. 36:19, 1943.

66. ————, C. E. Hall, and E. M. Rowley: Malignant hypertension produced by treatment with desoxycorticosterone acetate and sodium chloride, Canad. M. A. J. 49:88, 1943.

67. ————, J. Minzberg, and E. M. Rowley: Effect of various electrolytes upon toxicity of desoxycorticosterone acetate, J. Pharmacol. & Exper. Therap. 85:42, 1945.

68. ————, and E. I. Pentz: Pathogenetical correlations between periarteritis nodosa, renal hypertension and rheumatic lesions, Canad. M. A. J. 49:264, 1943.

69. ————, and H. Stone: Role of sodium chloride in production of nephrosclerosis by steroids, Proc. Soc. Exper. Biol. & Med. 52:190, 1943.

70. ————, H. Stone, K. Nielsen, and C. P. Leblond: Studies concerning effects of various hormones upon renal structure, Canad. M. A. J. 52:571, 1945.

71. ————, H. Stone, P. S. Timiras, and C. Schaffenburg: Influence of sodium chloride on the actions of desoxycorticosterone acetate, Am. Heart J. 37:1009, 1949.

72. Shorr, E.: Editorial, Seminars on hypertension, Am. J. Med. 5:783, 1948.

73. Skahen, J. G., and D. M. Green: Mechanisms of desoxycorticosterone actions: IV. Relationship of fluid intake and pressor responses to output of antidiuretic factor, Am. J. Physiol. 155:290, 1948.

74. Swingle, W. W., W. M. Parkins, and J. W. Remington: Effect of desoxycorticosterone acetate and of blood serum transfusions upon circulation of adrenalectomized dog, Am. J. Physiol. 134:503, 1941.

75. Wesson, L. G., W. P. Anslow, and H. W. Smith: Excretion of strong electrolytes, Bull. New York Acad. Med. 24:586, 1948.

76. Winter, H., and H. Selye: Factors influencing the diuretic effect of progesterone and desoxycorticosterone acetate, Federation Proc. 1:94, 1942.

77. Zweifach, B. W., and E. Shorr: Desoxycorticosterone hypertension in relation to hepatorenal mechanisms, Federation Proc. 9:141, 1950.

Sympatho-Adrenal Factors in Hypertension, by Mark Nickerson

1. E. Koch and H. Mies: Chronischer arterieller Hochdruck durch experimentelle Dauerausschaltung der Blutdruckzügler, Krankheitsforschung 7:241–256, 1929.

2. C. Heymans, J. J. Bouckaert, and P. Regniers: Le sinus carotidien et la zone homologue cardioaortique: Physiologie, pharmacologie, pathologie, clinique, Paris, G. Doin et Cie., 1933, pp. 332.

3. H. T. Wycis: Bilateral intracranial section of the glossopharyngeal nerve, Arch. Neurol. & Psychiat. 54:344–347, 1945.

4. W. Penfield: Diencephalic autonomic epilepsy, Arch. Neurol. & Psychiat. 22:358–374, 1929.

5. I. H. Page: Syndrome simulating diencephalic stimulation occurring in patients with essential hypertension, Am. J. M. Sc. 190:9–14, 1935.

6. I. L. Bennett and A. Heyman: Paroxysmal hypertension associated with tabes dorsalis; report of 3 cases, Am. J. Med. 5:729–735, 1948.

7. K. S. Grimson: Role of sympathetic nervous system in hypertension as revealed by the action of sympatholytic and depressor drugs, in Transactions of the Third Conference on Factors Regulating Blood Pressure, Josiah Macy, Jr., Foundation, New York, 1949, pp. 237–261.

8. M. de Jaegher and A. Van Bogaert: Hypertension hypothalamique expérimentale; sa nature, Compt. rend. Soc. de biol. 118:546–547, 1935.

9. C. W. Walter and M. J. Pijoan: Persistent hypertension due to hypothalamic injury, Surgery 1:282–283, 1937.

10. H. D. Green and E. C. Hoff: Effects of faradic stimulation of the cerebral cortex on limb and renal volumes in cat and monkey, Am. J. Physiol. 118:641–658, 1937.

11. E. C. Hoff, J. F. Kell, Jr., N. Hastings, E. H. Gray, and D. M. Sholes: Acute renal cortical ischemia produced by stimulation of the pressor area of the cerebral cortex, Federation Proc. 8:76, 1949.

12. H. G. Langford, J. W. Vester, and E. C. Hoff: Effect of electrical stimulation of the frontal cortex upon the production of renin by the kidneys, Am. J. Med. 8:394–395, 1950.

13. H. Cushing: Concerning a definite regulatory mechanism of the vaso-motor centre which controls blood pressure during cerebral compression, Bull. Johns Hopkins Hosp. 12:290–292, 1901.

14. W. E. Dixon and H. Heller: Experimentelle Hypertonie durch Erhöhung des intrakraniellen Druckes, Arch. f. exper. Path. u. Pharmakol. 166:265–275, 1932.

15. H. Cushing: The blood-pressure reaction of acute cerebral compression, illustrated by cases of intracranial hemorrhage, Am. J. M. Sc. 125:1017–1044, 1903.

16. A. C. Guyton: Acute hypertension in dogs with cerebral ischemia, Am. J. Physiol. 154:45–54, 1948.

17. C. Heymans and A. L. Delannois: Influences du débit artériel et de la pression artérielle sur l'activité des centres cardio-vasculaires et respiratoire, Arch. internat. de pharmacodyn. et de thérap. 72:444–456, 1946.

18. S. J. G. Nowak and Adli Samaan: The effect of adrenaline, anaemia and carbon dioxide on the vasomotor centre, Arch. internat. de pharmacodyn. et de thérap. 51:463–487, 1935.

19. W. Raab: Central vasomotor irritability; contribution to the problem of essential hypertension, Arch. Int. Med. 47:727–758, 1931.

20. C. Heymans and J. J. Bouckaert: Hypertension artérielle expérimentale et sympathectomie, Compt. rend. Soc. de biol. 120:82–84, 1935.

21. K. S. Grimson: The sympathetic nervous system in neurogenic and renal hypertension; experimental correlation and clinical consideration, Arch. Surg. 43:284–305, 1941.

22. C. B. Thomas: Experimental hypertension from section of moderator nerves; relationship to presence of kidney tissue, Proc. Soc. Exper. Biol. & Med. 48:24–27, 1941.

23. K. S. Grimson, J. J. Bouckaert, and C. Heymans: Production of a sustained neurogenic hypertension of renal origin, Proc. Soc. Exper. Biol. & Med. 42:225–226, 1939.

24. K. S. Grimson: Role of the sympathetic nervous system in experimental neurogenic hypertension, Proc. Soc. Exper. Biol. & Med. 44:219–221, 1940.

25. F. J. Kottke, W. G. Kubicek, and Donna Jeanne Laker: Physical and nervous factors in experimental hypertension, Arch. Phys. Med. 28:146–153, 1947.

26. S. Wolf, J. B. Pfeiffer, H. S. Ripley, O. S. Winter, and H. G. Wolff: Hypertension as a reaction pattern to stress; summary of experimental data on variations in blood pressure and renal blood flow, Ann. Int. Med. 29:1056–1076, 1948.

27. H. G. Wolff: Life stress and cardiovascular disorders, Circulation 1:187–203, 1950.

28. J. D. P. Graham: High blood-pressure after battle, Lancet 1:239–240, 1945.

29. M. Goldenberg, K. L. Pines, E. F. Baldwin, D. G. Greene, and C. E. Roh: The hemodynamic response of man to nor-epinephrine and epinephrine and its relation to the problem of hypertension, Am. J. Med. 5:792–806, 1948.

30. N. E. Freeman and W. A. Jeffers: Effect of progressive sympathectomy on hypertension produced by increased intracranial pressure, Am. J. Physiol. 128:662–671, 1940.

31. R. J. Bing and C. B. Thomas: The effect of two dioxane derivatives, 883 and 933F, on normal dogs and on animals with neurogenic and renal hypertension, J. Pharmacol. & Exper. Therap. 83:21–39, 1945.

32. M. Nickerson and J. W. Henry: Unpublished results.

33. C. Heymans and J. J. Bouckaert: Au sujet de l'action vasomotrice et vasculaire de l'ergotamine, Arch. internat. de pharmacodyn. et de thérap. 46:129–136, 1933.

34. C. Heymans and J. J. Bouckaert: Au sujet des influences du pipéridométhyl-3-benzodioxane (F. 933) sur le système circulatoire, Compt. rend. Soc. de biol. 120:79–82, 1935.

35. M. Nickerson: The pharmacology of adrenergic blockade, J. Pharmacol. & Exper. Therap. 95:27–101, 1949. (Part II, Pharmacol. Rev. vol. 1.)

36. M. Nickerson and L. S. Goodman: Pharmacological properties of a new adrenergic blocking agent: N,N-dibenzyl-β-chloroethylamine (Dibenamine), J. Pharmacol. & Exper. Therap. 89:167–185, 1947.

37. M. Nickerson and L. S. Goodman: Pharmacological and physiological aspects of adrenergic blockade, with special reference to Dibenamine, Federation Proc. 7:397–409, 1948.

38. R. D. Taylor, A. C. Corcoran, and I. H. Page: Effects of denervation on experimental renal hypertension, Federation Proc. 7:123, 1948.

39. J. Stamler, S. Rodbard, and L. N. Katz: Blood pressure and renal clearances in hypertensive dogs following tissue injury, Am. J. Physiol. 160:21–30, 1950.

40. L. K. Alpert, A. S. Alving, and K. S. Grimson: Effect of total sympathectomy on experimental renal hypertension in dogs, Proc. Soc. Exper. Biol. & Med. 37:1–3, 1937.

41. N. E. Freeman and I. H. Page: Hypertension produced by constriction of the renal artery in sympathectomized dogs, Am. Heart J. 14:405–414, 1937.

42. C. Heymans, J. J. Bouckaert, L. Elaut, F. Bayless, and A. Samaan: Hypertension artérielle chronique par ischémia rénale chez de chien totalement sympathectomisé, Compt. rend. Soc. de biol. 126:434–436, 1937.

43. E. B. Verney and Martha Vogt: An experimental investigation into hypertension of renal origin, with some observations on convulsive "uraemia," Quart. J. Exper. Physiol. 28:253–303, 1938.

44. J. Jacobs and F. F. Yonkman: Sympatholytic treatment of experimental hypertension, J. Lab. & Clin. Med. 29:1217–1221, 1944.

45. M. Nickerson, F. Bullock, and G. M. Nomaguchi: Effect of Dibenamine on renal hypertension in rats, Proc. Soc. Exper. Biol. & Med. 68:425–429, 1948.

46. M. Wilburne, L. N. Katz, S. Rodbard, and A. Surtshin: The action of N,N-dibenzyl-beta-chloroethylamine (Dibenamine) in hypertensive dogs, J. Pharmacol. & Exper. Therap. 90:213–223, 1947.

47. L. N. Katz and L. Friedberg: The hemodynamic effect of the dioxane derivative

933F on trained unanesthetized normal and renal hypertensive dogs and its effect on the pressor action of renin, Am. J. Physiol. 127:29–36, 1939.

48. Racheal K. Reed, L. A. Sapirstein, F. D. Southard, and E. Ogden: The effects of nembutal and yohimbine on chronic renal hypertension in the rat, Am. J. Physiol. 141:707–712, 1944.

49. L. A. Sapirstein and Racheal K. Reed: Effects of Fourneau 883 and Fourneau 933 on late renal hypertension in the rat, Proc. Soc. Exper. Biol. & Med. 57:135–136, 1944.

50. E. Ogden: The extra-renal sequel to experimental renal hypertension, Bull. New York Acad. Med. 23:643–660, 1947.

51. W. G. Moss and G. E. Wakerlin: Role of the nervous system in experimental renal hypertension, Am. J. Physiol. 161:435–441, 1950.

52. W. Dock: Vasoconstriction in renal hypertension abolished by pithing, Am. J. Physiol. 130:1–8, 1940.

53. W. Dock, F. Shidler, and B. Moy: The vasomotor center essential in maintaining renal hypertension, Am. Heart J. 23:513–521, 1942.

54. K. S. Grimson: Blood pressure of renal and of early and late neurogenic hypertension dogs after low cervical cord section, Ann. Surg. 122:990–995, 1945.

55. F. Glenn, C. G. Child, and I. Page: The effect of destruction of the spinal cord on hypertension artificially produced in dogs, Am. J. Physiol. 122:506–510, 1938.

56. F. Glenn and E. P. Lasher: The effect of destruction of the spinal cord on the artificial production of hypertension in dogs, Am. J. Physiol. 124:106–109, 1938.

57. M. Nickerson, J. W. Henry, and G. M. Nomaguchi: Blockade of responses to epinephrine and norepinephrine by Dibenamine congeners. To be published.

58. J. Flasher and D. R. Drury: Effects of removal of the "ischemic" kidney in rabbits with unilateral renal hypertension as compared to unilateral nephrectomy in normal rabbits, Am. J. Physiol. 158:438–443, 1949.

59. B. Friedman, J. Jarman, and P. Klemperer: Sustained hypertension following experimental unilateral renal injuries: Effects of nephrectomy, Am. J. M. Sc. 202:20–29, 1941.

60. A. Grollman: Experimental chronic hypertension in the rabbit, Am. J. Physiol. 142:666–670, 1944.

61. C. Wilson and F. B. Byrom: The vicious circle in chronic Bright's disease: Experimental evidence from the hypertensive rat, Quart. J. Med. 10:65–93, 1941.

62. N. H. Schwartz and S. Gross: Unilateral malignant nephrosclerosis, J. Urol. 62:426–435, 1949.

63. Béla Halpert and A. Grollman: Structural changes in the kidneys of rats with experimental chronic hypertension, Arch. Path. 43:559–565, 1947.

64. H. Selye and Helen Stone: Pathogenesis of the cardiovascular and renal changes which usually accompany malignant hypertension, J. Urol. 56:399–419, 1946.

65. F. B. Byrom and L. F. Dodson: The mechanism of the vicious circle in chronic hypertension, Clin. Sc. 8:1–10, 1949.

66. D. M. Green: Pheochromocytoma and chronic hypertension, J. A. M. A. 131:1260–1265, 1946.

67. G. F. Cahill: Pheochromocytomas, J. A. M. A. 138:180–186, 1948.

68. A. J. Barnett, R. B. Blacket, A. E. Depoorter, P. H. Sanderson, and G. M. Wilson: The action of noradrenaline in man and its relation to phaeochromocytoma and hypertension, Clin. Sc. 9:151–179, 1950.

69. H. Hamperl and H. Heller: Die Organveränderungen bei experimentellem Dauerhochdruck, Arch. f. exper. Path. u. Pharmakol. 174:517–531, 1934.

70. H. S. Medoff and A. M. Bongiovanni: Blood pressure in rats subjected to audiogenic stimulation, Am. J. Physiol. 143:300–305, 1945.

71. E. J. Farris, E. H. Yeakel, and H. S. Medoff: Development of hypertension in emotional gray Norway rats after air blasting, Am. J. Physiol. 144:331–333, 1945.

72. F. H. Smirk: Pathogenesis of essential hypertension, Brit. M. J. 1:791–799, 1949.

73. E. J. Farris and E. H. Yeakel: The susceptibility of albino and gray Norway rats to audiogenic seizures, J. Comp. Psychol. 35:73–80, 1943.

74. M. Goldenberg and H. Aranow, Jr.: Diagnosis of pheochromocytoma by the adrenergic blocking action of benzodioxan, J. A. M. A. 143:1139–1143, 1950.

75. E. A. Hines, Jr., and G. E. Brown: A standard test for measuring the variability of blood pressure: Its significance as a measure of the prehypertensive state, Ann. Int. Med. 7:209–217, 1933.

76. W. F. Rogers and R. S. Palmer: Transient nervous hypertension as a military risk; its relation to essential hypertension, New England J. Med. 230:39–42, 1944.

77. R. L. Levy, C. C. Hillman, W. D. Stroud, and P. D. White: Transient hypertension; its significance in terms of later development of sustained hypertension and cardiovascular-renal disease, J. A. M. A. 126:829–833, 1944.

78. R. L. Levy, P. D. White, W. D. Stroud, and C. C. Hillman: Transient tachycardia; prognostic significance alone and in association with transient hypertension, J. A. M. A. 129:585–588, 1945.

79. E. A. Hines, Jr.: Significance of vascular hyperreaction as measured by cold-pressor test, Am. Heart J. 19:408–416, 1940.

80. H. G. Armstrong and J. A. Rafferty: Cold pressor test follow-up study for seven years on 166 officers, Am. Heart J. 39:484–490, 1950.

Experimental Hypertension, by Eduardo Braun-Menendez

1. Alpert, L. K., A. S. Alving, and K. S. Grimson: Effect of total sympathectomy on experimental renal hypertension in dogs, Proc. Soc. Exper. Biol. & Med. 37:1, 1937.

2. Anderson, E., E. W. Page, C. H. Li, and E. Ogden: Restoration of renal hypertension in hypophysectomized rats by administration of adrenocorticotropic hormone, Am. J. Physiol. 141:393, 1944.

3. Bing, R. J.: Experimental renal hypertension and amino acid metabolism in the kidney, New York Acad. Sc. 3:168, 1946.

4. Blackman, S. S., Jr., C. B. Thomas, and J. E. Howard: Effect of testosterone propionate on arterial blood pressure, kidneys, urinary bladder and livers of growing dogs, Bull. Johns Hopkins Hosp. 74:321, 1944.

5. Blalock, A., and S. E. Levy: Studies on etiology of renal hypertension, Ann. Surg. 106:826, 1937.

6. Braun, L.: Experimentelle Untersuchungen über Blutdruck und Niere, Wien. klin. Wchnschr. 46:225, 1933.

7. ———, and B. Samet: Experimentelle Untersuchungen über Blutdruck und Niere, Wien. klin. Wchnschr. 47:65, 1934.

8. ———, and B. Samet: Experimentelle Untersuchungen über Blutdruck und Niere, Wien. klin. Wchnschr. 48:940, 1935.

9. ———, and B. Samet: Experimentelle Untersuchungen über die Beziehungen zwischen Blutdruck und Niere, Arch. f. exper. Path. u. Pharmakol. 177:662, 1935.

10. Braun-Menendez, E.: (a) La Presión arterial de los perros hipofisoprivos, Rev. Soc. argent. de biol. 8:463, 1932; (b) La Pression artérielle des chiens sans hypophyse, Compt. rend. Soc. de biol. 111:477, 1932.

11. ———, M. R. Covián, and C. E. Rapela: Presencia de renina en la sangre circulante de ratas normalese hipertensas, Rev. Soc. argent. de biol. 23:131, 1947.

12. ———, J. C. Fasciolo, L. F. Leloir, and J. M. Muñoz: (a) La substancia hipertensora de la sangre del riñón isquemiado, Rev. Soc. argent. de biol. 15:420, 1939; (b) Substance causing renal hypertension, J. Physiol. 98:283, 1940.

13. ———, J. C. Fasciolo, L. F. Leloir, J. M. Muñoz, and A. C. Taquini: Hipertensión arterial nefrógena, El Ateneo, Buenos Aires, 1943.

14. ——, J. C. Fasciolo, L. F. Leloir, J. M. Muñoz, and A. C. Taquini: Renal Hypertension, translated by Lewis Dexter and Charles C. Thomas, Springfield, Ill., 1946.
15. ——, and V. G. Foglia: Influencia de la hipófisis sobre la presión arterial de la rata, Rev. Soc. argent. de biol. 20:556, 1944.
16. ——, and J. L. Prado: Rev. Soc. argent. de biol. 26: 1950, in press.
17. Bülbring, E.: The methylation of noradrenaline by minced suprarenal tissue, Brit. J. Pharmacol. 4:234, 1949.
18. Collins, D. A.: Hypertension from constriction of arteries of denervated kidneys, Am. J. Physiol. 116:616, 1936.
19. Croxatto, H., and A. Muñoz: Características farmacológicas de fracciones vaso activas de plasmas y sueros sanguineos: I. Estudio sobre la preparación vascular de Loewen-Trendelenborg, Bol. Soc. biol., Chile 7:10, 1949.
20. Dell'Oro, R., and E. Braun-Menendez: Dosaje de renina en la sangre de perros hipertensos por isquemia renal, Rev. Soc. argent. de biol. 18:65, 1942.
21. Dexter, L., and F. W. Haynes: Relation of renin to human hypertension with particular reference to eclampsia, preeclampsia and acute glomerulonephritis, Proc. Soc. Exper. Biol. & Med. 55:288, 1944.
22. Dixon, W. E., and H. Heller: Experimentelle Hypertonie durch Erhöhung des intrakraniellen Drucks, Arch. f. exper. Path. u. Pharmakol. 166:265, 1932.
23. Dock, W.: The role of the central nervous system in experimental hypertension, J. Clin. Investigation 19:769, 1940.
24. ——: Vasoconstriction in renal hypertension abolished by pithing, Am. J. Physiol. 130:1, 1940.
25. Dontigny, P., E. C. Hay, J. L. Prado, and H. Selye: Hormonal hypertension and nephrosclerosis as influenced by diet, Am. J. M. Sc. 215:442, 1948.
26. Ellis, M. E., and A. Grollman: The antidiuretic hormone in the urine in experimental and clinical hypertension, Endocrinology 44:415, 1949.
27. von Euler, U. S., and U. Hamberg: L-noradrenaline in the suprarenal medulla, Nature, London 163:642, 1949.
28. Farris, E. J., E. H. Yeakel, and H. S. Medoff: Development of hypertension in emotional gray Norway rats after air blasting, Am. J. Physiol. 144:331, 1945.
29. Fasciolo, J. C.: (a) Acción del riñón sano sobre la hipertensión arterial por isquemia renal, Rev. Soc. argent. de biol. 14:15, 1938; (b) Action du rein sain sur l'hypertension artérielle par ischémie rénale, Compt. rend. Soc. de biol. 128:1129, 1938.
30. ——, and A. C. Taquini: Método para el reconocimiento de pequeñas cantidades de renins, Rev. Soc. argent. de biol. 23:138, 1947.
31. Fishback, H. R., F. R. Dutra, and E. T. MacCamy: Production of chronic hypertension in dogs by progressive ligation of arteries supplying the head, J. Lab. & Clin. Med. 28:1187, 1943.
32. Freeman, N. E., and I. H. Page: Hypertension produced by constriction of renal artery in sympathectomized dogs, Am. Heart J. 14:405, 1937.
33. Friedman, M., and A. Kaplan: Studies concerning site of renin formation in kidney; absence of renin in aglomerular kidney of midshipman fish, J. Exper. Med. 75:127, 1942.
34. ——: Studies concerning site of renin formation in kidney; renin content of mammalian kidney following specific necrosis of proximal convoluted tubular epithelium, J. Exper. Med. 77:65, 1943.
35. Gaudino, N. M.: La suprarrenal y el riñón en la hipertensión arterial nefrógena, Tesis Doct. Med., Buenos Aires, 1944.
36. Glenn, F., C. G. Child, and I. H. Page: Effect of destruction of spinal cord on hypertension artificially produced in dogs, Am. J. Physiol. 122:506, 1938.
37. ——, and E. P. Lasher: Effect of destruction of spinal cord on artificial production of hypertension in dogs, Am. J. Physiol. 124:106, 1938.
38. Goldblatt, H., J. Gross, and R. F. Hanzal: Studies on experimental hypertension;

effect of resection of splanchnic nerves on experimental renal hypertension, J. Exper. Med. 65:233, 1937.

39. ———, J. Lynch, R. F. Hanzal, and W. W. Summerville: Studies on experimental hypertension; production of persistent elevation of systolic pressure by means of renal ischemia, J. Exper. Med. 59:347, 1934.

40. ———, and W. B. Wartman: Studies on experimental hypertension; effect of section of anterior spinal nerve roots on experimental hypertension due to renal ischemia, J. Exper. Med. 66:527, 1937.

41. Goldenberg, M., K. L. Pines, E. de F. Baldwin, D. G. Greene, and C. E. Roch: The hemodynamic response of man to nor-epinephrine and epinephrine and its relation to the problem of hypertension, Am. J. Med. 5:792, 1948.

42. Gollan, F., E. Richardson, and H. Goldblatt: Hypertension in the systemic blood of animals with experimental renal hypertension, J. Exper. Med. 88:389, 1948.

43. Grimson, K. S.: Role of sympathetic nervous system in experimental neurogenic hypertension, Proc. Soc. Exper. Biol. & Med. 44:219, 1940.

44. ———, J. J. Bouckaert, and C. Heymans: Production of sustained neurogenic hypertension of renal origin, Proc. Soc. Exper. Biol. & Med. 42:225, 1939.

45. Grollman, A.: Experimental chronic hypertension: Its mechanism and amelioration by use of various blood-pressure reducing substances, Special Publications, New York Acad. Sc. 3:99, 1946.

46. ———, T. R. Harrison, and J. R. Williams: Effect of various sterol derivatives on blood pressure of rat, J. Pharmacol. & Exper. Therap. 69:149, 1940.

47. Hall, C. E., and H. Selye: Prevention of nephrosclerosis usually induced by anterior pituitary extract, Rev. canad. de biol. 4:197, 1945.

48. Hay, E. C., and P. Seguin: Assay of nephrosclerosis producing anterior pituitary preparations, Am. J. Physiol. 147:299, 1946.

49. Haynes, F. W., and L. Dexter: Renin, hypertensinogen, and hypertensinase concentration of blood of dogs during development of hypertension by constriction of renal artery, Am. J. Physiol. 150:190, 1947.

50. Heller, H.: Uber die zentrale Blutdruckzentren und die experimentelle Erzeugung zentral bedingten Hochdrucks, Klin. Wchnschr. 13:241, 1934.

51. Heymans, C., and J. J. Bouckaert: Au sujet de l'hypertension artérielle expérimentale, Bull. Acad. roy. de méd. de Belgique 4:441, 1939.

52. ———, J. J. Bouckaert, L. Elaut, F. Bayless, and A. Samaan: Hypertension artérielle chronique par ischémie rénale chez le chien totalement sympathectomisé, Compt. rend. de Soc. biol. 126:434, 1937.

53. Houssay, B. A., and J. C. Fasciolo: (a) Secreción hipertensora del riñón isquemiado, Rev. Soc. argent. de biol. 13:284, 1937; (b) Sécrétion hypertensive du rein ischémie, Compt. rend. de Soc. biol. 127:147, 1938.

54. Huidobro, F., and E. Braun-Menendez: Secretion of renin by intact kidney, Am. J. Physiol. 137:47, 1942.

55. Introzzi, A. S., A. N. Canonico, and J. A. Taiana: Hypertensión arterial; estudio experimental, tratamiento quirurgico, Semana méd. 1:841, 1938.

56. ———, J. Manrique, T. Raffaele, and M. I. O'Farrell: Efecto de la desnervación renal sobre el contenido de renina en la capa cortical del riñón, Rev. Soc. argent. de biol. 25:16, 1949.

57. ———, J. Manrique, T. Raffaele, M. I. O'Farrell, and C. Desgens: Estudios sobre la renina en el "shock" traumatico experimental: I. La fijacion de la renina, Medicina, Buenos Aires 9:262, 1949.

58. Katz, L. N., M. Friedman, S. Rodbard, and W. Weinstein: Observations on genesis of renal hypertension, Am. Heart J. 17:334, 1939.

59. Kernodle, C. E., H. C. Hill, and K. S. Grimson: Effect of activity, rest and natural sleep upon blood pressure of renal hypertensive dogs, Proc. Soc. Exper. Biol. & Med. 63:335, 1946.

60. Knowlton, A. I., E. N. Loeb, H. C. Stoerk, and B. C. Seegal: The development of hypertension and nephritis in normal and adrenalectomized rats with cortisone, Proc. Soc. Exper. Biol. & Med. 72:722, 1949.

61. Kohlstaedt, K. G., I. H. Page, and O. M. Helmer: Activation of renin by blood, Am. Heart J. 19:92, 1940.

62. Kottke, F. J., W. G. Kubicek, and M. B. Visscher: Production of arterial hypertension by chronic renal artery-nerve stimulation, Am. J. Physiol. 145:38, 1945.

63. Kuhlman, D., C. Ragan, J. W. Ferrebee, D. W. Atchley, and R. F. Loeb: Toxic effects of desoxycorticosterone esters in dogs, Science 90:496, 1939.

64. Leloir, L. F., J. M. Muñoz, E. Braun-Menendez, and J. C. Fasciolo: La secreción de renina y la formación de hipertensina, Rev. Soc. argent. de biol. 16:635, 1940.

65. Loeb, R. F., D. W. Atchley, J. W. Ferrebee, and C. Ragan: Observations on effects of desoxycorticosterone esters and progesterone in patients with Addison's disease, Tr. A. Am. Physicians 54:285, 1939.

66. Masson, G. M. C., A. C. Corcoran, and I. H. Page: Dietary and hormonal influences in experimental uremia, J. Lab. & Clin. Med. 34:1416, 1949.

67. Moss, W. G., and G. E. Wakerlin: Role of the nervous system in early and late hypertension in the dog, Federation Proc. 6:167, 1947; 7:82, 1948.

68. Nowak, S. J. G., and I. J. Walker: Experimental studies concerning nature of hypertension; their bearing on surgical treatment, New England J. Med. 220:269, 1939.

69. Ogden, E., W. D. Colling, A. N. Taylor, and E. Tripp: Production of neurohypertension by kidney, Texas Rep. Biol. & Med. 4:14, 1946.

70. Orías, O.: Hipófisis y presión arterial en el sapo, Rev. Soc. argent. de biol. 10:91, 1934.

71. Page, E. W., E. Ogden, and E. Anderson: Influence of steroids on restoration of hypertension in hypophysectomized rats, Am. J. Physiol. 147:471, 1946.

72. Page, I. H.: Relationship of extrinsic renal nerves to origin of experimental hypertension, Am. J. Physiol. 112:166, 1935.

73. ——: Effect of bilateral adrenalectomy on arterial blood pressure of dogs with experimental hypertension, Am. J. Physiol. 122:352, 1938.

74. ——, and O. M. Helmer: Crystalline pressor substance (angiotonin) resulting from reaction between renin and renin-activator, J. Exper. Med. 71:29, 1940.

75. ——, and R. D. Taylor: Variations of vascular reactivity in normal and hypertensive dogs, Am. J. Physiol. 156:412, 1949.

76. Perera, G. A.: The adrenal cortex and hypertension, Bull. New York Acad. Med. 26:75, 1950.

77. ——, and D. W. Blood: Pressor activity of desoxycorticosterone acetate in normotensive and hypertensive subjects, Ann. Int. Med. 27:401, 1947.

78. ——, and K. L. Pines: Simultaneous administration of adrenal cortical extract and desoxycorticosterone; effects on blood pressure of hypertensive patients, Proc. Soc. Exper. Biol. & Med. 71:443, 1949.

79. ——, K. L. Pines, H. B. Hamilton, and K. Vislocky: Clinical study of 11-dehydro-17-hydroxycorticosterone in hypertension, Addison's disease and diabetes, J. Clin. Investigation 28:803, 1949.

80. Pickering, G. W.: Circulation in arterial hypertension, Brit. M. J. 2:1, 31, 1943.

81. Prado, J. L., and P. Dontigny: Hipertensäo hormonal experimental, Rev. brasil. med. 5:5, 1948.

82. ——, P. Dontigny, E. C. Hay, and H. Selye: Further studies concerning the role of the diet in the production of nephrosclerosis and hypertension by anterior pituitary preparations, Federation Proc. 6:182, 1947.

83. Rogoff, J. M., E. Marcus, and P. Wasserman: Experiments on supposed relation of epinephrine secretion to hypertension, Proc. Soc. Exper. Biol. & Med. 38:199, 1938.

84. Sapeika, N.: Effect of stilboestrol on blood pressure of albino rat, Arch. internat. de pharmacodyn. et de thérap. 76:327, 1948.

85. Sapirstein, L. A., W. L. Brandt, and D. R. Drury: Production of hypertension in the rat by substituting hypertonic sodium chloride solutions for drinking water, Proc. Soc. Exper. Biol. & Med. 73:82, 1950.

86. Schroeder, H. A., M. L. Goldman, and N. S. Olsen: Pressor substances in hypertensive blood, Federation Proc. 7:110, 1948; J. Clin. Investigation 27:555, 1948.

87. Selye, H.: Production of nephrosclerosis by overdosage with desoxycorticosterone acetate, Canad. M. A. J. 47:515, 1942.

88. ———: Role of hypophysis in pathogenesis of diseases of adaptation, Canad. M. A. J. 50:426, 1944.

89. ———: Production of hypertension and hyalinosis by desoxycorticosterone, Brit. M. J. 1:203, 1950.

90. ———, E. Beland, and H. Stone: Effet des hormones hypophysaires, thyroidienne et cortico-surrénale sur la structure rénale, Rev. canad. de biol. 4:120, 1945.

91. ———, and E. M. Rowley: Prevention of experimental nephrosclerosis with methyl-testosterone, Federation Proc. 3:41, 1944.

92. ———, H. Stone, K. Nielsen, and C. P. Leblond: Studies concerning effects of various hormones upon renal structure, Canad. M. A. J. 52:571, 1945.

93. Shipley, R. E., and O. M. Helmer: Role of kidneys in modifying response to "sustained pressor principle," Am. J. Physiol. 151:606, 1947.

94. Shorr, E.: Editorial, Seminars on hypertension, Am. J. Med. 5:783, 1948.

95. ———, B. W. Zweifach, R. F. Furchgott, and S. Baez: Hepato-renal vasotropic factors in experimental shock and renal hypertension, Federation Proc. 6:200, 1947.

96. Skahen, J. G., and D. M. Green: Mechanisms of desoxycorticosterone action: IV. Relationship of fluid intake and pressor responses to output of antidiuretic factor, Am. J. Physiol. 155:290, 1948.

97. Sprague, R. G., et al.: Observations on the physiologic effects of cortisone and ACTH in man, Arch. Int. Med. 85:199, 1950.

98. Taquini, A. C., and J. C. Fasciolo: El papel de la renina circulante en la hipertensión arterial, Rev. argent. de cardiol. 14:1, 1947.

99. ———, and J. C. Fasciolo: Partial ischemia and renin content of the kidneys, Medicina, Buenos Aires 9:111, 1949.

100. ———, and J. C. Fasciolo: Medicina, Buenos Aires 10:1950, in press.

101. Taylor, R. D., A. C. Corcoran, and I. H. Page: Effects of denervation on experimental renal hypertension, Federation Proc. 7:123, 1948.

102. Tigerstedt, R., and P. G. von Bergmann: Niere und Kreislauf, Skandinav. Arch. f. Physiol. 8:223, 1898.

103. Trueta, J., A. E. Barclay, K. J. Franklin, P. M. Daniel, and M. M. L. Prichard: Studies of the Renal Circulation, Springfield, Ill., Charles C Thomas, 1947.

104. Vallery-Radot, P., S. Blondin, R. Israel, and C. Cachin: L'hypertension artérielle par ischémie rénale, Presse méd. 46:969, 1938.

105. Vaquez, H.: Hypertension, Congr. franç. méd. 1:338, 1904.

106. Yeakel, E. H., H. A. Shenkin, A. B. Rothballer, and S. M. McCann: Blood pressures of rats subjected to auditory stimulation, Am. J. Physiol. 155:118, 1948.

107. Zweifach, B. W., and E. Shorr: Desoxycorticosterone hypertension in relation to hepatorenal mechanisms, Federation Proc. 9:141, 1950.

Some Observations on Renal Vascular Disease in Hypertensive Patients Based on Biopsy Material Obtained at Operation,
by Reginald H. Smithwick and Benjamin Castleman

1. R. Bright: Reports of Medical Cases Selected with a View of Illustrating the Symptoms and Cure of Diseases by a Reference to Morbid Anatomy, London, Longman, Rees, Orne, Brown and Green, 1827, vol. 1, 231 pp.

2. R. Bright: Cases and observations illustrative of renal disease accompanied with secretion of albuminous urine, Guy's Hosp. Rep. 1:338–400, 1836.

3. W. W. Gull and H. G. Sutton: On the pathology of the morbid state commonly called chronic Bright's disease with contracted kidney ("arterio-capillary fibrosis"), Med.-Chir. Tr. 55:273–326, 1872.

4. A. R. Moritz and M. R. Oldt: Arteriolar sclerosis in hypertensive and non-hypertensive individuals, Am. J. Path. 13:679–728 (Sept.) 1937.

5. H. Goldblatt: Studies on experimental hypertension; experimental production and pathogenesis of hypertension due to renal ischemia, Am. J. Clin. Path. 10:40–72 (Jan.) 1940.

6. I. H. Page: Production of persistent arterial hypertension by cellophane perinephritis, J. A. M. A. 113:2046–2048 (Dec.) 1939.

7. B. Castleman and R. H. Smithwick: The relation of vascular disease to the hypertensive state, J. A. M. A. 121:1256–1261 (April) 1943.

8. B. Castleman and R. H. Smithwick: The relation of vascular disease to the hypertensive state: II. The adequacy of the renal biopsy as determined from a study of 500 patients, New England J. Med. 239:729–732 (Nov.) 1948.

9. H. Chasis and J. Redish: Effective renal blood flow in separate kidneys of subjects with essential hypertension, J. Clin. Investigation 20:655–661 (Nov.) 1941.

10. H. W. Smith: Studies in the Physiology of the Kidney, Lawrence, University of Kansas, University Extension Division, 1939.

11. E. A. Hines, Jr., and G. E. Brown: Standard test for measuring the variability of blood pressure: Its significance as an index of the prehypertensive state, Ann. Int. Med. 7:209–217 (Aug.) 1933.

12. J. H. Talbot, B. Castleman, R. H. Smithwick, R. S. Melville, and L. J. Pecora: Renal biopsy studies correlated with renal clearance observations in hypertensive patients treated by radical sympathectomy, J. Clin. Investigation 22:387–394 (May) 1943.

13. E. T. Bell and B. J. Clawson: Primary (essential) hypertension; a study of 420 cases, Arch. Path. 5:939–1002, 1928.

The Mechanism of Hypertension in Chronic Genuine Nephrosis,
by George E. Fahr

1. E. T. Bell and A. H. Pederson: Renal hypertension caused by clamping renal veins, Ann. Int. Med. 4:227, 1932.

2. H. Goldblatt, J. Lynch, R. Hanzal, and W. Summerville: Production of elevated blood pressure by means of renal ischaemia caused by clamping renal arteries, J. Exper. Med. 59:347, 1934.

3a. E. T. Bell: Pathology of nephritis and nephrosis, Am. J. Path. 14:691, 1938.

3b. ———: Renal Diseases, ed. 2, Philadelphia, Lea & Febiger, 1950, pp. 206–228.

Renal Hemodynamics in Essential Hypertension, by Herbert Chasis

1. Alving, A. S., W. Adams, K. S. Grimson, C. Scott, and I. Sandeford: The effect of bilateral sympathectomy on the cardio-renal system in essential hypertension, Proc. Central Soc. Clin. Research 13:39, 1940.

2. Bell, E. T.: Renal Diseases, Philadelphia, Lea & Febiger, 1946.

3. Bolomey, A. A., et al.: Simultaneous measurement of effective renal blood flow and cardiac output in resting normal subjects and patients with essential hypertension, J. Clin. Investigation 28:10, 1949.

4. Bradley, S. E.: Physiology of hypertension, Am. J. Med. 4:398, 1948.

5. Bradley, S. E., J. J. Curry, and G. P. Bradley: Renal extraction of p-aminohippurate in normal subjects and in essential hypertension and chronic diffuse glomerulonephritis, Federation Proc. 6:79, 1947.

6. Cargill, W. H.: The measurement of glomerular and tubular plasma flow in the normal and diseased human kidney, J. Clin. Investigation 28:533, 1949.

7. Cargill, W. H., and J. B. Hickam: The oxygen consumption of the normal and diseased human kidney, J. Clin. Investigation 28:526, 1949.

8. Chasis, H., and J. Redish: Effective renal blood flow in the separate kidneys of subjects with essential hypertension, J. Clin. Investigation 20:655, 1941.

9. Corcoran, A. C., and I. H. Page: Renal blood flow and sympathectomy in hypertension, Arch. Surg. 42:1072, 1941.

10. Foa, P. P., W. W. Wood, M. M. Peet, and N. L. Foa: Studies relative to physiological basis of splanchnicectomy in treatment of hypertension; preliminary report, Univ. Hosp. Bull., Ann. Arbor 8:9, 1942.

11. Goldring, W., and H. Chasis: Hypertension and Hypertensive Disease, New York, Commonwealth Press, 1944.

12. Goldring, W., and H. Chasis: Sympathectomy and unilateral nephrectomy in the treatment of hypertensive disease, M. Clin. North America, New York Number, May 1949, 751.

13. Goldring, W., H. Chasis, H. A. Ranges, and H. W. Smith: Effective renal blood flow in subjects with essential hypertension, J. Clin. Investigation 20:637, 1941.

14. Gomez, D. M.: Evaluation of Renal Vascular Characteristics in Normal Subjects and in Patients with Essential Hypertension. In preparation.

15. Lamport, H.: The effects on renal resistance to blood flow of renin, angiotonin, pitressin and atropine, hypertension, and toxemia of pregnancy, J. Clin. Investigation 21:685, 1942.

16. Maxwell, M. H., E. S. Breed, and H. W. Smith: Significance of the renal juxtamedullary circulation in man, Am. J. Med. 9:216, 1950.

17. Reubi, F. C., and H. A. Schroeder: Can vascular shunting be induced in the kidney by vasoactive drugs? J. Clin. Investigation 28:114, 1949.

18. Smith, H. W.: The Kidney: Structure and Function in Health and Disease, New York, Oxford University Press, in press.

19. Smith, H. W., H. Chasis, W. Goldring, and H. A. Ranges: Glomerular dynamics in the normal human kidney, J. Clin. Investigation 19:751, 1940.

20. Smith, H. W., W. Goldring, and H. Chasis: The measurement of the tubular excretory mass, effective blood flow and filtration rate in the normal human kidney, J. Clin. Investigation 17:263, 1938.

21. Smith, H. W., W. Goldring, H. Chasis, H. A. Ranges, and S. E. Bradley: The William Henry Welch Lectures: II. The application of saturation methods to the study of glomerular and tubular function in the human kidney, J. Mt. Sinai Hosp. 10:59, 1943.

22. Smith, H. W., E. A. Rovenstine, W. Goldring, H. Chasis, and H. A. Ranges: The effects of spinal anaesthesia on the circulation in normal, unoperated man with reference to the autonomy of the arterioles, and especially those of the renal circulation, J. Clin. Investigation 18:319, 1939.

23. Talbot, J. H., B. Castleman, R. Smithwick, R. S. Melville, and L. J. Pecora: Renal biopsy studies correlated with renal clearance observations in hypertensive subjects treated by radical sympathectomy, J. Clin. Investigation 22:387, 1943.

24. Trueta, J., A. E. Barclay, P. M. Daniel, K. J. Franklin, and M. M. L. Prichard: Studies of the Renal Circulation, Springfield, Ill., Charles C. Thomas, 1947.

The Heart in Essential Hypertension, by Benjamin J. Clawson

1. S. A. Levine: Clinical Heart Disease, Philadelphia, W. B. Saunders, 1937, p. 158.

2. R. L. Levy and W. C. Von Glahn: Cardiac hypertrophy of unknown cause, Am. Heart J. 28:714, 1944.

3. P. D. White: The hypertensive heart, New England J. Med. 225:571, 1941.

4. J. R. Kahn and E. S. Ingraham: Cardiac hypertrophy and coronary arteriosclerosis in hypertension, Arch. Path. 31:373, 1941.

5. J. C. Paterson: Capillary rupture with intimal hemorrhage as a causative factor in coronary thrombosis, Arch. Path. 25:474, 1938.

6. H. A. Edmondson and H. J. Hoxie: Hypertension and cardiac rupture, Am. Heart J. 24:719, 1942.

7. S. Friedman and P. D. White: Rupture of the heart in myocardial infarction, Ann. Int. Med. 21:778, 1944.

8. W. W. Jetter and P. D. White: Rupture of the heart in patients in mental institutions, Ann. Int. Med. 21:783, 1944.

Hepatorenal Factors in Essential Hypertension in Man, by Ephraim Shorr

1. E. Shorr, B. W. Zweifach, R. F. Furchgott, and S. Baez: Hepatorenal factors in experimental hypertension, in Transactions of the First Conference on Factors Regulating Blood Pressure, Josiah Macy, Jr., Foundation, New York, 1947, p. 32.

2. E. Shorr and B. W. Zweifach: Hepatorenal vasotropic factors in blood during chronic essential hypertension in man, Tr. A. Am. Physicians 61:350, 1948.

3. B. W. Zweifach, M. M. Black, and E. Shorr: Histochemical alterations revealed by tetrazolium chloride in hypertensive kidneys in relation to renal VEM mechanisms, Proc. Soc. Exper. Biol. & Med. 74:848, 1950.

4. R. E. Lee and E. A. Holze: The peripheral vascular system in the bulbar conjunctiva of young normotensive adults at rest, J. Clin. Investigation 29:146, 1950.

Pulmonary Hypertension, by Richard V. Ebert

1. R. A. Bloomfield, H. D. Lauson, A. Cournand, E. S. Breed, and D. W. Richards, Jr.: Recording of right heart pressures in normal subjects and in patients with chronic pulmonary disease and various types of cardiocirculatory disease, J. Clin. Investigation 25:639, 1946.

2. C. W. Borden: Fundamental and clinical aspects of pulmonary hypertension, Minnesota Med. 31:1216, 1948.

3. H. Lagerlöf and L. Werkö: Studies on the circulation in man: II. Normal values for cardiac output and pressure in the right auricle, right ventricle and pulmonary artery, Acta physiol. Scandinav. 16:75, 1948.

4. S. Rodbard, F. Brown, and L. N. Katz: The Pulmonary Arterial Pressure, Am. Heart J. 38:863, 1949.

5. W. F. Hamilton, R. A. Woodbury, and E. B. Woods: Relation between systemic and pulmonary blood pressures in the fetus, Am. J. Physiol. 119:206, 1937.

6. L. Werkö and H. Lagerlöf: Studies on the circulation in man: IV. Cardiac output and pressure in the right auricle, right ventricle, and pulmonary artery in patients with hypertensive cardiovascular disease, Acta med. Scandinav. 133:427, 1949.

7. C. W. Borden, R. H. Wilson, R. V. Ebert, and H. S. Wells: Pulmonary hypertension in chronic pulmonary emphysema, Am. J. Med. 8:701, 1950.

8. J. B. Johnson, M. I. Fener, J. R. West, and A. Cournand: The relation between electrocardiographic evidence of right ventricular hypertrophy and pulmonary arterial pressure in patients with chronic pulmonary disease, Circulation 1:536, 1950.

9. A. Cournand: Recent observations on the dynamics of the pulmonary circulation, Bull. New York Acad. Med. 23:27, 1947.

10. C. W. Borden and J. W. LaBree: Primary Pulmonary Hypertension. To be published.

11. R. L. Riley, A. Himmelstein, H. L. Motley, H. M. Weiner, and A. Cournand: Circulation at rest and during exercise in normal individuals and patients with chronic pulmonary disease, Am. J. Physiol. 152:372, 1948.

12. J. B. Hickam and W. H. Cargill: Effect of exercise on cardiac output and pul-

Bibliography 563

monary arterial pressure in normal persons and in patients with cardiovascular disease
and pulmonary emphysema, J. Clin. Investigation 27:10, 1948.

13. L. Dexter et al.: Studies of congenital heart disease: III. Venous catheterization
as a diagnostic aid in patent ductus arteriosus, tetralogy of fallot, ventricular septal
defect and auricular septal defect, J. Clin. Investigation 26:561, 1947.

14. J. C. Handlesman, R. J. Bing, J. A. Campbell, and H. E. Griswold: Physiological
studies in congenital heart disease: V. The circulation in patients with isolated septal
defects, Bull. Johns Hopkins Hosp. 82:615, 1948.

15. A. Cournand, J. S. Baldwin, and A. Himmelstein: Cardiac catheterization in
congenital heart disease, New York, The Commonwealth Fund, 1949.

16. H. B. Burchell: Variations in the clinical and pathologic picture of patent ductus
arteriosus, M. Clin. North America 32:911, 1948.

17. H. E. Griswold, R. J. Bing, J. C. Handlesman, J. A. Campbell, and E. Le Brun:
Physiological studies in congenital heart disease: VII. Pulmonary arterial hypertension
in congenital heart disease, Bull. Johns Hopkins Hosp. 84:76, 1949.

18. J. B. Hickam: Atrial septal defect; a study of intracardiac shunts, ventricular
outputs, and pulmonary pressure gradient, Am. Heart J. 38:801, 1949.

19. R. J. Bing, L. D. Vandam, and F. D. Gray, Jr.: Physiological studies in congenital heart disease: III. Results obtained in five cases of Eisenmenger's complex,
Bull. Johns Hopkins Hosp. 80:323, 1947.

20. H. B. Burchell, B. E. Taylor, J. R. B. Knutson, and E. H. Wood: Circulatory
adjustments to the hypoxemia of congenital heart disease of the cyanotic type, Circulation 1:404, 1950.

21. G. W. Campbell, F. J. Haddy, W. L. Adams, and M. B. Visscher: Circulatory
changes and pulmonary lesions in dogs following increased intracranial pressure and
effect of atropine upon such changes, Am. J. Physiol. 158:96, 1949.

22. C. W. Borden, R. V. Ebert, R. H. Wilson, and H. S. Wells: Pulmonary hypertension in heart disease, New England J. Med. 242:529, 1950.

23. L. Dexter et al.: Studies of the pulmonary circulation in man at rest: Normal
variations and interrelations between increased pulmonary blood flow, elevated pulmonary artery pressures and high pulmonary "capillary" pressures, J. Clin. Investigation 29:602, 1950.

24. H. L. Motley, A. Cournand, L. Werkö, A. Himmelstein, and D. Dresdale: Influence of short periods of induced acute anoxia upon pulmonary artery pressures in
man, Am. J. Physiol. 150:315, 1947.

25. G. Liljestrand: Regulation of pulmonary arterial blood pressure, Arch. Int. Med.
81:162, 1948.

26. M. N. J. Dirken and H. Heemstra: Alveolar oxygen tension and lung circulation,
Quart. J. Exper. Physiol. 34:193, 1948.

*A Summary of Experimental Evidence Relating Life Stress to the
Pathogenesis of Essential Hypertension in Man,*
by Stewart Wolf and Harold G. Wolff

1. J. P. O'Hare: Vascular reactions in vascular hypertension, Am. J. M. Sc. 159:371,
1920.

2. T. H. Holmes, H. Goodell, Stewart Wolf, and H. G. Wolff: The Nose: An Experimental Study of Reactions within the Nose in Human Subjects during Varying
Life Experiences, New York, Charles C. Thomas, 1950.

3. Stewart Wolf and H. G. Wolff: Human Gastric Function: An Experimental
Study of a Man and His Stomach, New York, Oxford University Press, 1943. Rev.
1947.

4. W. J. Grace, Stewart Wolf, and H. G. Wolff: The Human Colon, New York, Paul
Hoeber, 1950.

5. L. E. Hinkle, G. Conger, and Stewart Wolf: Studies on diabetes mellitus: The relation of stressful life situations to the concentration of ketone bodies in the blood of diabetic and nondiabetic humans, J. Clin. Investigation 29:754, 1950.

6. D. Graham and Stewart Wolf: The pathogenesis of hives: Experimental study of life situations, emotions and cutaneous vascular reactions, J. A. M. A. 143:1396, 1950.

7. L. R. Straub, H. S. Ripley, and Stewart Wolf: Disturbances in bladder function in association with varying life situations and emotional states, J. A. M. A. 141:1139, 1949.

8. H. G. Wolff: Protective reaction patterns and disease, Ann. Int. Med. 27:944, 1947.

9. Stewart Wolf and E. M. Shepard: An appraisal of factors that evoke and modify the hypertensive reaction pattern, Proc. A. Research Nerv. & Ment. Dis. 29:976, 1950.

10. Stewart Wolf, J. B. Pfeiffer, H. S. Ripley, O. S. Winter, and H. G. Wolff: Hypertension as a reaction pattern to stress: Summary of experimental data on variations in blood pressure and renal blood flow, Ann. Int. Med. 29:1056, 1948.

11. William H. Sheldon: Personal communication.

12. F. Alexander: Emotional factors in essential hypertension, Psychosom. Med. 1:173, 1939.

13. L. J. Saul: Hostility in cases of essential hypertension, Psychosom. Med. 1:153, 1939.

14. E. Weiss: Psychosomatic aspects of hypertension, J. A. M. A. 120:1081, 1942.

15. C. Binger, N. Ackerman, A. Cohn, H. A. Schroeder, and J. M. Steele: Personality in arterial hypertension, Monograph, Psychosom. Med., 1945.

16. I. P. Stevenson, C. H. Duncan, and Stewart Wolf: Hypertension as a reaction pattern to stress: Observations on variations in peripheral resistance with changes in the emotional state. In press.

17. J. L. Nickerson, J. V. Warren, and E. S. Brannon: The cardiac output in man: Studies with the low frequency, critically-damped ballistocardiograph, and the method of right atrial catheterization, J. Clin. Investigation 26:1, 1947.

18. I. P. Stevenson, C. H. Duncan, and H. G. Wolff: Circulatory dynamics before and after exercise in subjects with and without structural heart disease during anxiety and relaxation, J. Clin. Investigation 28:1534, 1949.

19. H. L. Taylor, A. Henschel, J. Brozek, and A. Keys: Relationship between the blood pressure increase in exercise, carbon dioxide inhalation and cold pressor test, Federation Proc. 8:154, 1949.

20. John T. Flynn: Data to be published.

21. R. A. Schneider: Variations in clotting time, relative viscosity and certain other physio-chemical changes in the blood accompanying physical and emotional stress in the normotensive and hypertensive subject, Psychosom. Med., in press.

22. H. Y. T'ang and S. H. Wang: Clinical application of plasma viscosity determination: Description of pipette viscosimeter and the report of findings in tuberculosis, Chinese M. J. 57:546, 1940.

23. N. W. Barker and H. Margulies: Coagulation time of blood in silicone tubes in patients on dicoumarol, Am. J. M. Sc. 218:52, 1949.

24. E. A. Hines, Jr.: Technique of the cold pressor test, Proc. Staff Meet., Mayo Clin. 14:185, 1939.

25. Stewart Wolf and J. D. Hardy: Studies on pain: Observations on pain due to local cooling and on factors involved in the "cold pressor" effect, Proc. A. Research Nerv. & Ment. Dis. 23:123, 1943.

26. R. A. Schneider: The relation of stress to clotting time, relative viscosity and certain other biophysical alterations of the blood in the normotensive and hypertensive subject, Proc. A. Research Nerv. & Ment. Dis. 29:818, 1950.

27. W. B. Cannon and W. L. Mendenhall: The factors effecting the coagulation time of blood, Am. J. Physiol. 34:225, 1914.

28. H. W. Smith: Physiology of the renal circulation, Harvey Lectures, 1939–1940, Series 35, p. 204.

29. J. B. Pfeiffer and H. G. Wolff: Studies in renal circulation during periods of life stress and accompanying emotional reactions in subjects with and without essential hypertension; observations on the role of neural activity in regulation of renal blood flow, Proc. A. Research Nerv. & Ment. Dis. 29:929, 1950.

30. H. Goldblatt: The renal origin of hypertension, Physiol. Rev. 27:1, 1947.

31. W. Goldring and H. Chasis: Hypertension and Hypertensive Disease, New York, The Commonwealth Fund, 1944.

32. H. Lamport: Formulae for afferent and efferent arteriolar resistance in the human kidney, J. Clin. Investigation 20:535, 1941.

———: Relative change in afferent and efferent arteriolar resistance in the normal human kidney, J. Clin. Investigation 20:545, 1941.

———: Effect on renal resistance to blood flow of renin, angiotonin, pitressin, atropin, hypertension and pregnancy, J. Clin. Investigation 21:685, 1942.

———: Improvement of calculation of renal resistance to blood flow: Charts for osmotic pressure and viscosity of blood, J. Clin. Investigation 22:461, 1943.

33. D. M. Gomez: Hemodynamics of the renal circulation, Revue Scientifique, numéro 3272:451, 1947.

———: Calculation of effective efferent and afferent arteriolar resistance, Federation Proc. 7:41, 1948.

34. J. T. Flynn, M. A. K. Kennedy, and Stewart Wolf: Essential hypertension in one of identical twins: An experimental study of cardiovascular reactions in the Y twins, Proc. A. Research Nerv. & Ment. Dis. 29:954, 1950.

35. W. H. Sheldon and R. Ball: Physical characteristics of the Y twins and their relation to hypertension, Proc. A. Research Nerv. & Ment. Dis. 29:962, 1950.

36. C. L. Evans and Y. Matsuoka: The effect of various mechanical conditions on the gaseous metabolism and efficiency of the mammalian heart, J. Physiol. 49:378, 1915.

37. R. W. Tibbetts: Leucotomy and hypertension, Brit. M. J. 11:1452, 1949.

38. W. P. Chapman, R. B. Livingston, K. E. Livingston, and W. B. Sweet: Possible cortical areas involved in arterial hypertension, Proc. A. Research Nerv. & Ment. Dis. 29:775, 1950.

39. E. A. Spiegel: Personal communication.

40. L. J. Pool and R. G. Heath: Bilateral fractional resection of frontal cortex for the treatment of psychoses, J. Nerv. & Ment. Dis. 107:411, 1948.

41. W. Freeman and J. W. Watts: Psychosurgery, Springfield, Ill., Charles C. Thomas, 1942.

Vascular Reactivity and Hypertensive Disease, by Edgar A. Hines, Jr.

1. E. A. Hines, Jr.: Technic of the cold-pressor test, Proc. Staff Meet., Mayo Clin. 14:185–187 (Mar. 22) 1939.

2. E. A. Hines, Jr.: The significance of vascular hyperreaction as measured by the cold-pressor test, Am. Heart J. 19:408–416 (Apr.) 1940.

3. E. A. Hines, Jr.: Range of normal blood pressure and subsequent development of hypertension: A follow-up study of 1,522 patients, J. A. M. A. 115:271–274 (July 27) 1940.

4. H. S. Diehl and M. B. Hesdorffer: Changes in blood pressure of young men over a seven year period, Arch. Int. Med. 52:948–953 (Dec.) 1933.

5. S. C. Robinson and Marshall Brucer: Range of normal blood pressure: A statistical and clinical study of 11,383 persons, Arch. Int. Med. 64:409–444 (Sept.) 1939.

6. R. L. Levy, P. D. White, W. D. Stroud, and C. C. Hillman: Transient hypertension: The relative importance of various systolic and diastolic levels, J. A. M. A. 128:1059–1061 (Aug. 11) 1945.

7. E. A. Hines, Jr.: The hereditary factor in essential hypertension, Ann. Int. Med. 11:593–601 (Oct.) 1937.

8. J. F. Briggs and Harry Oerting: Vasomotor response of normal and hypertensive individuals to thermal stimulus (cold), Minnesota Med. 16:481–486 (July) 1933.

9. W. J. Dieckmann and H. L. Michel: Thermal study of vasomotor lability in pregnancy; preliminary report, Arch. Int. Med. 55:420–430 (Mar.) 1935.

10. M. R. Yates and J. E. Wood, Jr.: Vasomotor response of non-hypertensive individuals to a standard cold stimulus, Proc. Soc. Exper. Biol. & Med. 34:560–562 (May) 1936.

11. E. H. Schwab, D. L. Curb, J. L. Matthews, and V. E. Schulze: Blood pressure response to a standard stimulus in the white and Negro races, Proc. Soc. Exper. Biol. & Med. 32:583–585 (Jan.) 1935.

12. Norman Reider: Blood pressure studies on psychiatric patients, Bull. Menninger Clin. 2:65–73 (May) 1938.

13. B. V. White, Jr., and E. F. Gildea: "Cold pressor test" in tension and anxiety: A cardiochronographic study, Arch. Neurol. & Psychiat. 38:964–984 (Nov.) 1937.

14. M. F. Reiser and E. B. Ferris, Jr.: The nature of the cold pressor test and its significance in relation to neurogenic and humoral mechanisms in hypertension, J. Clin. Investigation 27:156–163 (Jan.) 1948.

15. E. A. Hines, Jr., and H. H. Lander: Factors contributing to the development of hypertension in patients suffering from renal disease, J. A. M. A. 116:1050–1052 (Mar. 15) 1941.

Cerebral Attacks in Hypertension, by George W. Pickering

1. F. Volhard and Th. Fahr: Die Brightsche Nierenkrankheit, Berlin, 1914.

2. B. S. Oppenheimer and A. M. Fishberg: Arch. Int. Med. 41:264, 1928.

3. F. M. R. Walshe: Diseases of the Nervous System, ed. 6, Edinburgh, p. 99.

4. C. S. Roy and C. S. Sherrington: J. Physiol. 11:85, 1890.

5. L. Hill and J. J. R. MacLeod: J. Physiol. 26:394, 1900.

6. H. W. Florey: Brain 48:23, 1925.

7. H. S. Forbes and H. G. Wolff: Arch. Neurol. & Psychiat. 19:1057, 1928.

8. H. S. Forbes, K. H. Finley, and G. I. Nason: Arch. Neurol. & Psychiat. 30:957, 1933.

9. T. Lewis, G. W. Pickering, and T. Rothschild: Heart 16:1, 1931.

10. C. E. Beevor: Phil. Trans. R. S. Lond. S. B. 200:1, 1909.

11. J. T. Shepherd: Clin. Sci. 9:1950.

12. G. W. Pickering: J. A. M. A. 137:423, 1948.

13. E. F. Rosenberg: Arch. Int. Med. 65:545, 1940.

14. K. Westphal and R. Bär: Deutsche Arch. f. klin. Med. 131:1, 1926.

15. W. Spielmayer: Monatschr. f. Psychiat. u. Neurol. 68:605, 1928.

16. L. Traube: Gesammette Beiträge zur Pathologie und Physiologie, Berlin, 1871, vol. 2, p. 551.

17. H. Gorke and G. Topplich: Ztschr. f. klin. Med. 92:113, 1921.

18. K. D. Blackfan and B. Hamilton: Boston M. & S. J. 193:617, 1925.

19. F. Volhard, in L. Mohr and R. Staehelin: Handbuch der inneren Medizin, ed. z, Berlin, vol. 6, pt. 1.

20. G. W. Pickering: Clin. Sci. 1:193.

21. D. McAlpine: Quart. J. Med. 2:463, 1933.

Blood Lipid Transport in Hypertensive Patients and Its Relation to Atherosclerotic Complications, by John W. Gofman

1. J. Gofman, F. T. Lindgren, and H. Elliott: Ultracentrifugal studies of lipoproteins of human serum, J. Biol. Chem. 179:973, 1949.

2. J. Gofman, F. T. Lindgren, T. P. Lyon, et al.: The role of lipids and lipoproteins in atherosclerosis, Science 111:166, 1950.

3. J. Gofman, H. B. Jones, F. T. Lindgren, et al.: Blood lipids and human atherosclerosis, Circulation 2:161, 1950.

4. W. Hueper: Experimental approaches to the problem of arteriosclerosis, Geriatrics 2:293, 1947.

5. E. F. Hirsch and S. Weinhouse: The role of lipids in atherosclerosis, Physiol. Rev. 23:3, 1943.

The Hemodynamic Effects of Various Types of
Therapy in Hypertensive Patients,
by Robert W. Wilkins

1. R. H. Smithwick: Surgery of the Autonomic Nervous System: Cole's Operative Technic in Specialty Surgery, New York, Appleton-Century-Crofts, 1949, pp. 553–598.

2. J. A. Evans and C. C. Bartels: Results of high dorsolumbar sympathectomy for hypertension, Ann. Int. Med. 30:307, 1949.

3. R. W. Wilkins, J. W. Culbertson, and R. H. Smithwick: The effects of various types of sympathectomy upon vasopressor responses in hypertensive patients, Surg., Gynec. & Obst. 87:661, 1948.

4. W. E. Judson, J. W. Culbertson, C. M. Tinsley, J. Litter, and R. W. Wilkins: The comparative effects of small intravenous doses of epinephrine upon arterial pressure and pulse rate in normotensive subjects and in hypertensive patients before and after thoracolumbar sympathectomy, J. Clin. Investigation, in press.

5. W. E. Judson, F. H. Epstein, and R. W. Wilkins: The comparative effects of small intravenous doses of l-nor-epinephrine upon arterial pressure and pulse rate in normotensive subjects and in hypertensive patients before and after thoracolumbar sympathectomy, J. Clin. Investigation, in press.

6. A. M. DiMare, F. H. Epstein, and R. W. Wilkins: Unpublished studies.

7. R. W. Wilkins, J. W. Culbertson, and M. H. Halperin: The hemodynamic effects of sympathectomy in essential hypertension, Ann. Int. Med. 30:291, 1949.

8. H. A. Shenkin, J. H. Hafkenschiel, and S. S. Kety: The effects of sympathectomy on the cerebral circulation of hypertensive patients, Arch. Surg. 61:319, 1950.

9. R. W. Wilkins, J. W. Culbertson, and F. J. Ingelfinger: The effect of splanchnic sympathectomy in hypertensive patients upon estimated hepatic blood flow in the upright as contrasted with the horizontal position, J. Clin. Investigation, in press.

10. R. W. Wilkins, E. D. Freis, and J. R. Stanton: Essential hypertension: Laboratory studies in human beings with drugs recently introduced, J. A. M. A. 140:261, 1949.

11. E. D. Freis et al.: The hemodynamic effects of hypotensive drugs in man: II. Dihydroergocornine, J. Clin. Investigation 28:1387, 1949.

12. F. C. Moister, J. R. Stanton, and E. D. Freis: Observations on the development of tolerance during prolonged oral administration of dihydroergocornine, J. Pharmacol. & Exper. Therap. 96:21, 1949.

13. J. H. Hafkenschiel, C. W. Crumpton, J. H. Moyer, and W. A. Jeffers: The effects of dihydroergocornine on the cerebral circulation of patients with essential hypertension, J. Clin. Investigation 29:408, 1950.

14. E. D. Freis et al.: The hemodynamic effects of hypotensive drugs in man: I. Veratrum viride, J. Clin. Investigation 28:353, 1949.

15. J. R. Stanton, W. E. Judson, and R. W. Wilkins: Unpublished studies.

16. M. H. Halperin, F. H. Epstein, W. E. Judson, and R. W. Wilkins: Unpublished studies.

17. C. W. Crumpton, J. H. Hafkenschiel, and W. A. Jeffers: Personal communication.

Sympathetic Blockade in the Therapy of Hypertension,
by Mark Nickerson

1. M. Goldenberg, C. H. Snyder, and H. Aranow, Jr.: New test for hypertension due to circulating epinephrine, J. A. M. A. 135:971–976, 1947.

2. M. Nickerson: The pharmacology of adrenergic blockade, J. Pharmacol. & Exper. Therap. 95:27–101, 1949. (Part II, Pharmacol. Rev., vol. 1.)

3. V. A. Drill: Reactions from the use of benzodioxane (933 F) in diagnosis of pheochromocytoma, New England J. Med. 241:777–779, 1949.

4. M. Nickerson and L. S. Goodman: Pharmacological properties of a new adrenergic blocking agent: N, N-dibenzyl-β-chloroethylamine (Dibenamine), J. Pharmacol. & Exper. Therap. 89:167–185, 1947.

5. M. Nickerson and G. M. Nomaguchi: Locus of the adrenergic blocking action of Dibenamine, J. Pharmacol. & Exper. Therap. 93:40–51, 1948.

6. H. C. Spear and D. Griswold: The use of Dibenamine in pheochromocytoma, New England J. Med. 239:736–739, 1948.

7. N. N. Litman and D. State: Pheochromocytoma: Use of N, N-dibenzyl-β-chloroethylamine (Dibenamine) and piperidino-methyl-benzodioxane (benzodioxane) in surgical therapy, Pediatrics 4:735–743, 1949.

8. O. Spühler, H. Walther, and W. Brunner: Zur Diagnose, Klinik und operativen Therapie des Phäochromocytoms: Histamintest und Dibenamin, Schweiz. med. Wchnschr. 79:357–361, 1949.

9. K. S. Grimson, F. H. Longino, C. E. Kernodle, and H. B. O'Rear: Treatment of a patient with a pheochromocytoma: Use of an adrenolytic drug before and during operation, J. A. M. A. 140:1273–1274, 1949.

10. H. Haimovici and H. E. Medinets: Effect of Dibenamine on blood pressure in normotensive and hypertensive subjects, Proc. Soc. Exper. Biol. & Med. 67:163–166, 1948.

11. G. de Takats and E. F. Fowler: The surgical treatment of hypertension: III. The "neurogenic" versus renal hypertension from the standpoint of operability, Surgery 21:773–799, 1947.

12. W. B. Cannon, H. F. Newton, E. M. Bright, V. Menkin, and R. M. Moore: Some aspects of the physiology of animals surviving complete exclusion of the sympathetic nerve impulses, Am. J. Physiol. 89:84–107, 1929.

13. Z. M. Bacq, L. Brouha, and C. Heymans: Recherches sur la physiologie et la pharmacologie du système nerveux autonome: VIII. Réflexes vasomoteurs d'origine sino-carotidienne et actions pharmacologiques chez le chat et chez le chien sympathectomisés, Arch. internat. de pharmacodyn. et de thérap. 48:429–456, 1934.

14. K. S. Grimson, E. S. Orgain, B. Anderson, R. A. Broome, and F. H. Longino: Results of treatment of patients with hypertension by total thoracic and partial to total lumbar sympathectomy, splanchnicectomy and celiac ganglionectomy, Ann. Surg. 129:850–871, 1949.

15. B. S. Ray and A. D. Console: Evaluation of total sympathectomy, Ann. Surg. 130:652–673, 1949.

16. L. K. Alpert, A. S. Alving, and K. S. Grimson: Effect of total sympathectomy on experimental renal hypertension in dogs, Proc. Soc. Exper. Biol. & Med. 37:1–3, 1937.

17. N. E. Freeman and I. H. Page: Hypertension produced by constriction of the renal artery in sympathectomized dogs, Am. Heart J. 14:405–414, 1937.

18. C. Heymans, J. J. Bouckaert, L. Elaut, F. Bayless, and A. Samaan: Hypertension artérielle chronique par ischémia rénale chez le chien totalement sympathectomisé, Compt. rend. Soc. de biol. 126:434–436, 1937.

19. E. B. Verney and Martha Vogt: An experimental investigation into hypertension of renal origin, with some observations on convulsive "uraemia," Quart. J. Exper. Physiol. 28:253–303, 1938.

20. B. S. Ray and A. D. Console: Residual sympathetic pathways after paravertebral sympathectomy, J. Neurosurg. 5:23–50, 1948.

21. J. D. Boyd and P. A. G. Monro: Partial retention of autonomic function after paravertebral sympathectomy; intermediate lumbar sympathetic ganglia as the probable explanation, Lancet 2:892–895, 1949.

22. W. C. Randall, W. F. Alexander, A. B. Hertzman, J. W. Cox, and W. P. Henderson: Functional significance of residual sympathetic pathways following verified lumbar sympathectomy, Am. J. Physiol. 160:441–450, 1950.

23. K. S. Grimson, H. Wilson, and D. B. Phemister: The early and remote effects of total and partial paravertebral sympathectomy on blood pressure, Ann. Surg. 106:801–825, 1937.

24. K. S. Grimson: Role of sympathetic nervous system in hypertension as revealed by the action of sympatholytic and depressor drugs, in Transactions of the Third Conference on Factors Regulating Blood Pressure, Josiah Macy, Jr., Foundation, New York, 1949, pp. 237–261.

25. H. Hermann, J. F. Cier, J. Chatonnet, and J. Vial: Les conditions de la "vie sans moelle" chez le rat, Compt. rend. Soc. de biol. 141:934–936, 1947.

26. F. Glenn, C. G. Child, and I. Page: The effect of destruction of the spinal cord on hypertension artificially produced in dogs, Am. J. Physiol. 122:506–510, 1938.

27. F. Glenn and E. P. Lasher: The effect of destruction of the spinal cord on the artificial production of hypertension in dogs, Am. J. Physiol. 124:106–109, 1938.

28. H. Hermann, G. Morin, and J. Vial: Les régulations périphériques chez le chien sans moelle: II. Évolution de la pression artérielle après la destruction de la moelle dorso-lombo-sacrée, Arch. internat. de physiol. 44:125–138, 1937.

29. M. Wilburne, L. N. Katz, S. Rodbard, and A. Surtshin: The action of N,N-dibenzyl-beta-chloroethylamine (Dibenamine) in hypertensive dogs, J. Pharmacol. & Exper. Therap. 90:215–223, 1947.

30. M. Nickerson and J. W. Henry: Unpublished results.

31. M. Nickerson: Unpublished results.

32. P. De la Barreda, C. Jimenez Diaz, and A. F. De Molina: Estudio acerca de la regularización neuroquímica de la presión arterial (función endocrina de las arteries), Rev. españ. de card. 1:1–22, 1947.

33. A. Blalock, E. L. Sanford, and R. D. Cressman: Experimental hypertension: The effects of unilateral renal ischemia combined with intestinal ischemia on the arterial blood pressure. J. Exper. Med. 69:833–846, 1939.

34. E. Ogden, G. J. Hildebrand, and E. W. Page: Rise of blood pressure during ischemia of the gravid uterus, Proc. Soc. Exper. Biol. & Med. 43:49–51, 1940.

35. H. E. Essex, J. F. Herrick, E. J. Baldes, and E. C. Mann: Observations on the circulation in the hind limbs of a dog ten years following left lumbar sympathetic ganglionectomy, Am. J. Physiol. 139:351–355, 1943.

36. H. Barcroft and A. J. Walker: Return of tone in blood vessels of the upper limb after sympathectomy, Lancet 1:1035–1039, 1949.

37. J. F. Perkins, Jr., M. Li, F. Hoffman, and E. Hoffman: Sudden vasoconstriction in denervated or sympathectomized paws exposed to cold, Am. J. Physiol. 155:165–178, 1948.

38. H. Barcroft, W. M. Bonnar, and O. G. Edholm: Reflex vasodilatation in human skeletal muscle in response to heating the body, J. Physiol. 106:271–278, 1947.

39. E. R. Clark and Eleanor L. Clark: Observations on living preformed blood vessels as seen in a transparent chamber inserted into the rabbit's ear, Am. J. Anat. 49:441–477, 1932.

40. L. M. N. Bach: The reflex activation of the vasodilator fibers of the dorsal roots and their role in vasodilator tone, Am. J. Physiol. 145:474–477, 1946.

41. M. Nickerson, F. Bullock, and G. M. Nomaguchi: Effect of Dibenamine on renal hypertension in rats, Proc. Soc. Exper. Biol. & Med. 68:425–429, 1948.

42. H. J. Bein: Änderung der Carotis-Sinus-Reflexe bei Blutdrucksteigerung aus verschiedener Ursache, Helvet. physiol. et pharmacol. acta 5:169–177, 1947.

43. J. J. Bouckaert, L. Elaut, and C. Heymans: Vaso-motor carotid sinus reflexes in experimental hypertension produced by renal ischemia, J. Physiol. 89:3P–4P, 1937.

44. W. Dock, F. Shidler, and B. Moy: The vasomotor center essential in maintaining renal hypertension, Am. Heart J. 23:513–521, 1942.

45. F. von Brücke and F. Kaindl: Zur Frage der Pressorischen Carotis-Sinus-Reflexe bei Hochdruck durch einengung der Nierenarterien, Arch. internat. de pharmacodyn. et de thérap. 79:32–34, 1949.

46. M. Prinzmetal and C. Wilson: The nature of the peripheral resistance in arterial hypertension with special reference to the vaso-motor system, J. Clin. Investigation 15:63–83, 1936.

47. G. D. Gammon: The carotid sinus reflex in patients with hypertension, J. Clin. Investigation 15:153–156, 1936.

48. E. A. Stead, Jr., and P. Kunkel: Nature of peripheral resistance in arterial hypertension, J. Clin. Investigation 19:25–33, 1940.

49. R. D. Taylor, A. C. Corcoran, and I. H. Page: Effects of denervation on experimental renal hypertension, Federation Proc. 7:123, 1948.

50. J. Stamler, S. Rodbard, and L. N. Katz: Blood pressure and renal clearances in hypertensive dogs following tissue injury, Am. J. Physiol. 160:21–30, 1950.

51. A. C. Corcoran and I. H. Page: Renal blood flow and sympathectomy in hypertension, Arch. Surg. 42:1072–1082, 1941.

52. H. J. Bluntschli and R. H. Goetz: The effect of a new sympathicolytic drug (dihydroergocornine) on blood pressure with special reference to hypertension, South African M. J. 21:382–401, 1947.

53. E. D. Freis, J. R. Stanton, and R .W. Wilkins: The effects of certain dihydrogenated alkaloids of ergot in hypertensive patients, Am. J. M. Sc. 216:163–171, 1948.

54. R. H. Goetz: The action of dihydroergocornine on the circulation with special reference to hypertension, Lancet 1:510–514, 1949.

55. F. C. Moister, J. R. Stanton, and E. D. Freis: Observations on the development of tolerance during prolonged oral administration of dihydroergocornine, J. Pharmacol. & Exper. Therap. 96:21–30, 1949.

56. D. W. Hayes, K. G. Wakim, B. T. Horton, and G. A. Peters: The effects of dihydroergocornine on the circulation in the extremities of man, J. Clin. Investigation 28:615–620, 1949.

57. G. Schimert, Jr., and H. Zickgraf: Therapy of angina pectoris with dihydrogenated ergot alkaloids (CCK 179), Klin. Wchnschr. 27:59–63, 1949.

58. E. D. Freis et al.: Hemodynamic effects of hypotensive agents in man, Am. J. Med. 7:414–415, 1949.

59. A. P. Crosley, Jr., A. J. Cummins, H. G. Barker, and J. K. Clark: The renal hemodynamic effects of dihydroergocornine (DHO-180) in man, J. Pharmacol. & Exper. Therap. 98:138–143, 1950.

60. C. T. Bello, W. G. Moss, and E. Weiss: Effect of orally administered dihydroergocornine (D.H.O. 180) on hypertension, Am. J. Med. 8:634–639, 1950.

61. R. P. Ahlquist, R. A. Huggins, and R. A. Woodbury: The pharmacology of benzylimidazoline (Priscol), J. Pharmacol. & Exper. Therap. 89:271–288, 1947.

62. K. S. Grimson, M. J. Reardon, F. A. Marzoni, and J. P. Hendrix: The effects of Priscol (2-benzyl-4, 5-imidazoline HCl) on peripheral vascular diseases, hypertension and circulation in patients, Ann. Surg. 127:968–991, 1948.

63. E. Moller: Forgiftning med Vasodil (Priscol): Kasuistisk Meddelelse, Nord. med. 33:610–611, 1947.

64. H. Bietendüfel: Akute Blutdrucksteigerung nach Priscol, München. med. Wchnschr. 88:888–889, 1941.

65. F. H. Longino, K. S. Grimson, J. R. Chittum, and B. H. Metcalf: Effects of a

new quaternary amine and a new imidazoline derivative on the autonomic nervous system, Surgery 26:421–434, 1949.

66. R. E. Wunsch, R. D. Warnke, and G. B. Myers: The effects of Dibenamine on severe hypertension, Ann. Int. Med. 33:613–628, 1950.

67. W. C. Bridges and P. D. White: The treatment of diastolic hypertension, M. Clin. North America 31:1106–1120, 1947.

The Effect of Sympathectomy upon Mortality and Survival Rates of Patients with Hypertensive Cardiovascular Disease,
by Reginald H. Smithwick

1. T. C. Janeway: A clinical study of hypertensive cardiovascular disease, Arch. Int. Med. 12:755–798 (Dec.) 1913.

2. J. M. Blackford, J. M. Bowers, and J. W. Baker: Follow-up study of hypertension, J. A. M. A. 94:328–333 (Feb.) 1930.

3. N. M. Keith, H. P. Wagener, and N. W. Barker: Some different types of essential hypertension; their course and prognosis, Am. J. M. Sc. 197:332–343 (Mar.) 1939.

4. H. Rasmussen and J. Boe: Prognosis of essential hypertension, with remarks respecting indications for operative treatment, Acta med. Scandinav. 120:12–31, 1945.

5. P. Bechgaard: Arterial hypertension; follow-up study of 1000 hypertonics, Acta med. Scandinav. supp. 172:3–358, 1946.

6. R. S. Palmer, D. Loofbourow, and C. R. Doering: Prognosis in essential hypertension: Eight year follow-up study of 430 patients on conventional medical treatment, New England J. Med. 239:990–994 (Dec.) 1948.

7. G. A. Perera: Diagnosis and natural history of hypertensive vascular disease, Am. J. Med. 4:416–422 (Mar.) 1948.

8. S. Hammarström and P. Bechgaard: Progress in arterial hypertension: Comparison between 251 patients after sympathectomy and a selected series of 435 non-operated patients, Am. J. Med. 8:53–56 (Jan.) 1950.

9. S. Hammarström: Arterial hypertension; variability of blood pressure; neurosurgical treatment, indications and results, Acta med. Scandinav. supp. 192:1–301, 1947.

The Management of Hypertensive Patients,
by Harold G. Wolff and Stewart Wolf

1. H. P. Wagener and N. M. Keith: Diffuse arteriolar disease with hypertension and the associated retinal lesions, Medicine 18:317, 1939.

2. R. H. Smithwick: Surgical treatment of hypertension: The effect of radical splanchnicectomy on the hypertensive state of 156 patients followed for one to five years, Arch. Surg. 49:180, 1944.

3. H. Rasmussen and J. Boe: Prognosis of essential hypertension with remarks on indications for operative treatment, Acta med. Scandinav. 120:12, 1945.

4. R. Frant and J. Groen: Prognosis of vascular hypertension: A nine year follow-up study of 418 cases, Arch. Int. Med. 85:727, 1950.

5. K. A. Evelyn, F. Alexander, and S. R. Cooper: Effect of sympathectomy on blood pressure in hypertension, J. A. M. A. 140:592, 1949.

6. R. L. Levy, P. D. White, W. D. Stroud, and C. C. Hillman: Sustained hypertension: Predisposing factors and causes of disability and death, J. A. M. A. 135:77, 1947.

7. E. A. Hines, Jr.: Range of normal blood pressure and subsequent development of hypertension: A follow-up study of 1522 patients, J. A. M. A. 115:271, 1940.

8. T. Holmes and H. G. Wolff: Life situations, emotions and backache, Proc. A. Research Nerv. & Ment. Dis. 29:750, 1950.

9. T. Lewis: Pain, New York, Macmillan, 1942.

10. D. J. Simons, Emerson Day, Helen Goodell, and Harold G. Wolff: Experimental studies on headache: Muscles of the scalp and neck as sources of pain, Proc. A. Research Nerv. & Ment. Dis. 23:228, 1943.

11. W. H. Robey: Headache, Philadelphia, J. B. Lippincott, 1931.

12. A. M. Sutherland and H. G. Wolff: Experimental studies on headache: Further analysis of the mechanism of headache in migraine, hypertension and fever, Arch. Neurol. & Psychiat. 44:929, 1940.

13. G. A. Wolf, Jr., and H. G. Wolff: Studies on the nature of certain symptoms associated with cardiovascular disorders, Psychosom. Med. 8:293, 1946.

14. Stewart Wolf: Sustained contraction of the diaphragm; the mechanism of a common type of dyspnea and precordial pain, J. Clin. Investigation 26:1201, 1947.

15. Harold N. Willard, Roy C. Swan, and George A. Wolf, Jr.: Life situations, emotions and dyspnea, Proc. A. Research Nerv. & Ment. Dis. 29:583, 1950.

16. G. A. Wolf, Jr.: The effect of pain on renal function, Proc. Research Nerv. & Ment. Dis. 23:358, 1943.

17. I. Stevenson, C. H. Duncan, and H. G. Wolff: Circulatory dynamics before and after exercise in subjects with and without structural heart disease during anxiety and relaxation, J. Clin. Investigation 28:1534, 1949.

18. C. H. Duncan, I. Stevenson, and H. S. Ripley: Life situations, emotions and paroxysmal auricular arrhythmias, Psychosom. Med. 12:23, 1950.

19. I. Stevenson, C. H. Duncan, and H. S. Ripley: Variations in the electrocardiogram with changes in emotional state. To be published.

20. W. J. Grace, S. Wolf, and H. G. Wolff: The Human Colon, New York, Paul B. Hoeber, 1950, in press.

21. H. G. Wolff: Protective reaction patterns and disease, Ann. Int. Med. 27:944, 1947.

22. S. Wolf and E. M. Shepard: An appraisal of factors that evoke and modify the hypertensive reaction pattern, Proc. A. Research Nerv. & Ment. Dis. 29:976, 1950.

23. H. Ripley, S. Wolf, and H. G. Wolff: Treatment in a psychosomatic clinic: Preliminary report, J. A. M. A. 138:949, 1948.

24. B. Berle and R. Pinsky: Data to be published.

25. Solomon Garb: Personal communication.

26. S. Wolf: Effects of suggestion and conditioning on the action of chemical agents in human subjects: The pharmacology of placebos, J. Clin. Investigation 29:100, 1950.

27. J. T. Flynn, M. A. K. Kennedy, and S. Wolf: Essential hypertension in one of identical twins: An experimental study of cardiovascular reactions in the Y twins, Proc. A. Research Nerv. & Ment. Dis. 29:944, 1950.

Some Effects of the Rice-Fruit Diet in Patients with Essential Hypertension, by Carleton B. Chapman

1. L. Ambard and E. Beaujard: Causes de l'hypertension artérielle, Arch. gén. de méd. 1:520–533, 1904.

2. W. Redtenbacher: Beobachtungen am Harne bei Lungenentzündungen, Ztschr. Gesellschaft der Ärzte zu Wien 1:373–375, 1850.

3. E. Salkowski: Untersuchungen über die Ausscheidung der Alkalisalze, Virchows Arch. f. path. Anat. 53:209–234, 1871.

4. A. von Koranyi: Physiologische und klinische Untersuchungen über den osmotischen Druck thierischer Flussigkeiten, Ztschr. f. klin. Med. 34:1–52, 1898.

5. Carrion and Hallion: Contribution expérimentale à la pathogénie des oedèmes, Compt. rend. Soc. de biol. 51:156–158, 1899.

6. F. Widal and Lemierre: Rôle du chlorure de sodium dans la pathogénie de certains oedèmes, Semaine méd. 23:199, 1903.

7. F. M. Allen and J. W. Sherrill: The treatment of arterial hypertension, J. Metabol. Research 2:429–545, 1922.

8. W. Kempner: Treatment of kidney disease and hypertensive vascular disease with rice diet, North Carolina M. J. 5:125–133, 1944.

9. W. Kempner: Treatment of hypertensive vascular disease with rice diet, Am. J. Med. 4:545–577, 1948.

10. W. Schwartz and J. Merlis: Nitrogen balance studies on the Kempner rice diet, J. Clin. Investigation 27:406–411, 1948.

11. A. R. Behnke, Jr., B. G. Feen, and W. C. Welham: The specific gravity of healthy men: Body weight ÷ Volume as an index of obesity, J. A. M. A. 118:495–498, 1942.

12. E. N. Rathbun and N. Pace: Studies on body composition: I. The determination of total body fat by means of the body specific gravity, J. Biol. Chem. 158:667–676, 1945.

13. N. Pace and E. N. Rathbun: Studies on body composition: III. The body water and chemically combined nitrogen content in relation to fat content, J. Biol. Chem. 158:685–691, 1945.

14. M. F. Morales, E. N. Rathbun, R. E. Smith, and N. Pace: Studies on body composition: II. Theoretical considerations regarding the major body tissue components, with suggestions for application to man, J. Biol. Chem. 158:677–684, 1945.

15. A. Keys, J. Brozek, A. Henschel, O. Mickelsen, and H. L. Taylor: The Biology of Human Starvation, Minneapolis, University of Minnesota Press, 1950.

Pyrogens in the Treatment of Malignant Hypertension, by Irvine H. Page, Robert D. Taylor, and A. C. Corcoran

1. I. H. Page and G. J. Heuer: Treatment of essential and malignant hypertension by section of anterior nerve roots, Arch. Int. Med. 59:245, 1937.

2. I. H. Page: Medical aspects of surgical treatment of hypertension, J. A. M. A. 110:1161, 1938.

3. A. C. Corcoran, R. D. Taylor, and I. H. Page: Controlled observations on the effect of low sodium dietotherapy in essential hypertension, Circulation, in press.

4. A. C. Corcoran and I. H. Page: The effect on renal function of renal extracts which lower arterial blood pressure in patients with essential and malignant hypertension and in dogs with experimental hypertension, Proc. Central Soc. Clin. Research 13:38, 1940.

5. J. Stamler, A. P. Fishman, L. N. Katz, and S. Rodbard: Circulatory dynamics in spontaneous and nephrogenic hypertensive dogs during the depressor response to acute inflammation, Circulation 2:392, 1950.

6. H. Chasis, W. Goldring, and H. W. Smith: Reduction of blood pressure associated with the pyrogenic reaction in hypertensive subjects, J. Clin. Investigation 21:369, 1942.

7. S. E. Bradley, H. Chasis, W. Goldring, and H. W. Smith: Hemodynamic alterations in normotensive and hypertensive subjects during the pyrogenic reaction, J. Clin. Investigation 24:749, 1945.

8. A. Grollman: Variations in the cardiac output of man: V. The cardiac output of man during the malaise and pyrexia following the injection of typhoid vaccine, J. Clin. Investigation 8:25, 1929.

9. R. D. Taylor and I. H. Page: Studies in the mechanism of the hypotensive effect of substances eliciting leucocytosis and fever, Am. J. M. Sc. 208:281, 1944.

10. R. D. Taylor, A. C. Corcoran, and I. H. Page: Further experience with bacterial pyrogens in the treatment of malignant hypertension, Proc. Central Soc. Clin. Research 22:83, 1949.

11. I. H. Page and R. D. Taylor: Pyrogens in the treatment of malignant hypertension, Mod. Concepts Cardiovas. Dis. 18:51, 1949.